Study Guide
to accompany

Whaley & Wong's
Nursing Care of Infants and Children

Sixth Edition

Anne Rath Rentfro, MSN, RN, CS, CDE
Associate Professor
BSN Completion Program
The University of Texas at Brownsville
    in Partnership with Texas Southmost College
Brownsville, Texas

Linda Sawyer McCampbell, MSN, RN, CS, FNP
Family Nurse Practitioner
Rural Clinics of South Texas
Port Isabel Health Clinic
Port Isabel, Texas

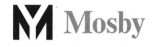 Mosby

St. Louis Baltimore Boston Carlsbad Chicago Minneapolis New York Philadelphia Portland
London Milan Sydney Tokyo Toronto

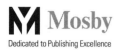
Mosby
Dedicated to Publishing Excellence

Publisher: Sally Schrefer
Developmental Editor: Michele D. Hayden
Project Manager: Gayle May Morris
Manufacturing Manager: Linda Ierardi
Cover Design: Pati Pye
Cover Photograhs: Arthur Tilley/FPG International LLC
                         Rob Gage/FPG International LLC

Printed in the United States of America
Composition by DBT Communications, Inc.
Printing/binding by Plus Communications

Mosby, Inc.
11830 Westline Industrial Drive
St. Louis, Missouri 63146

International Standard Book Number 0-323-00104-1

99 00 01 02 / 9 8 7 6 5 4 3 2

Reviewers

Elizabeth Ahmann, ScD, RN
Senior Lecturer,
Columbia University,
School of Nursing,
New York, New York;
Consultant, Child and Family Health,
Washington, D.C.

Pamela A. DiVito-Thomas, MS, RN
Instructor,
Oral Roberts University,
Anna Vaughn School of Nursing,
Tulsa, Oklahoma

Marilyn Hockenberry-Eaton, PhD, RN, CS, PNP, FAAN
Associate Professor,
Department of Pediatrics,
Baylor College of Medicine;
Director of Nurse Practitioners,
Texas Children's Hospital,
Houston, Texas

David Wilson, MS, RNC
Clinical Instructor,
Oral Roberts University,
Anna Vaughn School of Nursing,
Tulsa, Oklahoma

Marilyn L. Winkelstein, PhD, RN
Associate Professor,
University of Maryland,
School of Nursing,
Baltimore, Maryland

Preface

This Study Guide accompanies the sixth edition of *Whaley & Wong's Nursing Care of Infants and Children*. Students may use the Study Guide not only to review content but also to enhance their learning through critical thinking. The Study Guide's purpose is to assist students in mastering the content presented in the text, developing problem-solving skills, and applying their knowledge to nursing practice.

The Study Guide includes questions that will assist the student to meet the objectives of each corresponding textbook chapter. Because most students using this Study Guide will also be preparing to pass the nursing examination (NCLEX), we have primarily used a multiple-choice format. A Critical Thinking section is included for each chapter. The questions in the Critical Thinking section help students analyze the chapter's content and address their own attitudes about pediatric nursing practice. Case Studies were used in many of the Critical Thinking sections to help students address specific practice issues. All case presentations are fictitious but designed to address situations that are frequently encountered by the nurse in practice. This new edition includes features to help students learn and retain pediatric terminology used in each chapter.

How to Use the Study Guide

We intend for the student to use this Study Guide while he or she studies a chapter in the textbook, processing the material chapter by chapter and section by section. For this reason we chose to present the questions in an order that follows the textbook's content. The student will find the answers to the questions for each chapter at the end of the Study Guide. Page numbers from the textbook have been included to facilitate finding content related to the answers.

It is our hope that this Study Guide will function as both an aid to learning and a means for measuring progress in the mastery of pediatric nursing practice.

Anne Rath Rentfro
Linda Sawyer McCampbell

Contents

CHAPTER 1
Perspectives of Pediatric Nursing

1. Terms—Health During Childhood

A. health
B. mortality
C. morbidity
D. National Health Promotion and Disease Prevention Objectives
E. vital statistics
F. mortality statistics
G. National Center of Health Statistics (NCHS)
H. infant mortality rate
I. neonatal mortality
J. post neonatal mortality
K. birth weight
L. low birth weight (LBW)

M. Family Medical Leave Act of 1993
N. perinatal mortality rate
O. violent deaths
P. suicide
Q. morbidity statistics
R. acute illness
S. disability
T. new morbidity
U. accident
V. injury
W. host
X. environment
Y. agent

Z. passive injury
AA. active injury
BB. Consumer Product Safety Commission (CPSC)
CC. financial barriers
DD. system barriers
EE. information barriers
FF. prospective payment system
GG. diagnosis related groups
HH. health maintenance organization (HMO)

___HH___ companies that provide health care within a managed care framework

___R___ symptoms severe enough to limit activity or require medical attention

___P___ a form of self violence; the third leading cause of death among teenagers and young adults 15 to 24 years of age

___N___ commonly defined as the number of fetal deaths (fetuses of 28 weeks or more gestation) and deaths in infants under 7 days per 100 live births.

___G___ responsible for the collection analysis and dissemination of data on the health of American people

___B___ death

___Y___ the object that is the direct cause of an injury

___FF___ a major change in health care delivery in the U.S. where payment is based on pretreatment billing

___F___ describes the incidence or number of individuals who have died over a specific period of time

___C___ illness

___I___ the number of deaths during the first 28 days of life

___GG___ categories that define prospective billing for almost all U.S. hospitals reimbursed by Medicare

___A___ a state of complete physical, mental, and social well-being and not merely the absence of disease

___L___ a key factor in the U.S. higher neonatal mortality rates when compared with other countries

___K___ the major determinant of neonatal death in technologically developed countries

___U___ a chaotic, random event that is luck or chance

___m___ the legislation that determines eligibility to take leave from work to care for infants

___S___ measured in days off from school or days confined to bed

___W___ the person affected by an injury

___O___ recent steady increases have occurred among young people ages 10 through 25 years especially blacks and males

X	the time and place of an injury
D	increase the span of health life for Americans; reduce health disparities among Americans and achieve access to preventive services for all Americans
BB	established by the U.S. government to protect the public against unreasonable risks of injuries and death associated with products
V	connotes a sense of responsibility and control; the preferred term to use when discussing the leading cause of death in children over age 1
EE	examples are lack of understanding about the need or value of prenatal or child health supervision or an unawareness of the services that are available
CC	examples are not having insurance, having insurance that does not cover certain services, or being unable to pay for services
T	pediatric social illness; behavioral, social, family and educational problems
AA	prevention strategies used to persuade individuals to change their behavior for increased self protection, such as seat belts
Q	the prevalence of a specific illness in the population at a particular time, generally presented as rates per 1000 population
Z	prevention strategies provide automatic protection by product and environment design; air bags
DD	examples are having to travel great distance for health care or state to state variations in Medicaid benefits
H	the number of deaths during the first year of life per 1000 live births
J	the number of deaths that occur in infants from the first 28 days to the first 11 months of life
E	figures describing rates of occurrence of events such as death in children

2. Terms—Pediatric Nursing Care

A. definition of nursing
B. family-centered care
C. enabling
D. empowerment
E. parent-professional partnership
F. atraumatic care
G. therapeutic care
H. setting
I. personnel
J. interventions
K. psychological distress
L. physical distress

M. clinical practice guidelines
N. Agency for Health Care Policy and Research (AHCPR)
O. therapeutic relationship
P. nontherapeutic
Q. caring
R. Pediatric Nurse Practitioner (PNP)
S. Clinical Nurse Specialist
T. Advanced Nurse Practitioner

U. autonomy
V. nonmaleficence
W. beneficence
X. justice
Y. nursing process
Z. community-based health driven system
AA. standard of practice
BB. provider of care
CC. manager of care
DD. unlicensed assistive personnel

B	recognizes the family as the constant in a child's life
E	a mechanism for enabling and empowering families where parents serve as respected equals with professionals and have the rightful role in deciding what is important for themselves and their family. The professional's role is to support and strengthen the family's ability to nurture and promote its members' development in a way that is both enabling and empowering.
A	the diagnosis and treatment of human responses to actual or potential health problems
U	the patient's right to be self-governing
F	the provision of therapeutic care in settings by personnel and through the use of interventions that eliminate or minimize the psychological and physical distress experienced by children and their families in the health care system
Y	a systematic problem-solving method used routinely by nurses

_C_ creating opportunities and means for all family members to display their present abilities and competencies and to acquire new ones that are necessary to meet the needs of the child and family

_I_ include anyone directly involved in providing therapeutic care

_D_ describes the interaction of professionals with families in such a way that families maintain or acquire a sense of control over their family lives

_DD_ individuals who are trained to function in an assistive role to the registered professional nurse in the provision of care activities as delegated by and under the supervision of the registered professional nurse

_K_ may include anxiety, fear, anger, disappointment, sadness, shame, or guilt

_G_ encompasses the prevention, diagnosis, treatment, or palliation of chronic or acute conditions

_M_ reflect the research that has been conducted relative to a specific disease or illness

_H_ refers to the place in which care is given

_O_ a meaningful relationship with children and their families that has well-defined boundaries that separate the nurse from the child and family

_AA_ the level of performance that is expected of a professional

_P_ a relationship where boundaries that separate the nurse from the child and family are blurred

_T_ a role that combines the Clinical Nurse Specialist and Nurse Practitioner into one

_R_ a specialized ambulatory or primary care role for pediatric nurses

_L_ may range from sleeplessness and immobilization to the experience of disturbing sensory stimuli such as pain, temperature extremes, loud noises, bright lights, or darkness

_Q_ expressing compassion and empathy for others

_J_ approaches that range from psychological, such as preparing children for procedures, to physical interventions, such as providing space for a parent to room in

_N_ a U.S. federal agency that was founded in 1989 for the purpose of developing national guidelines and enhancing the quality, appropriateness, and effectiveness of care

_S_ a role that has been developed in an attempt to provide expert nursing care; serves as a role model, a researcher, a change agent, and a consultant.

_V_ the obligation to minimize or prevent harm

_BB_ the traditional role of the nurse in the which the focus is promotion, maintenance, and restoration of health

_Z_ the system of the future in which the nurse's role will expand to health care planning, particularly on a political or legislative level

_W_ the obligation to promote the patient's well being

_X_ the concept of fairness

_CC_ a role of the nurse that requires a shift in thinking and different skills from those needed for health promotion, health maintenance, and health restoration; a shift from performing tasks to collaborative practice.

3. Terms—Critical Thinking and the Process of Nursing

A. critical thinking
B. nursing diagnosis
C. problem statement
D. risk factor
E. etiology
F. signs and symptoms

G. dependent activities
H. interdependent activities
I. independent activities
J. outcome
K. standard care plans
L. individualized care plans

M. Joint Commission on Accreditation of Healthcare Organizations (JCAHO)
N. continuous quality improvement (CQI)

___D___ signs indicating a potential health problem

___m___ the accrediting body for many types of health care providers such as hospitals, nursing homes, ambulatory services, and home health agencies. This accreditation status is required for the agency to receive federal funds, such as Medicare or Medicaid.

___B___ a clinical judgment about individual family or community responses to actual and potential health problems/life process

___F___ refers to a cluster of cues and/or defining characteristics that are derived from patient assessment and indicate actual health problems

___A___ purposeful, goal-directed thinking that assists individuals to make judgments based on evidence rather than guesswork

___G___ those areas of nursing practice that hold the nurse accountable for implementing the prescribed treatment

___N___ the process of ongoing review of systems, problem identification, and resolution; allows the institution to establish and maintain quality care

___C___ the first component of the nursing diagnosis; describes the response to health pattern deficits

___H___ those areas of nursing practice in which nursing responsibility and accountability overlap with other disciplines, such as medicine and require collaboration between the two disciplines

___K___ plans that are sufficiently broad to account for situations that may develop in patients with particular problems

___E___ the second component of the nursing diagnosis; describes the physiologic, situational, and maturational factors that cause the problem or influence its development

___I___ those areas of nursing practice that are the direct responsibility of the nurse

___L___ care plans that are concerned with only those diagnoses that apply to the particular patient situation

___J___ the projected change in a patient's health status, clinical condition, or behavior that occurs after nursing interventions have been instituted

4. Which one of the following objectives would NOT be considered a "Healthy People 2000" priority area for the 1990's?
   A. Improve nutritional and infant health
   B. Eradicate acute respiratory disorders in infants
   C. Reduce violent and abusive behavior
   D. Expand community based health promotion programs

5. Which one of the following statements is TRUE about infant mortality in the United States?
   A. Infant mortality is at an all-time high in the U.S.
   B. The U.S. currently holds its lowest infant mortality rate ever.
   C. Infant mortality rates in the U.S. are significantly lower than in other well-developed countries.
   D. The U.S. ranks lower than Canada in regard to mortality rate.

6. Which one of the following risks for neonatal mortality increased in 1991 and is considered a key factor in the higher U.S. neonatal mortality rates when compared with other countries?
   A. Birth weight less than 2500 grams
   B. Short or long gestation
   C. Race and gender
   D. Lower level of maternal education

7. Which one of the following causes of death accounts for the most deaths in infants under 1 year of age?
   A. Pneumonia and influenza
   B. Infections specific to the perinatal period
   C. Accidents and adverse effects
   D. Congenital anomalies

8. Neural tube defects are expected to decrease as much as 50% with the current recommendation by the American Academy of Pediatrics for all women of childbearing age to receive ____folic acid____ supplementation.

9. Which one of the following differences is seen when infant death rates are categorized according to race? Infant mortality for:
   A. Native Americans has decreased due to post neonatal mortality.
   B. Hispanics may not include all Hispanic subgroups.
   C. blacks is five times the rate for whites.
   D. whites is the same as for other races.

10. After a child reaches the age of one, the leading cause of death is from:
    A. Human Immunodeficiency Virus (HIV).
    B. congenital anomalies.
    C. cancer.
    D. accidents.

11. Causes of violence against children can usually be attributed to:
    A. the presence of firearms in the household.
    B. numerous socioeconomic influences.
    C. depression.
    D. poor safety devices on firearms.

12. Which two diseases are becoming more prominent on the list of leading causes of death during childhood?
    A. Neoplasm and tuberculosis
    B. Tuberculosis and Acquired Immunodeficiency Syndrome (AIDS)
    C. Neoplasm and AIDS
    D. Infectious diseases and AIDS

13. Morbidity statistics which depict the prevalence of a specific illness in the population are:
    A. presented as rates per 100 population.
    B. difficult to define.
    C. denoting acute illness only.
    D. denoting chronic disease only.

14. Fifty percent of all acute conditions of childhood can be accounted for by:
    A. injuries and accidents.
    B. bacterial infections.
    C. parasitic disease.
    D. respiratory illness.

15. Identify one major category of disease that children tend contract in infancy and early childhood.

    _____Resp. illnesses_____

16. List three factors that contribute to increasing the morbidity of any disorder in children.

    homelessness, poverty, LBW

    chronic illnesses, adoption

    day care centers

17. The degree of disability in children can be measured by:
    A. days of hospitalization.
    B. developmental stages.
    C. days off from school or confined to bed.
    D. physical growth patterns.

18. Another term for the *new morbidity* is:
    A. pediatric social illness.
    B. pediatric noncompliance.
    C. learning disorder.
    D. dyslexia.

19. Which one of the following statements about injuries in childhood is FALSE?
    A. Developmental stage determines the prevalence of injuries at a given age.
    B. Most fatal injuries occur in children under the age of nine.
    C. Developmental stage helps to direct preventive measures.
    D. The highest incidence of injury occurs in children under the age of nine.

20. An important nursing consideration when an injury occurs in children is to:
    A. provide anticipatory guidance.
    B. judge whether this injury could have been prevented.
    C. analyze the specific type of injury in regard to age.
    D. decide whether the cause of injury was intentional.

21. Identify the following strategies as either *passive* or *active* prevention measures.

    _____A_____   A. child proof medicine caps

    _____P_____   B. airbags

    _____A_____   C. smoke detectors

    _____A_____   D. seat belts

    _____A_____   E. safety restraints

_____P_____	F. automatic seat belts
_____A_____	G. warning labels
_____P_____	H. automatic fire sprinklers
_____A_____	I. education about firearms
_____A_____	J. anticipatory guidance
_____P_____	K. window guards
_____A_____	L. mandatory seat belt laws
_____A_____	M. bicycle helmet laws
_____P_____	N. childproof cigarette lighters
_____A_____	O. swimming pool fences
_____A_____	P. swimming pool surface alarm

22. Which one of the following statements about injury prevention in children is TRUE?
   A. Including only the mother may be the most effective teaching strategy with the Hispanic population.
   B. Less than 30% of pediatric nurse practitioners routinely give advice about child car restraints.
   C. Most pediatric nurse practitioners routinely give advice about child car restraints.
   D. Parents are usually aware of their child's developmental progress and capabilities.

23. ___Anticipatory___ ___Guidance___ is the term used for teaching and counseling of parents and others about developmental expectations that serve to alert the parents to the issues that are most likely to arise at a given age.

24. Child health care in the United States has evolved from the colonial era with its many hazards and epidemics, to the advances of the twentieth century when studies of economic and social factors stimulated the creation of better standards of care for mothers and children.

   Indicate whether each statement better reflects *colonial* times or modern (*industrial*) times:

   A. _____I_____ nurses needing to be aware of economics
   B. _____I_____ milk stations
   C. _____C_____ illiterate parents
   D. _____I_____ knowledge barriers (such as not knowing about available services)
   E. _____I_____ rooming in, sibling visitation, child life (play) programs
   F. _____C_____ scarcity of books
   G. _____I_____ the dawn of improved health care
   H. _____I_____ Maternal and Child Health, Crippled Children's Services and child welfare services
   I. _____C_____ Quackery is common.
   J. _____I_____ Lina Rogers became the first full-time school nurse.

K. _____1_____ decline in infant mortality

L. _____c_____ Exposure to new fatal diseases is common.

M. _____1_____ prevention and health promotion measures

N. _____1_____ Lillian Wald founded the Henry Street Settlement.

O. _____1_____ Spitz and Robertson demonstrated the effects of isolation and maternal deprivation.

P. _____c_____ statistics on childhood mortality unavailable

Q. _____1_____ parents prohibited from visiting sick children

R. _____1_____ isolation and maternal deprivation

S. _____c_____ training based on past experiences

T. _____1_____ Lillian Wald, the founder of community nursing

U. _____1_____ parent education

V. _____1_____ hospital schooling

W. _____c_____ epidemic diseases

X. _____1_____ cow's milk as the chief source of bovine tuberculosis

Y. _____1_____ financial barriers such as not having insurance

Z. _____c_____ smallpox, measles, mumps, chickenpox and influenza

AA. _____1_____ School health helped to develop pediatric courses.

BB. _____1_____ Diagnosis Related Groups (DRG's)

CC. _____c_____ diphtheria, yellow fever, cholera, and whooping cough

DD. _____1_____ cow's milk as the chief source of infantile diarrhea

EE. _____1_____ Nurses were employed to teach parents and children.

FF. _____1_____ prehospitalization preparation

GG. _____c_____ dysentery

HH. _____1_____ Abraham Jacobi, the Father of Pediatrics

II. _____c_____ unknown control for diseases

JJ. _____1_____ sanitation and pasteurization of cow's milk

KK. _____1_____ system barriers such as state-to-state variations

LL. _____1_____ American Medical Association opposes the Maternity and Infancy Act.

MM. _____1_____ American Academy of Pediatrics is created.

NN. _____c_____ medical care limited to the wealthy

OO. _____1_____ Title V of the Social Security Act passes.

PP. _____c_____ physician shortage

QQ. _____1_____ White House Conference on Children

25. Match the federal program with the impact it has on maternal and child health.

A. Education of the Handicapped Act Amendments of 1986 (P.I. 99-457)
B. Social Services Block Grant
C. Alcohol, Drug Abuse, and Mental Health Block Grants
D. Education for All Handicapped Children Act (P.I. 94-1432)
E. Medicaid
F. Family and Medical Leave Act (FMLA)
G. Aid to Families with Dependent Children (AFDC)
H. MCH Service Block Grant
I. Women Infants and Children (WIC)

  __E__ Created in 1965, the largest maternal-child health program. The Child Health Assessment Program (CHAP) provides services for children and pregnant women under this program. Eligibility varies from state to state.

  __G__ created in 1935 as a cash grant to aid needy children without fathers

  __H__ provides services to reduce infant mortality, disease and handicaps and to increase access to care

  __C__ established in 1981 to fund projects related to substance abuse and treat mentally disturbed children

  __B__ provides funds for child protective services, family planning and foster care

  __I__ started in 1974 to provide nutritious food and education to low income childbearing women, infants and children up to age 5 years

  __D__ passed in 1975 to provide free public education to handicapped children

  __A__ provides funding for multidisciplinary programs for handicapped infants and toddlers

  __F__ allows employees to take unpaid leave (1993)

26. List three barriers to health care in the U.S. and give an example of each one.

Financial - ∅ ins., ins. that doesn't cover certain services; inability to pay

System - need to travel great distances or state-to-state variations in benefits

Information - lack of knowledge @ prenatal or child health supervision, or being unaware of available services

27. Define the following components of prospective payment.

Diagnosis Related Groups: a prospective payment system that allows for pretreatment billing for hospitals reimbursed by Medicare

Health Maintenance Organizations: health services that use a network of specific providers for a set fee

Managed care: a way to efficiently coordinate delivery of health services c̄ the intent to provide an integrated approach to health care delivery

28. Two basic concepts in the philosophy of family-centered pediatric nursing care are:
   (A) enabling and empowerment.
   B. empowerment and bias.
   C. enabling and curing.
   D. empowerment and self control.

29. The role of the nurse in the parent professional partnership is to:
   A. decide what is most important for the family.
   B. decide what is most important for the child.
   (C) strengthen the family's ability to nurture.
   D. manipulate the available resources.

30. An example of atraumatic care would be to:
   A. eliminate all traumatic procedures.
   B. restrict visiting hours to adults only.
   (C) perform invasive procedures only in the treatment room.
   D. remove parents from the room during painful procedures.

31. A care delivery system that balances quality and cost that has been shown to improve satisfaction, decrease fragmentation, and measure patient outcomes would best describe _Case management_.

32. As the movement for providing care based on guidelines continues, nurses will be using:
   A. Agency for Health Care Policy and Research (AHCPR) guidelines in place of guidelines developed locally.
   B. guidelines that are based on traditional practice.
   (C) timelines that are developed locally.
   D. guidelines that reflect current research but decrease job satisfaction.

33. Match the role of the pediatric nurse with its description.

   A. family advocacy/caring   F. restorative care
   B. disease prevention/health promotion   G. coordination/collaboration
   C. health teaching   H. ethical decision making
   D. support   I. research
   E. counseling   J. health care planning

   ___E___ a mutual exchange of ideas and opinions
   ___J___ extending to include the community or society as a whole
   ___B___ health maintenance strategies
   ___G___ working together as a member of the health team
   ___F___ providing physical and emotional care (feeding/bathing)
   ___I___ systematically recording and analyzing observations
   ___D___ attention to emotional needs (listening/physical presence)
   ___C___ transmitting information
   ___H___ using patient/family/societal values in care
   ___A___ acting in the child's best interest

Marisa Gutierrez arrives with her infant, Sara, in the Well Baby Clinic. Sara, who is 14 months old, is the youngest of three children. Her mother has brought her to the clinic for well child care. Sara's two brothers, who are seven and eight years old, have come along. As you are interviewing her mother, Sara explores the examination room. She reaches for her older brother's marbles and puts one in her mouth.

34. After organizing the data into similar categories, the nurse makes which one of the following decisions?
    A. No dysfunctional health problems are evident.
    B. High risk for dysfunctional health problems exist.
    C. Actual dysfunctional health problems are evident.
    D. Potential complications are evident.

35. The nurse then identifies a possible human response pattern to further classify the data. Which one of the following functional health patterns would be BEST for the nurse to select?
    A. Role-Relationship Pattern
    B. Nutritional-Metabolic Pattern
    C. Coping-Stress Tolerance Pattern
    D. Self-Perception-Self Concept Pattern

36. Based on the data collected, which one of the following nursing diagnoses would be most appropriate?
    A. Altered Family Process
    B. Altered Family Coping
    C. Altered Individual Coping
    D. Altered Parenting

37. Which one of the following patient outcomes are individualized for Sara?
    A. Sara will receive her immunizations on time.
    B. Sara will demonstrate adherence to the nurses recommendations.
    C. Marisa Gutierrez will verbalize the need to keep small objects away from Sara to avoid aspiration.
    D. Sara's brothers will verbalize the need to discontinue playing with small objects.

38. During the evaluation phase, which one of the following responses by Sara's mother would indicate that the expected outcomes have been met?
    A. "I will have to go through all of the boys things when we get home to be sure there aren't any other small objects that could hurt Sara."
    B. "I had forgotten how curious babies are. It has been many years since the boys were babies and they didn't have an older child's toys around."
    C. "I will have to start to discipline Sara now so that she knows not to play with the older children's belongings."
    D. "I am afraid she cannot receive her immunizations. She had a fever after her last one."

39. At Sara's next well baby visit, what information would be most important to document in the chart?
    A. Written evidence of progress toward outcomes
    B. The standard care plan
    C. Broad based goals
    D. Interventions applicable to patients like Sara

CHAPTER 2

Social, Cultural, and Religious Influences on Child Health Promotion

1. Chapter Terms—Matching

A. transcultural nursing orientation	G. subcultures	M. visible poverty
B. culture	H. roles	N. invisible poverty
C. race	I. primary group	O. relative standard of poverty
D. socialization	J. secondary group	
E. material overt/manifest culture	K. ethnic stereotyping	P. episodically poor
F. nonmaterial covert culture	L. absolute standard of poverty	Q. chronically poor
		R. parens patriae

_J_ have limited intermittent contact; generally less concern for members' behavior; usually offer little in terms of support or pressure toward conformity except in rigidly limited areas

_C_ a division of mankind possessing traits that are transmissible by descent and sufficient to characterize it as distinct human type

_A_ an awareness of the nurse's own frame of reference with a conscious effort to recognize and appreciate the views and beliefs of the health care recipients

_D_ the process by which children acquire the beliefs, values, and behaviors of a given society in order to function within that group

_G_ related to the large culture; each has an identity of its own

_P_ income falls below the official poverty line from time to time reflecting short term fluctuations in household composition or economic circumstances

_F_ refers to those aspects that cannot be observed directly such as ideas, beliefs, customs, and feeling of the culture

_N_ refers to social and cultural deprivation such as limited employment opportunities, inferior educational opportunities, lack of, or inferior medical services/health care facilities and absence of public services

_K_ labeling that stems from ethnocentric views

_I_ characterized by intimate, continued, face-to-face contact, mutual support of the members, and the ability to order or constrain a considerable proportion of individual members' behavior in which roles are carried out; examples are the family and the peer group

_B_ a pattern of assumptions, beliefs, and practices that unconsciously frames or guides the outlook of a group of people

_H_ patterns of behavior for persons in a variety of social positions that are cultural creations

_L_ delineates a basic set of resources needed for adequate existence

_O_ reflects the median standard of living in a society; term used to refer to childhood poverty in the U.S.

_R_ the legal principle that says the state has an overriding interest in the health and welfare of its citizens

_M_ refers to lack of money or material resources such as insufficient clothing, poor sanitation, and deteriorating housing

_Q_ incomes below the poverty line year after year

_E_ the observable components of a culture such as material objects and actions

2. Cultural Terms—Matching

A. biculturation
B. cultural diversity
C. blacks
D. Asian/Pacific Islander
E. American Indian/Alaska Native
F. Hispanics
G. cultural shock
H. cultural sensitivity
I. culturally competent care
J. acculturation
K. assimilation
L. cultural pluralism
M. cultural relativity

___D___ any person who has origins in any of the original peoples of the Far East, Southeast Asia, the Indian subcontinent or the Pacific Islands

___B___ the differences that exist as the minority population increases and the majority white population decreases

___E___ persons having the origins in the original peoples of North America and who maintain cultural identification through tribal affiliations or community recognition

___C___ any persons whose lineage includes ancestors who originated from any of the black racial groups of Africa

___I___ care that goes beyond the awareness of similarities and differences to implementing care that is sensitive

___K___ the process of developing a new cultural identity

___F___ persons of Mexican, Puerto Rican, Cuban, Central or South American or other Spanish culture or origin regardless of race

___H___ an awareness of cultural similarities and differences

___M___ the concept that any behavior must be judged first in relation to the context of the culture in which it occurs

___G___ the feelings of helplessness and discomfort and state of disorientation experienced by an outsider attempting to comprehend or effectively adapt to a different cultural group because of difference in cultural practices and values and beliefs

___L___ the attitude that supports the rights of group differences and promotes a mutual respect for the existence of cultural differences

___J___ gradual changes produced in a culture by the influence of another culture that cause one or both cultures to be more similar to the other

___A___ the straddling of two cultures; involves the ability to efficiently bridge the gap between and individual culture of origin and the dominant culture

3. Cultural/Religious Influences on Health Care—Matching

A. miseries
B. locked bowels
C. caidal de la molera
D. susto
E. dolor/duels/lele
F. la diarrhea
G. chi
H. mal ojo
I. yin/yang
J. curandero/curandera
K. acupuncture
L. acupressure
M. moxibustion
N. kakunas
O ho oponopono
P. asafetida

___F___ the term for diarrhea used by some Hispanic people

___H___ the term for evil eye used by some Hispanic people

___C___ the term for fallen fontanel from dehydration used by some Hispanic people

___E___ the term for pain used by some Hispanic people

___A___ the term for pain used by some black people

___L___ application of pressure to cure maladies

___G___ the Chinese term for the innate energy that leaves the body through the mouth, nose, and ears and flows through the body in definite pathways or meridians at specific time and locations

___N___ Hawaiian folk healers

___D___ the term for fright used by some Hispanic people

___K___ insertion of needles to cure maladies

___O___ the practice of healing family imbalances or disputes among Native Hawaiians

___I___ the Chinese terms for the forces of hot and cold that are believed to be out of balance when a person is ill

___B___ the term used for constipation by some black people

___m___ application of heat to cure maladies

___P___ a piece of rotten flesh that looks like a dried sponge that is worn around the neck to prevent contagious diseases

___J___ the Mexican-American folk healer

4. Folk Medicine Practices that May be Harmful—Matching

A. coining
B. force kneeling
C. female genital mutilation (female circumcision)
D. topical garlic application
E. greta/azarcon, paylooah, surma
F. azogue
G. lok

___E___ traditional remedies that contain lead

___G___ Haitian folk medicine practice used to rid the newborn of meconium. A mixture of castor oil, grated nutmeg, sour orange juice, garlic, unrefined sugar, and water; may result in dehydration

___C___ removal or injury to any part of the female genital organ; practiced in Africa, the Middle East, Latin America, India, the Far East, North America, Australia, and Western Europe

___B___ child discipline measure of some Caribbean groups

___D___ a practice of Yemenite Jews; applied to the wrist to treat infectious disease; can result in blisters or burns

___A___ Vietnamese practice; may produce weltlike lesions on the child's back

___F___ a mercury compound commonly used in Mexico and sometimes sold illegally to low income Hispanic families in the United States as a remedy for diarrhea, can cause permanent central nervous system damage

5. When considering the impact of culture on the pediatric client, the nurse recognizes that culture:
   A. is synonymous with race.
   B. affects the development of health beliefs.
   C. refers to a group of people with similar physical characteristics.
   D. refers to the universal manner and sequence of growth and development.

6. Which of the following social groups is an example of a primary group?
   A. Six inseparable teenagers
   B. A second grade class
   C. The members of a national church
   D. The city garden club

7. The use of guilt and shame by a culture provides:
   A. feelings of comfort about wrongdoing.
   B. an outlet following wrongdoing.
   C. rewards for culturally acceptable social behavior.
   D. internalization of the cultural norms.

8. Match the following subcultural influences with the phrase or sentence that describes the word or its influence on a child's cultural development.

A. ethnicity
B. ethnocentrism
C. social class
D. poverty
E. homelessness
F. migrant families
G. affluence
H. religion
I. school
J. peers
K. biculture

____G____ Purchased surrogates may provide the adult authority.

____K____ Language is a often a major educational controversy.

____E____ occurs when there is a lack of resources for adequate shelter

____I____ After family this subcultural influence has the most impact on a child's socialization.

____A____ differentiation by similar distinguishing factors

____D____ limit of resources needed for adequate existence

____B____ belief that one's own ethnic group is superior to others

____F____ lack of continuity in education and health care

____H____ dictates the code of morality

____C____ synonymous with occupation in the United States

____J____ increase in influence as child moves through school

9. Currently in North America there is less reliance on tradition, families are fragmented, and transmission of customs is limited because of:
A. a growing proportion of ethnic minorities.
B. more emphasis on ethnic diversity.
C. the frontier background of the American culture.
D. increasing geographic and economic mobility.

10. Which country has more racial, ethnic, and religious minority groups than any other country?
A. United States
B. Mexico
C. Canada
D. India

11. Which of the following groups is the largest minority group in the United States?
A. Spanish/Hispanic
B. black
C. Asian
D. Latino

12. A child has become acculturated when:
A. a gradual process of ethnic blending occurs.
B. the child identifies with traditional heritage.
C. ethnic and racial pride emerge.
D. counteraggressive behavior is eliminated.

13. Which of the following strategies would be likely to produce the most conflict when considering the concept of cultural shock?
A. Teaching the family some of the dominant culture's customs
B. Utilizing an older sibling to translate a health history
C. Identifying some of the usual family customs
D. Learning tolerance of other's values and beliefs

14. Cultural beliefs and practices are an important part of nursing assessment, because when analyzed and incorporated into the nursing process beliefs:
    A. may sometimes expedite the plan of care.
    B. can be manipulated more easily if known.
    C. must be in unison with standard health practices.
    D. are very similar from one culture to another.

15. An innate susceptibility is acquired through:
    A. the child's general physical status.
    B. exposure to environmental factors.
    C. long term proximity to disease.
    D. generations of evolutionary changes.

16. Match the racial/ethnic group and its commonly associated diseases.

    A. Tay-Sachs disease   F   Greeks
    B. cystic fibrosis   I   Middle Eastern people
    C. sickle cell disease   E   Japanese
    D. neural tube defects   A   Jewish
    E. cleft lip/palate   D   Irish
    F. beta-Thalassemia   G   Polynesians
    G. clubfoot   H   Navaho Indians
    H. ear anomalies   C   African blacks
    I. Werdnig-Hoffman disease   B   whites

17. In which of the following ethnic groups would the finding of phenylketonuria be considered unusual?
    A. Scandinavian
    B. Scottish/Irish
    C. Mediterranean
    D. Middle Eastern

18. Lactose intolerance symptoms usually become problematic at around the age of:
    A. 1 to 3 years old.
    B. 3 to 5 years old.
    C. 1 to 3 months old.
    D. 3 to 5 months old.

19. Sickle cell anemia is an example of selective advantage against which of the following diseases?
    A. Phenylketonuria
    B. Diphtheria
    C. Tuberculosis
    D. Malaria

20. When considering social, cultural, and religious factors in a child's development, the nurse recognizes that the most overwhelming influence on health is the individual's:
    A. genetic background.
    B. proximity to the disease.
    C. socioeconomic status.
    D. health beliefs and practices.

21. The concept that any behavior must be judged first in relation to the context of the culture in which it occurs is called:
   A. cultural relativity.
   B. cultural stereotyping.
   C. nonverbal communication.
   D. culturally sensitive interaction.

22. Match the custom with the ethnic group.

   A. Jewish   _F_ eye contact considered a sign of hostility
   B. United States (dominant   _E_ Nonverbal communication is a practiced art.
       culture)   _D_ seek to avoid disharmony
   C. Hispanic   _B_ focus on time; use the expression "time flies"
   D. Oriental   _A_ believe that the male child will take care of his
   E. American Indian   parents in their old age
   F. Asian   _C_ believe infants can develop symptoms of the "evil
                                                eye"

23. Which of the following strategies would NOT be considered culturally sensitive?
   A. Active listening
   B. Slow and careful speaking
   C. Loud and clear speaking
   D. Repetition and clarification

24. Which of the following groups of food would be common to most cultures?
   A. Chicken, milk, tomatoes, rice, apples
   B. Pork, milk, broccoli, noodles, bananas
   C. Sausage, milk, carrots, dry cereal, oranges
   D. Beef, milk, green beans, oatmeal, pears

25. Match the food with the ethnic group that food is associated with.

   A. black   _F_ curry
   B. Hispanic   _C_ raw tuna
   C. Japanese   _E_ lychee
   D. Chinese   _B_ nopales
   E. Vietnamese   _D_ bok choy
   F. Eastern Indian   _A_ chitterlings

26. All of the following factors have been shown to affect food preferences and traditions EXCEPT
   A. age.
   B. availability.
   C. religion.
   D. gender.

27. Voodoo is an example of an influence that would be considered:
   A. a supernatural force.
   B. a natural force.
   C. an imbalance of the forces.
   D. an imbalance of the four humors.

28. Adopting a multicultural perspective means that the nurse:
    A. explains that biomedical measures are usually more effective.
    B. uses the client's traditional health cultural beliefs.
    C. realizes that most folk remedies have a scientific basis.
    D. uses aspects of the cultural beliefs to develop a plan.

29. Which of the following terms is NOT used to describe a kind of folk healer?
    A. Asafetida
    B. Curandera
    C. Curandero
    D. Kahuna

30. Which of the following health practices may compromise the health and well-being of either mother or fetus?
    A. The mother reaching her arms above her head
    B. The practice of eating clay
    C. The use of asafetida
    D. The practice of ho'oponopono

31. To provide culturally sensitive care to children and their families, the nurse should:
    A. disregard ones own cultural values.
    B. identify behavior that is abnormal.
    C. recognize characteristic behaviors of certain cultures.
    D. rely on one's own feelings and experiences for guidance.

32. In planning and implementing transcultural patient care nurses need to strive to:
    A. adapt the family's ethnic practices to the health need.
    B. change the family's long standing beliefs.
    C. use traditional ethnic practices in every client's care.
    D. teach the family only how to treat the health problem.

33. Generalizations about cultural groups are important for nurses to know, because this information helps the nurse to:
    A. learn the similarities between all cultures.
    B. learn the unique practices of various groups.
    C. stereotype groups' characteristics.
    D. categorize groups according to their similarities.

34. During assessment the client reveals that her family uses an acupuncturist occasionally. Based on this information, the nurse would realize that another health practice commonly found from the same cultural group would be:
    A. voodoo.
    B. moxibustion.
    C. santeria.
    D. kampo.

35. Cultural assessment data would be MOST important for which of the following nursing diagnoses?
    A. Decreased cardiac output
    B. Impaired skin integrity
    C. Ineffective airway clearance
    D. Altered nutrition

36. In planning any meal for the client whose family holds beliefs of the Black Muslims, the nurse could include which of the following food?
    A. Pork
    B. Corn bread
    C. Rice
    D. Collard greens

37. Using a framework to evaluate transcultural nursing care, the nurse would identify which of the following health practices as typical?
    A. A Japanese family cares for a disabled family member in their home.
    B. An American black family uses amulets as a shield from witchcraft.
    C. A Puerto Rican family seeks help from a curandera.
    D. A Mexican American family seeks help from santeros.

CHAPTER 3
Family Influences on Child Health Promotion

1. Match the term with its description.

   A. family
   B. structure
   C. consanguineous
   D. coping strategies
   E. discipline
   F. limit-setting
   G. time-out
   H. divided, split custody
   I. joint custody
   J. function
   K. adoption
   L. step-family
   M. household

   __F__ establishment of the rules or guidelines for behavior

   __J__ family interaction

   __M__ persons sharing a common dwelling

   __A__ a group of people, living together or in close contact, who take care of one another and provide guidance for their dependent members

   __C__ blood relationships

   __E__ a system of rules governing conduct

   __H__ family situation in which each parent is awarded custody of one or more of the children, thereby separating siblings

   __D__ resources for dealing with stress such as community services, social support, and the adoption of a future orientation

   __B__ composition of the family

   __G__ a refinement of the practice of "sending the child to his/her room"; based on the premise of removing the reinforcer and using the strategy of unrelated consequences

   __I__ family situation in which the children reside with one parent, with both parents acting as legal guardians and both participating in childrearing

   __K__ establishment of a legal relationship of parent and child between persons not related by birth

   __L__ one or both married adults have children from a previous marriage residing in the household

2. Which one of the following descriptions would NOT be correct in defining the term *family* as it is viewed today?
   A. The family is what the client considers it to be.
   B. The family may be related or unrelated.
   C. The family is always related by legal ties or genetic relationships and live in the same household.
   D. The family members share a sense of belonging to their own family.

3. Match the family theory with its description. (Some theories may be used more than once.)

A. Family Systems theory
B. Family Stress theory
C. Developmental theory
D. Structural-Functional theory

_B_ employs crisis intervention strategies with the focus on helping members cope with the challenging event

_A_ continual interaction between family members and the environment

_A_ A problem or dysfunction is not viewed as lying in any one family member but rather in the interactions used by the family; focus is on interactions of members rather than on an individual member.

_B_ uses concepts of basic attributes, resources, perception, and coping behaviors or strategies in assessing family crisis management

_C_ addresses family change over time based on the predictable changes in the structure, function, and roles of the family, with the age of the oldest child as the marker for stage transition

_C_ Both the family and each individual member must achieve developmental tasks as part of each family life cycle stage.

_D_ views the major goal of the family as socialization of its members into society

4. In working with children, nurses include family members in their plan of care. Which one of the following statements does the nurse recognize as FALSE when planning nursing interventions for the family?
   A. A complete family assessment is needed to discover family dynamics, family strengths, and family weaknesses.
   B. recognition of situations where referral of the family to specialized services is not a nursing responsibility
   C. The intervention used with families will depend on the nurse's view of the theoretic model of the family.
   D. The level of assistance a family needs will depend on the type of crisis, factors affecting family adjustment, and the family's level of functioning.

5. Debbie is 2 years old and lives with her brother Mark, her sister Mary, and her mother. Her father and mother recently divorced and now her father lives one hour away. Debbie sees her father once a month for a day's visit. Her mother retains custody of Debbie. Debbie's grandparents live in a different state but she visits them each year. Debbie's family represents which one of the following?
   A. Binuclear family
   B. Extended family
   C. Single-parent family
   D. Reconstituted family

6. Three major objectives of the family in relation to children are:

   Caregiving

   Nurturing

   Training

7. Which one of the following is an effective approach for working with vulnerable families?
   A. Identify and emphasize family deficits
   B. Offer single-purpose services with responses aimed at solving emergencies
   C. Emphasize and focus on the troubled individual child or family member
   D. Identify cultural differences, treating families with respect and honoring their traditions

8. Identify the following statements as TRUE or FALSE.
   ___T___ Roles are learned through the socialization process.
   ___F___ Role continuity is described as role behavior that is expected of children conflicting with desirable adult behavior.
   ___T___ All families have strengths and vulnerabilities.
   ___T___ Each family has its own standards for interaction within and outside the family.
   ___F___ Role definitions are changing as a result of the changing economy and women's liberation movement. Marital roles, however, are still most segregated among the middle classes.

9. Identify the type of role that is related to fantasy and important in childhood as a means of adjustment and socialization. In this role, the child uses the environment as a primary resource for learning the conduct that befits position or status.
   A. Ascribed role
   B. Achieved role
   C. Adopted role
   D. Assumed role

10. Children learn role behavior and to perform in an expected way within the family at a very early age. One influence of the role each sibling is assigned within the family structure is the
    _____birth_____ _____order_____.

11. Parenting practices differ between small and large families. Which one of the following characteristics is NOT found in small families?
    A. Emphasis is placed on the individual development of the child with constant pressure to measure up to family expectations.
    B. Adolescents identify more strongly with their parents and rely more on their parents for advice.
    C. Emphasis is placed on the group and less on the individual.
    D. Children's development and achievement is measured against children in the neighborhood and social class.

12. Because age differences between siblings affect the childhood environment, the nurse recognizes that there is more affection, less rivalry and hostility between children that are spaced how many years apart?
    A. 4 or more years
    B. 4 or fewer years
    C. 3 or fewer years
    D. 2 or fewer years

13. Johnny has always been viewed by his parents as being less dependent than his brother, Tommy, or his sister, Julie. Johnny is described as affectionate, good-natured, and flexible in his thinking. He identifies with his peer group and is very popular with classmates. His parents tend to place fewer demands on Johnny for household help. From this description, the nurse would expect Johnny to have what birth position within the family?
    A. Firstborn child
    B. Middle child
    C. Youngest child
    D. Any of the above; birth position does not affect personality.

14. Monozygotic twins are:
    A. the result of fertilization of two ova.
    B. the result of fertilization of one ovum that became separated early in development.
    C. different physically and genetically.
    D. of dissimilar behaviors with greater sibling rivalry.

15. The MOST essential component of successful parenting is which one of the following?
    A. Strong religious and cultural ties to the community
    B. Previous experience with childcare, usually during adolescence as an older sibling or babysitter
    C. An understanding of childhood growth and development
    D. One person responsible for providing childcare within the family structure

16. Which one of the following does NOT identify a method to promote separation-individuation among twins?
    A. Parents discipline and praise twins as a unit.
    B. Parents foster feeling of separateness among twins.
    C. Parents avoid the term "the twins."
    D. Parents foster opportunities to build one-to-one relationships with each twin.

17. Development of a parental sense can be divided into four phases. Briefly describe each phase.

    A. Anticipation: _looking forward to parenthood_

    B. Honeymoon: _transition to parent role is made._

    C. Plateau: _parental development parallels child development_

    D. Disengagement: _end of active parental role_

18. The parenting behavior of warmth-hostility is best described by which one of the following?
    A. The degree of autonomy that parents allow their children
    B. The degree of open or frequent parental affection combined with the degree of affection, mixed with feelings of rejection or hostility that is expressed by the parents to their children
    C. The degree of restrictive control the parents impose on their children, combined with the degree of active survey of their children's behavior
    D. The degree to which the parents allow their children to openly display feelings of rejection and hostility, combined with the acceptance of this behavior

19. Match the parenting style with its description.

A. authoritarian/dictatorial

B. permissive/laissez-faire

C. authoritative/democratic

___B___ allows children to regulate their own activity; sees the parenting role as being a resource rather than a role model

___A___ establishes rules, regulations, and standards of conduct for the child that are to be followed without question

___C___ respects the child's individuality; directs the child's behavior by emphasizing the reason for rules

20. Child misbehavior requires parental implementation of appropriate disciplinary action. Identify which one of the following would NOT be a correct guideline for implementing discipline.

A. Focus on child and misbehavior utilizing "you" messages rather than "I" messages

B. Maintain consistency with disciplinary action

C. Make sure all caregivers maintain unity of plan by agreeing on plan and being familiar with details before implementation

D. Maintain flexibility by planning disciplinary actions appropriate to child's age, temperament, and severity of misbehavior

21. Which one of the following is a correct interpretation in the use of reasoning as a form of discipline?

A. Used for older children when moral issues are involved

B. Used for younger children to "see the other side" of an issue

C. Used only in combination with scolding and criticism

D. Used to allow children to obtain lengthy explanations and a greater degree of attention from parents

22. Which one of the following is NOT a description of the discipline "time out"?

A. Allows the reinforcer to be maintained

B. No physical punishment is involved.

C. Offers both parents and child "cooling off" time

D. Facilitates the parent's ability to consistently apply the punishment

23. Johnny spilled his milk on the living room rug. His mother smacks him on the bottom and says, "you are a messy, bad boy, Johnny." The discipline strategies utilized are:

1. Consequence
2. Corporal punishment
3. Scolding
4. Behavior modification
5. Ignoring

A. 1, 2, and 3

B. 2 and 3

C. 3 and 5

D. 2, 3, and 4

24. Areas of concern for parents of adoptive children include:
    A. the initial attachment process.
    B. telling the children that they are adopted.
    C. identity formation of children during adolescence.
    D. all of the above.

25. Identify the following statements about the impact of divorce on children as TRUE or FALSE.

    __F__ Research has shown that children of divorce suffer no lasting psychologic and social difficulties.

    __T__ One outcome found in children of divorce is a heightened anxiety about forming enduring relationships as young adults.

    __F__ Children of divorce cope better with their feelings of abandonment when there is continuing conflict between parents.

    __T__ Preschoolers assume themselves to be the cause of the divorce and interpret the separation as punishment.

    __T__ School-age children's teachers and school counselors should be informed because these children will often display altered behaviors.

    __T__ Adolescents have concerns and heightened anxiety about their own future as a marital partner and the availability of money for future needs.

26. Which one of the following is NOT considered important by parents when telling their children about the decision to divorce?
    A. Initial disclosure should include both parents and siblings.
    B. Time should be allowed for discussion with each child individually.
    C. The initial disclosure should be kept simple and reasons for divorce should not be included.
    D. Parents should physically hold or touch their child to provide feelings of warmth and reassurance.

27. List and describe the two major phases that children go through when adjusting to a divorce.

    Crisis phase - usually lasts 1 yr or longer & is characterized by an emotional upheaval affecting the relationship c̄ the parent granted custody

    adjustment - child settling ↓ + beginning to adapt to life in a single-parent home

28. Single-parenting, step-parenting, and dual-earner family parenting adds stress to the parental role. Match the family type with an expected stressor or concern.

    A. single-parenting
    B. step-parenting
    C. dual-earner families

    __A__ Managing shortages of money, time, and energy are major concerns.

    __C__ Overload is a common source of stress, and social activities are significantly curtailed with time demands and scheduling seen as major problems.

    __B__ Competition is a major area of concern among adults with reduction of power conflicts a necessity.

Ester and Roberto Garcia are the proud new parents of twin boys Timothy and Thomas. Ester and Roberto Garcia have been married less than one year. Ester is 17 years old and plans to return to finish school next year. Roberto finished high school and works with his father in a local auto repair shop. He is taking a week off from work to help Ester at home with Timothy and Thomas. Neither attended child parenting classes. You are making a home visit to the couple one day after they have brought Timothy and Thomas home from the hospital. As you arrive at the house you see that both Timothy and Thomas are crying. Ester is trying to give Timothy his bath while Roberto is busy trying to get Thomas to take his formula. Both new parents appear tired and Roberto admits they have been up all night with the infants and that either Timothy or Thomas seems to be crying "all the time" and that "something must be terribly wrong with them."

29. As you begin your assessment of the family, you know that the Garcia family are in stage II, families with infants, according to Duvall's developmental stages of the family. Which one of the following is a developmental task of this stage?
    A. Reestablish couple identity
    B. Socialize children
    C. Make decisions regarding parenthood
    D. Accommodate to parenting role

30. A priority nursing diagnosis for this family would be:
    A. altered family process related to gain of family members.
    B. growth and development altered, related to inadequate caretaking.
    C. fear related to new parental role.
    D. injury, high risk for, related to unsafe environment.

31. As the nurse developing the plan for this new family, your priority intervention would be which one of the following?
    A. Teaching the parents about Duvall's developmental stages so they will understand that what they are experiencing is normal transition into parenthood
    B. Reassuring the parents that you will examine each of the infants but that they appear to be healthy and that the parents are doing a good job
    C. Take over the feeding and bathing of the infants, explaining to the parents the necessity of child parenting classes
    D. Check the infant supplies and environment to make sure the home has been made safe for children

32. Both Thomas and Timothy are now sleeping and you have completed your family assessment with Roberto and Ester Garcia. As a nurse you decide to use the family stress theory to promote adaptation to the family's new role. Which one of the following does the nurse know is NOT a capability the family can use to manage the crisis?
    A. Basic attributes of the family
    B. Resources within the family
    C. Perception of family to the situation
    D. Closed boundary within the family system

33. Identify a long-term goal for the family and discuss nursing interventions that would foster achievement of this long-term goal.

Establish a healthy family unit

_____

_____

_____

_____

34. Compare and contrast the following types of consequences and give an example of a discipline technique for each type.

A. Natural

_____

_____

B. Logical

_____

_____

C. Unrelated

_____

_____

35. Discuss the use and concerns of using corporal punishment as a form of discipline to stop or decrease certain behaviors.

_____

_____

_____

_____

_____

CHAPTER 4
Growth and Development of Children

1. Terms—Foundations

A. growth	F. standards or norms	K. epigenisis
B. development	G. cross-sectional method	L. saltatory pattern of growth
C. maturation	H. longitudinal method	
D. differentiation	I. cephalocaudal	M. sensitive periods
E. developmental task	J. proximodistal	N. terminal points

___N___ the time when growth ceases

___B___ a gradual change and expansion; advancement from a lower to a more advanced stage of complexity; the emerging and expanding of the individual's capabilities through growth, maturation, and learning

___H___ used to determine growth trends and rates; useful in assessing the long term or delayed effects of early experiences

___J___ near to far direction (midline to periphery); early embryonic development of limb buds followed by rudimentary fingers and toes

___E.___ a set of skills and competencies unique to each developmental stage, which children must accomplish or master in order to deal effectively with their environment

___A___ an increase in the number and size of cells as they divide and synthesize new proteins; results in increased size and weight of the whole or any of its parts

___I___ head to tail directional trend; the head end of the organism develops first and is very large and complex; the lower end is small and simple and takes shape at a later period

___C___ an increase in competence and adaptability; aging; usually used to describe a qualitative change; change in the complexity of a structure that makes it possible for that structure to begin functioning; to function at a higher level

___D___ the process by which early cells and structures are systematically modified and altered to achieve specific and characteristic physical and chemical properties; sometimes used to describe the trend of mass to specific, development from simple to more complex activities

___G___ tests or measures the characteristics of a number of children representing the various ages or stages of development; the more commonly used method of comparing groups of children

___F___ the average age for expected parameters to appear, such as height, weight, and motor skills

___L___ follows no regular cycle and can occur after "quiet" periods that last as long as 4 weeks; negative influences

___K___ continuity with the past development; new biologic parts and behaviors arise out of and build on those already established

___M___ critical, vulnerable, and optimal periods in an organism's lifetime in which the organism is more susceptible to positive or negative influence

2. Terms—Biologic Growth and Development

A. lordosis
B. height
C. weight
D. bone age
E. dentition
F. diaphysis
G. epiphysis
H. epiphyseal cartilage plate
I. metaphysis
J. brain growth
K. spinal cord growth
L. cauda equina
M. basal metabolic rate (BMR)
N. reflexive/rudimentary movements
O. general fundamental skills
P. specific skills
Q. specialized skills
R. active sleep (REM sleep)
S. quiet sleep (non-REM sleep)
T. sleep stage 1
U. sleep stage 2
V. sleep stage 3
W. sleep stage 4
X. sleep cycle
Y. partial waking
Z. temperament
AA. the easy child
BB. the difficult child
CC. the slow to warm up child
DD. degree of fit

__DD__ the match between the amount of demand for change with the child's capacities

__E__ used as an indicator of growth because of its relative regularity; does not correlate well with bone age and is less reliable as an index of biologic age

__D__ used as an indicator of growth; correlates more closely with measures of physiologic maturity than with chronologic age or height

__N__ present at birth and forms the foundation of all other movements, including sitting, crawling, creeping, reaching, standing, and walking

__B__ occurs as a result of skeletal growth; considered a stable measure of general growth

__C__ a variable measure of growth; at birth it is considered a reflection of intrauterine environment

__A__ exaggerated lumbar curvature

__K__ demonstrates alterations relative to the vertebral column during prenatal and early postnatal growth, but ends at the level of the third and fourth lumbar vertebrae in the newborn

__J__ reflected in head circumference which increases six times as much during the first year of life as it does in the second year

__P__ develop during later childhood; greater emphasis on form, accuracy, and adaptability; children begin to apply these skills to sports and other activities that require body movement.

__I__ the spongy tissue that unites the diaphysis and the epiphyseal cartilage in bone

__M__ the rate of metabolism when the body is at rest

__F__ the long central portion of the bone

__CC__ the New York Longitudinal Study category for children; typically react negatively and with mild intensity to new stimuli and, unless pressured, adapt slowly with repeated contact; respond with mild but passive resistance to novelty or changes in routine.

__G__ the end portion of the bone

__L__ the arrangement of the sacral and coccygeal nerves that resemble the hairs on a horse's tail

__O__ develop during early childhood and include activities such as running, jumping, balancing, catching, and throwing

__H__ situated between the diaphysis and the epiphysis; unites with the diaphysis by columns of spongy tissue

__X__ the time between two consecutive appearances of the same sleep state

__R__ characterized by irregular pulse, expirations, many body movements and rapid eye movements

_BB_ the New York Longitudinal Study category for children who are highly active, irritable and irregular in their habits; negative withdrawal responses typical; require a more structured environment; adapt slowly to new routines, people or situations; mood expressions are usually intense and primarily negative.

_S_ sleep in which breathing and the heartbeat are regular and body and eye movements are absent

_T_ consists of drowsiness with decreasing awareness of the external world

_Q_ evolve slowly from late childhood through adolescence and depend on training and repetition

_Y_ characteristic of normal sleep; after about 1 hour of stage 4 sleep, the child arouses for a brief period that lasts a few seconds or up to several minutes; sleepwalking and bed wetting occur in this stage.

_U_ a sleeping person can be easily wakened, and, if wakened, may not admit to having been asleep

_Z_ the manner of thinking, behaving, or reacting characteristic of an individual; refers to the way a person deals with life

_V_ sleep becomes increasingly deep; breathing and the heart rate are very stable; the muscles are relaxed and the brain waves are very slow

_AA_ the New York Longitudinal Study category for even tempered; regular and predictable in their habits; and they have a positive approach to new stimuli

_W_ the deepest sleep; from this stage it is difficult to be roused except by strong stimuli

3. Terms—Mental Function and Personality

A. id	L. inductive reasoning	U. interactional proponent's theory of language development
B. the ego	M. preconventional level	V. role
C. superego	N. conventional level	W. self-concept
D. psychosexual	O. postconventional level	X. body image
E. psychosocial development	P. phonology	Y. self-esteem
F. autonomy	Q. semantics	Z. high self-esteem
G. permanence	R. pragmatics	AA. identification
H. egocentrism	S. learning theorist's theory of language development	BB. Consumer Product Safety Commission (CPSC)/Canadian Toy Testing Council
I. intuitive reasoning	T. nativist's theory of language development	
J. transductive reasoning		
K. conservation		

_Y_ the value that an individual places on oneself; refers to an overall evaluation of oneself

_H_ the predominant characteristic of the preoperational stage of intellectual development according to Piaget; the inability to put oneself in the place of another; does not mean selfishness or self-centeredness

_Z_ a feeling based on unconditional acceptance of oneself as a worthy and important being

_AA_ the process by which children style themselves after their parent of the same sex and internalize that parent's values and outlook

_C_ the conscience, functions as the moral arbitrator and represents the ideal; mechanism that prevents individuals from expressing undesirable instincts that might threaten the social order.

_BB_ government agencies that maintain information on a variety of recalled products; these agencies do not inspect or police all toys on the market

_A_ the unconscious mind; the inborn component that is driven by instincts

_O_ the term used by Freud to describe any sexual pleasure

_K_ a concept of permanence; the child realizes that physical factors such as volume, weight, and number remain the same even though outward appearances are changed; occurs during Piaget's stage of concrete operations

_B_ the conscious mind; serves the reality principle; functions as the conscious or controlling self that is able to find a realistic means for gratifying instincts while blocking the irrational thinking of the id

_J_ the idea that because two events occur together, they cause each other; occurs during Piaget's preoperational stage

_E_ the most widely accepted theory of personality development advanced by Erikson; built on Freudian theory; emphasizes a healthy personality as opposed to a pathologic approach.

_M_ the level of morality according to Kohlberg that parallels the preconceptual level of cognitive development and intuitive thought; children at this level conform to rules imposed by authority figures.

_G_ the awareness that objects exist even when they are no longer visible

_I_ the ability to make simple associations between ideas; occurs during the beginning of Piaget's preoperational stage

_L_ problems are solved in a concrete, systematic fashion based on what the child can perceive; occurs during Piaget's stage of concrete operations

_O_ the autonomous or principled level of morality according to Kohlberg; children at this level have reached the cognitive formal operational stage and they endeavor to define moral values and principles that are valid and applicable beyond the authority of the groups and persons holding these principles.

_Q_ that words and sentences convey an expressed meaning syntax; the form or structure of language

_N_ the level of morality according to Kohlberg in which children are concerned with conformity and loyalty; actively maintaining, supporting, and justifying the social order and the personal expectations of those significant in their lives

_V_ a set of duties, rights, obligations, and expected behaviors that accompanies a given position in a social structure

_R_ the principles specifying how language is to be used in different social contexts and situations

_P_ refers to the basic units of sound that are combining to produce words

_S_ language is acquired as children hear and respond to the speech of their companions

_T_ propose that human beings have an inborn linguistic processor or language acquisition mechanism that is specialized for language learning

_W_ how an individual describes himself or herself; comprises all the notions, beliefs, and convictions that constitute children's knowledge of themselves and influence their relationships with others

_U_ acknowledge that children are biologically prepared to acquire language but suggest that what may be innate is the development and maturation of the nervous system rather than a special linguistic processor

_X_ refers to the subjective concepts and attitudes that individuals have toward their own bodies

_F_ symbolized by holding onto and letting go of sphincter muscles; corresponds to Freud's anal stage

4. Terms—Selected Influences on Growth and Development

A. Dietary Guidelines for Americans
B. Food Guide Pyramid
C. malnutrition
D. masked deprivation
E. emotional bank
F. coping strategies
G. coping styles
H. fear
I. anxiety
J. resilience

___I___ a general uneasiness, apprehension, or feeling of impending doom

___E___ a concept to help parents and care givers maintain a proper perspective regarding the effects of stress and coping

___D___ the term used to describe children who are reared in homes in which there is a distorted parent-child relationship or otherwise disordered home environment

___J___ the ability of an individual to resist, recover, or "spring back" from adversity

___C___ the term usually used to describe under nutrition, primarily that resulting from insufficient caloric intake

___G___ relatively unchanging personality characteristics or outcomes of coping

___H___ an emotional reaction to a specific real or unreal threat or danger

___A___ the most well known published dietary advice that encourages eating a variety of food, maintaining ideal body weight, consuming adequate starch and fiber, and limiting the intake of fat, cholesterol, sugar, salt, and alcohol

___F___ the specific ways in which children cope with stressors

___B___ a visual companion to the Dietary Guidelines for Americans that is intended to help consumers understand more about the food they need

5. Categorizing growth and behavior into approximate age stages:
   A. helps to account for individual differences in children.
   B. can be applied to all children with some degree of precision.
   C. provides a convenient means to describe the majority of children.
   D. determines the speed of each child's growth.

6. Which of the following terms is the correct term to use to describe the period of rapid growth rate and total dependency between 8 weeks after conception until birth?
   A. Prenatal
   B. Germinal
   C. Embryonic
   D. Fetal

7. Which of the following is an example of a cephalocaudal directional trend in development?
   A. Infants stand after they are able to hold their back erect.
   B. Fingers and toes develop after embryonic limb buds.
   C. Infants manipulate fingers after they are able to use the whole hand as a unit.
   D. Infants begin to have fine muscle control after gross random muscle movement is established.

8. The directional trend that predicts an orderly and continuous development is known as:
   A. cephalocaudal.
   B. proximodistal.
   C. sequential.
   D. differentiation.

9. Which of the following traits of development is fixed and precise?
   A. The pace and rate of development
   B. The order of development
   C. Physical growth, in particular height
   D. Growth during the vulnerable period

10. During a sensitive period in development, the child is:
    A. more likely to respond to stimulation.
    B. more likely to require specific stimulation for physical growth.
    C. less likely to acquire a specific skill if it is not learned during this time.
    D. less likely to be harmed by external conditions.

11. Which of the following statements about individual differences in growth and development is FALSE?
    A. The pubescent growth spurt begins early in some children.
    B. Females reach their terminal height before males.
    C. Males reach their terminal height before females.
    D. Males reach their terminal weight after females.

12. Match the developmental trend in external proportions to the correct age group.

    A. fetal
    B. newborn
    C. infancy
    D. childhood
    E. adolescent
    F. adult

    __C__ Rapid growth and growth of the trunk with a high center of gravity predominates in this age group.

    __F__ The lower limbs constitute one half of the total body weight and 30% of the total body weight.

    __A__ The head is the fastest growing part of the body; at one point during this stage the head constitutes 50% of the total body length.

    __D__ The legs are the most rapidly growing part of the body, and the slender, long-legged build is characteristic of both sexes during this stage.

    __B__ The lower limbs are one third of the total body length, but only 15% of the total body weight in this age group.

    __E__ A large portion of the increase in height during this stage is the result of trunk elongation. The feet and hands also grow rapidly and may appear large and ungainly in proportion to the rest of the body.

13. Which of the following growth patterns is considerably greater in the male adolescent when compared to the female adolescent?
    A. Shoulder and hip growth
    B. Anterior hip diameter
    C. The width of the pelvis
    D. The deposition of body fat

14. The lordosis that a 15-month-old infant develops would be considered a secondary curvature that is:
    A. located in the cervical region.
    B. fused and permanently fixed.
    C. a sign of a developmental delay.
    D. a compensatory lumbar curve exaggeration.

15. The maximum skeletal growth measure by linear growth or weight occurs:
    A. between age 3 and 9 years.
    B. between age 2 and 4 years.
    C. in the newborn stage.
    D. before birth.

16. If the height of a 2 year old is measured as 88 cm., his height at adulthood may be estimated to be:
    A. 132 cm.
    B. 176 cm.
    C. 172 cm.
    D. 190 cm.

17. If a newborn measures 19 inches at birth, the expected length at age 4 years would be approximately:
    A. 28.5 inches.
    B. 38 inches.
    C. 43.5 inches.
    D. 48 inches.

18. At 17 years of age, a girl will be considered to be at her:
    A. midgrowth height.
    B. terminal height.
    C. growth spurt.
    D. transitory height.

19. The 6 year molar is often used as a criterion for:
    A. developmental assessment.
    B. bone age.
    C. biologic age.
    D. certain endocrine problems.

20. The BEST estimate of biologic age can be made using measurement obtained from:
    A. nasal bone height.
    B. facial bone radiography.
    C. hand and wrist radiography.
    D. mandibular size.

21. At birth, the infant brain has achieved _____ of its adult size.
    A. 90%
    B. 50%
    C. 25%
    D. 98%

22. Increasingly complex movement and neurologic changes in the infant can be attributed to the:
    A. persistence of primitive reflexes after birth.
    B. dramatic increase in the number of neurons immediately after birth.
    C. new nerve cells that appear after the sixth month of life.
    D. increasing control over reflex activity.

23. The acquisition of motor skills depends primarily on the:
   A. myelinization and maturation of the nerve tracts.
   B. amount of stimulation the nerve tracts receive.
   C. influences of the environmental stimuli.
   D. persistence of primitive reflexes.

24. One probable reason for large lymph node development in the child is that lymph tissues growth patterns reflect the:
   A. parallel development of the nervous system.
   B. general growth patterns of the child.
   C. repeated exposure to new infectious agents.
   D. parallel development of the thymus gland.

25. When a child has experienced a secondary cause of growth deficiency such as prematurity they usually lag behind age mates in their developmental milestones until about the age of:
   A. 6 months.
   B. 2 years.
   C. 4 years.
   D. 6 years.

26. The daily requirement for dietary protein intake is lowest for which one of the following groups?
   A. Adult males
   B. Infants over 6 months of age
   C. School aged children
   D. Infants under 6 months of age

27. The nurse determines that a 7-month-old infant who weighs 10 kg needs about:
   A. 450 kcal per day.
   B. 700 kcal per day.
   C. 1000 kcal per day.
   D. 1200 kcal per day.

28. The basal metabolic rate (BMR) is highest in the:
   A. adult male.
   B. infant over 6 months of age.
   C. school-age child.
   D. infant under 6 months of age.

29. The energy requirement to build tissue:
   A. fluctuates randomly.
   B. fluctuates based on need.
   C. steadily decreases with age.
   D. steadily increases with age.

30. One of the most important body responses in the transition from intrauterine life for the newborn is:
   A. general fundamental motor skills.
   B. thermoregulation.
   C. basal metabolic rate.
   D. reflexive movements.

31. Body temperature in young children and infants responds to:
    A. changes in the environment.
    B. exercise.
    C. emotional upset.
    D. all of the above.

32. Which one of the following motor behaviors is considered a general fundamental skill?
    A. Jumping
    B. Maturation of muscles
    C. Rudimentary movement
    D. All of the above

33. Infants with which one of the following disorders is at highest risk for motor disability?
    A. Cerebral palsy
    B. Myleodysplasia
    C. Limb deficiency
    D. Severe muscle disease

34. The length of time spent in sleep increases somewhat:
    A. throughout childhood.
    B. during the pubertal growth spurt.
    C. by age 3 years.
    D. by age of 18 months.

35. The rapid eye movement (REM) sleep of newborns consists of __50__ percent of their sleep time.

36. A mother asks whether her child's sleep behavior is abnormal because he usually arouses during the night, looks around, and speaks unintelligibly. The nurse's response would be based on the knowledge that periodic wakening indicates that the child:
    A. has normal sleep behavior.
    B. has periods of sleeplessness.
    C. is slow to return to sleep.
    D. was very fatigued.

37. If parenting skills are lacking, the child's behavior may be perceived by the parent as:
    A. less difficult.
    B. easier.
    C. more distracted.
    D. more difficult.

38. Match the attribute of temperament with its description.

A. activity
B. rhythmicity
C. approach-withdrawal
D. adaptability
E. threshold of responsiveness
F. intensity of reaction
G. mood
H. distractibility
I. attention span and persistence

___E___ amount of stimulation required to evoke a response

___C___ nature of initial responses to a new stimulus: positive or negative

___B___ regularity in the timing of physiologic functions such as hunger, sleep, and elimination

___F___ energy level of the child's reactions

___A___ level of physical motion during activity

___D___ ease or difficulty with which the child adapts or adjusts to new situations

___I___ length of time a child pursues a given activity and continues

___H___ ease with which attention can be diverted

___G___ amount of pleasant behavior compared with the unpleasant

39. The term "difficult child" is a category derived by the individual's overall pattern of temperamental attributes that may:
A. be used to categorize about 40% of all children.
B. indicate that the child is even-tempered.
C. indicate that the child has a poor "fit" with his/her environment.
D. affect the child's adjustment throughout childhood.

40. Assessment of temperament provides useful information for anticipating probable areas of:
A. maladaptive functioning.
B. developmental risk.
C. demand for adaptation.
D. parental dissonance.

41. The BEST strategy for the nurse to use to promote mastery motivation is to:
A. assist the infant during play.
B. correct errors immediately.
C. initiate activities for the infant.
D. control feedback during play.

42. Personality development as viewed by Freud focuses on:
A. the desire to satisfy biological needs.
B. the suppression of psychosexual instincts.
C. direct observations of adults
D. retrospective studies of children.

43. Erikson's theory provides a framework for:
A. clearly indicating the experience needed to resolve crises.
B. emphasizing pathologic development.
C. coping with extraordinary events.
D. explaining children's behavior in mastering developmental tasks.

44. Erikson's stage trust vs. mistrust corresponds to Freud's:
    A. anal stage.
    B. oral stage.
    C. phallic stage.
    D. guilt stage.

45. For adolescents, their struggle to fit the roles they have played and those they hope to play is best outlined by:
    A. Freud's latency period.
    B. Freud's phallic stage.
    C. Erikson's identity vs. role confusion.
    D. Erikson's intimacy vs. isolation.

46. Sullivan's theory of interpersonal development:
    A. recognizes the importance of the biologic maturation process.
    B. recognizes the interpersonal relationships between children.
    C. explains the importance of social approval in developing self-concept.
    D. explains how children acquire feelings of security.

47. The best known theory regarding cognitive development was developed by:
    A. Sullivan.
    B. Kohlberg.
    C. Erikson.
    D. Piaget.

48. A schema according to Piaget is a:
    A. skill of organizing new knowledge.
    B. cognitive developmental stage.
    C. mechanism to move from one stage to the next.
    D. pattern of action or thought.

49. An important prerequisite for all other mental activity is the child's awareness that an object exists even though it is no longer visible. According to Piaget, this awareness is called:
    A. object permanence.
    B. logical thinking.
    C. egocentricity.
    D. reversibility.

50. The predominant characteristic of Piaget's preoperational period is egocentricity, which according to Piaget means:
    A. concrete and tangible reasoning.
    B. selfishness and self-centeredness.
    C. inability to see another's perspective.
    D. ability to make deduction and generalize.

51. The stages of moral development which allow for prediction of behavior but not for individual differences are outlined in the moral development theory according to:
    A. Fowler.
    B. Holstein.
    C. Gilligan.
    D. Kohlberg.

52. The difference between religion and spirituality is that spirituality:
    A. requires an organized set of practices.
    B. affects the whole person: mind, body and spirit.
    C. assures the individual's desire to differentiate right from wrong.
    D. assures rational moral decision making.

53. Children learn most of the syntax structures of their native language by the age of:
    A. 2 years.
    B. 3 years.
    C. 5 years.
    D. 7 years

54. According to the theories of learning theorists, language is acquired:
    A. as children hear simplified versions of adult speech.
    B. through the maturation of the nervous system.
    C. through the assistance of an inborn language acquisition mechanism.
    D. as children hear and respond to the speech of their companions.

55. Match the concept with its description.

    A. classical conditioning   G   gender identity
       where two events evoke   B   operant conditioning
       the same response
                                     D   self concept
    B. use of rewards to   A   Pavlovian conditioning
       encourage specific
       behavior   E   body image
    C. role modeling   F   self esteem
    D. knowledge of oneself   C   Bandura's observational learning
       that influences
       relationships with others
    E. a component of self
       concept that encompasses
       the individual's attitude
       toward his/her own body
    F. the affective component
       of self concept
    G. the process by which
       children internalize the
       same sex parent's values
       and outlook

56. The gender label:
    A. is achieved early and subtly through imitation.
    B. should not be assigned until at least 3 years of age.
    C. is affected primarily by the chromosomal determination of sex.
    D. is only a small component of the child's total identity.

57. Match the type of play with the example of that type of play.

A. sense pleasure   __G__ coloring a picture

B. skill play   __D__ rocking a doll

C. unoccupied behavior   __C__ daydreaming

D. dramatic play   __E__ peekaboo/pattycake

E. games   __F__ watching *Sesame Street* on television

F. onlooker play   __J__ putting on a puppet show

G. solitary play   __B__ learning to ride a bicycle

H. parallel play   __A__ swinging

I. associative play   __I__ playing with dolls

J. cooperative play   __H__ toddlers playing blocks in the same room

58. Which of the following functions of play may be hindered by increasing the early academic achievements of a child?
A. Intellectual development
B. Creative development
C. Sensorimotor development
D. Moral development

59. Match the stage with the example of an appropriate toy for that stage.

A. exploratory stage   __C__ a deck of cards

B. toy stage   __D__ popular magazines to browse through

C. play stage   __B__ a tool box and tools

D. daydreaming stage   __A__ a busy box

60. The influence of heredity on behavior characteristics and intelligence is based on the:
A. action of environment on heredity.
B. action of heredity on environment.
C. interaction between the environment and heredity.
D. influence of environmental stimulation on achievement.

61. Based on documented research, which one of the following behaviors can be attributed more to girls than to boys during childhood?
A. More analytic
B. Lower self esteem
C. Physical aggressiveness
D. Verbal aggressiveness

62. Based on documented research which one of the following behaviors can be attributed more to boys than to girls?
A. More analytic
B. Lower self esteem
C. Physical aggressiveness
D. Verbal aggressiveness

63. Altered growth and development would be LEAST likely to be noteworthy in which one of the following disorders?
    A. Chromosome abnormalities
    B. Acute appendicitis
    C. Chronic hepatitis
    D. Cystic fibrosis

64. Match the growth and developmental influences with the example or description.

    A. prenatal influences   __I__ protects children from dangers
    B. altitude   __C__ lead, pollution, radiation
    C. environmental hazards   __J__ There are often great fluctuations in the
    D. socioeconomic level   development of this ability.
    E. nutrition   __F__ the single most important emotional need for
    F. love   growth
    G. significant others   __E__ the single most important influence on growth
    H. security   __G__ play an important role in personality and
    I. discipline   intellectual development
    J. independence   __B__ hypoxia may limit development
    K. emotional deprivation   __K__ occurs in homes with disorganized distorted
                                         parental child relationships
                                  __D__ general health and nutrition vary
                                  __H__ Most childhood behavior problems are associated
                                         with each of these influencing factors.
                                  __A__ smoking/fetal alcohol

65. In relation to stress in childhood, it is MOST desirable to:
    A. identify all of the possible childhood stressors.
    B. provide children with interpersonal security.
    C. protect children from stressors.
    D. realize that most children are not vulnerable to stress.

66. The medium that has the MOST impact on children in America today is:
    A. television.
    B. movies.
    C. comic books.
    D. newspapers.

Brian Adams, who is 8 years old, arrives at the clinic for a check up for school. He has historically been in the 50th percentile for both height and weight and is generally considered healthy. He has a family history of heart disease.

Mrs. Adams is concerned about an increase in her son's physical aggressiveness lately. Today Brian's height is noted to be in the 50th percentile, but his weight is in the 90th percentile. His mother states that he watches television each day. His cholesterol is elevated.

67. Based on the information in the case study above, the nurse would estimate that:
    A. Brian is exposed to only the positive effects of television.
    B. using family history of heart disease is an excellent screening indicator for cholesterol testing.
    C. Brian probably watches more than 2 hours of television per day.
    D. there is no link between Brian's television viewing and his increased physical aggression.

68. Based on the assessment information presented about Brian in the case study, which one of the following nursing diagnoses would be MOST appropriate?
    A. Altered growth and development
    B. Altered nutrition less than body requirements
    C. Fluid volume excess
    D. Altered parenting

69. Which one of the following interventions in regard to Brian's television viewing would be LEAST appropriate for the nurse to suggest?
    A. Restrict Brian's viewing of violent programs.
    B. Watch Brian's favorite shows with him each day.
    C. Help Brian to correlate consequences with actions and point out subtle messages.
    D. Explore alternatives to aggressive conflict resolution.

70. Which of the following outcomes would be BEST to expect in regard to Brian?
    A. Brian's aggressive behavior decreases significantly, his intake of cholesterol snacks decreases and his television viewing time decreases.
    B. Brian is able to explain the television programs that he watches.
    C. Brian selects more healthful snacks and watches television about one hour per day.
    D. Brian's cholesterol decreases to within normal level, his weight is at the 50th percentile and his mother reports that his aggressive behavior is decreased.

CHAPTER 5
Hereditary Influences on Health Promotion of the Child and Family

1. Terms—Genetic Influences on Health

A. genes
B. chromosomes
C. major structural abnormalities
D. minor anomalies
E. syndrome
F. association
G. aberration
H. chromosome aberrations
I. structural aberration
J. ring chromosome
K. somy
L. monosomy
M. trisomy

N. gamete formation
O. postzygotic cell division
P. non-disjunction
Q. sister chromatid
R. partial chromosome abnormalities
S. classic deletion syndromes
T. contiguous gene syndromes
U. X inactivation
V. consanguinity
W. mutation
X. variable expression

Y. premutations
Z. genetic anticipation
AA. genomic imprinting
BB. Prader-Willi syndrome
CC. Angelman syndrome
DD. uniparental disomy
EE. mitochondria
FF. karyotyping
GG. in situ hybridization
HH. mapped
II. multifactorial disorders
JJ. human leukocyte antigen HLA system
KK. teratogens

_____C_____ malformations that can result from genetic and/or prenatal environmental causes that have serious medical, surgical, or quality of life consequences

_____E_____ a recognized pattern of malformations that is due to a single specific cause

_____A_____ the genetic material responsible for programing the body's physiologic process and characteristics

_____F_____ a non-random pattern of malformations for which an etiology has not been determined, such as VATER, vertebral defects, imperforate anus, tracheoesophageal fistula and radial-renal defects

_____B_____ structures that are organized from genes and visible only during certain stages of cell division

_____G_____ a deviation from that which is normal or typical

_____D_____ normal variants with non-serious consequences such as a sacral dimple, an extra nipple, or an umbilical hernia

_____I_____ loss, addition, rearrangement, or exchange of some of the genes of a chromosome

_____K_____ the suffix used to designate that deviation of chromosome involves the gain or loss of a chromosome

_____H_____ cytogenic disorders; deviations in structure or number of chromosomes

_____J_____ a relatively rare structural abnormality/structural alteration in the chromosome where a break occurs in the terminal end of both arms of a chromosome

_____P_____ failure of separation of homologous chromosomes during meiosis or of sister chromosomes during meiosis II or mitosis

_____R_____ involve a missing (deletion) or extra (duplication) segment of a chromosome

_____N_____ meiosis

_____V_____ selecting a mate because of geographic, ethnic, or religious restrictions

_____M_____ a cell that contains one more than the total number of chromosomes resulting in the addition of an extra member to a normal pair

_T_ disorders characterized by a microdeletion or micro duplication of smaller chromosome segments which may require special analysis techniques or molecular testing to detect

_L_ a cell that contains one less than the total number of chromosomes; loss of one member of a chromosome pair

_O_ mitosis

_Q_ refers to the pair of chromosome strands that constitute a metaphase (a stage of mitosis) chromosome

_X_ the concept that describes differences in the extent and/or severity of manifestations of genetic diseases

_S_ can be detected on a routine chromosome analysis and include cri-du-chat, Wolf Hirschhorn, and chromosome 18 deletions

_Z_ the concept that certain dominantly inherited disorders tend to worsen or have an earlier age of onset with succeeding generations

_U_ Lyon hypothesis; explains the milder physical and mental deficiencies of children with sex chromosome abnormalities compared to children with autosomal abnormalities

_W_ any heritable change in the DNA sequence of a gene

_Y_ containing a large number of DNA nucleotide repeats which are unstable and can undergo amplification

_BB_ characterized by central hypotonia, cognitive dysfunction, dysmorphic appearance, behavioral disturbances, hypothalamic hypogonadism, short stature, and obesity, as well as abnormally low body temperature, an increased tolerance to pain, and diminished salivation

_AA_ modification in some instances of genetic material resulting in phenotypic differences based on whether the genes/chromosomes were from the mother or the father

_II_ diseases and defects that show an increased incidence in some families, but have no clear cut affected/unaffected classification with no specific mode of inheritance; environmental factors; prenatal, environment appear to play an important role; examples are neural tube defects, cleft lip, congenital hip dislocation and pyloric stenosis.

_CC_ called happy puppet syndrome; includes severe mental retardation, characteristic facies, abnormal gait, and paroxysms of inappropriate laughter

_GG_ a new technique of chromosome analysis that uses radioactive or fluorescent probes in a variety of ways to identify chromosome and DNA abnormalities

_EE_ components of the cell cytoplasm involved in energy production

_DD_ cases where both copies of a chromosome pair are determined to have come from one parent, instead of one from each

_JJ_ the inherited histocompatability (tissue) antigens similar to the blood group antigens that may be implicated in the development of many diseases; present on the cell membrane of almost all body cells and occur in linked pairs; inherited in the same manner as the blood group antigens.

_FF_ a pictorial representation of chromosomal analysis

_HH_ the ability to locate a gene on a specific chromosome or segment of a chromosome

_KK_ agents that cause birth defects when present in the prenatal environment

2. Terms—Impact of Hereditary Disorders on the Family

A. presymptomatic testing
B. false positive
C. false negative
D. screening tests
E. diagnostic tests
F. maternal serum alpha-fetoprotein (MSAFP) testing
G. percutaneous umbilical blood sampling (PUBS)
H. fetal biopsy (FB)
I. fetal echocardiography
J. fetal in situ hybridization(FISH)
K. preimplantation genetic diagnosis
L. gentetic counseling
M. proband
N. empiric risks
O. theoretic risks
P. pedigree chart
Q. burden of a genetic defect
R. chronic sorrow

___B___ test results indicate a problem exists when it does not

___D___ the test only indicates a higher risk than expected in the general population

___P___ family tree; genogram

___E___ tests that determine with a high degree of accuracy the presence or absence of a birth defect or genetic disorder

___G___ prenatal genetic testing that can be performed after 18 weeks gestation

___I___ may be performed for further diagnosis when a cardiac defect is noted; ultrasound

___C___ test results indicate a problem does not exist when it does

___A___ refers to the process of screening for disease in high risk populations who are currently asymptomatic

___F___ indicates the presence of an open neural tube defect or ventral wall defect in the fetus

___H___ used to diagnose certain genetic skin disorders and metabolic disorders when DNA studies are unavailable or uninformative

___M___ the genetic counseling term for the affected person or index case

___J___ use chromosome specific probes; results could be available in 48-72 hours but the test is specific only for the most common disorders 21, 18, 13, X, and Y

___Q___ the total amount of distress, economic and emotional that is placed on persons, their families, and society by the birth of an affected child

___O___ risks based on Mendelian inheritance patterns

___L___ a communication process that deals with the human problems associated with the risk of occurrence of a genetic disorder in a family

___K___ through the technique of in vitro (test tube) fertilization, the embryo can be tested at the six to the cell stage for the presence of the specific genetic disorder and the embryo can be implanted if normal or an unaffected carrier

___N___ risks based on observations of recurrence in similar situations

___R___ the grieving process that has delayed resolution while a child with a disability is alive

3. Trisomy 21 or Down syndrome is an example of a:
   A. congenital chromosomal association.
   B. sex chromosome abnormality.
   C. autoimmune aberration.
   D. autosomal structural aberration.

4. All of the following chromosomal disorders are considered sex chromosome abnormalities EXCEPT:
   A. Turner syndrome.
   B. Klinefelter syndrome.
   C. Cri-du-chat syndrome.
   D. Triple X syndrome.

5. The Lyon hypothesis helps to explain why children with sex chromosome abnormalities when compared to children with autosomal abnormalities:
   A. usually have milder physical and mental deficiencies.
   B. are shorter in stature with poor coordination.
   C. are more easily identified at birth.
   D. usually have more severe handicaps.

6. Match disorder with inheritance pattern. (Inheritance patterns may be used more than once.)

   A.   autosomal dominant   B.   autosomal recessive   C.   sex linked (dominant or recessive)

   __B__ Wilson disease   __A__ achondroplasia
   __B__ Tay Sachs disease   __B__ cystic fibrosis
   __A__ osteogenesis imperfecta   __B__ galactosemia
   __A__ neurofibromatosis   __B__ familial hypothyroidism
   __C__ Duchenne Muscular Dystrophy   __A__ Marfan syndrome
   __B__ maple syrup urine disease   __A__ myotonic dystrophy
   __C__ hemophilia A   __A__ Noonan syndrome
   __C__ fragile X syndrome   __B__ phenylketonuria
   __B__ ocular albinism   __B__ thalassemias

7. A disease or defect that is encountered frequently in the population without a clear cut inheritance pattern would be classified as:
   A. mutation.
   B. mosaicism.
   C. uniparental disomy.
   D. multifactorial.

8. Which one of the following disorders has no clear relationship to the HLA (human leukocyte antigen)?
   A. Type 1 diabetes
   B. Rheumatoid arthritis
   C. Fetal alcohol syndrome
   D. Myasthenia gravis

9. Fetal surgery has been used in particular to treat congenital:
   A. urinary tract abnormalities.
   B. heart disease.
   C. facial and limb deformities.
   D. pyloric stenosis.

10. Phenylketonuria is usually treated by:
    A. diet modification.
    B. hormone replacement.
    C. surgical repair.
    D. vitamin supplement.

11. Most genetic centers recommend that genetic testing should be reserved for children:
    A. prior to their adoption.
    B. when clear medical benefits exist.
    C. who have deleterious recessive genes.
    D. who have deleterious dominant genes.

12. Careful counseling is necessary when screening an individual for carrier status of hereditary disorders because:
    A. this type of screening is controversial.
    B. of possible ethical dilemmas.
    C. this type of screening is expensive.
    D. the emotional threat for the child is always devastating.

13. Which one of the following statements is NOT a part of the controversial aspect of mass genetic screening programs?
    A. Health professionals sometimes lack knowledge about the purpose of the testing.
    B. The public cost of testing does not always outweigh the benefits.
    C. Many well organized programs have been successful in preventing disease.
    D. The psychological implications of the carrier states can be handled improperly.

14. Match the type of prenatal genetic test with its purpose.

    A. maternal serum alpha-fetoprotein (MS-AFP)   __C__ to perform chromosome and biochemical analysis

    B. ultrasonography   __B__ to estimate gestational age and identify structural abnormalities

    C. amniocentesis   __D__ to perform chromosomal analysis at the earliest possible point during pregnancy

    D. chorionic villus sampling (CVS)   __A__ to screen for neural tube defects

15. Preimplantation genetic diagnosis has been used for parents at risk of having a child with:
    A. Down syndrome.
    B. a neural tube defect.
    C. a congenital heart defect.
    D. cystic fibrosis.

16. Which of the following actions would NOT be considered an appropriate nursing responsibility in genetic counseling?
    A. Choose the best course of action for the family
    B. Identify families who would benefit from genetic evaluation
    C. Become familiar with community resources for genetic evaluation
    D. Learn basic genetic principles

17. The most efficient genetic counseling service provided by a group of genetic screening specialists may:
    A. predict the outcome of the disease.
    B. take less than two hours.
    C. evaluate the affected child only.
    D. be inaccessible to the people who need it most.

18. *Proband* is the term used in genetic counseling that means the:
    A. affected person.
    B. genetic history.
    C. clinical manifestations.
    D. mode of inheritance.

19. When teaching families about genetic risks and probabilities the nurse may need to:
    A. make specific recommendations.
    B. use games such as flipping coins and horse racing.
    C. realize that most people have a basic understanding of biology.
    D. Recognize that each pregnancy's probabilities build on the previous pregnancy's probabilities.

20. Which one of the following assessment findings would alert the nurse to the need for genetic counseling?
    A. Individuals with a family history of tuberculosis
    B. Parents who had an infant born at 42 weeks gestation
    C. Couples with a history of infertility
    D. Pregnant adolescents

21. Which one of the following assessment findings in an infant would indicate to the nurse that there is a need for genetic referral?
    A. Vernix caseosa
    B. Acrocyanosis
    C. Mongolian spots
    D. Odorous breath

22. When drawing a pedigree genogram, which one of the following facts would be LEAST significant? The proband's:
    A. paternal grandmother had two stillbirth pregnancies.
    B. sibling died as an infant in a motor vehicle accident.
    C. paternal grandfather was a carrier for sickle cell disease.
    D. half brother carries the sickle cell trait.

23. Which one of the following statements in regard to genetic counseling is FALSE?
    A. Families have a tendency to be more ashamed of a hereditary disorder than other illness.
    B. The nurse's role in genetic counseling involves sympathy and supportive listening.
    C. The nurse ensures that clients have accurate and complete information to make decisions.
    D. Most couples will choose not to have a child if there is any risk of disability.

Mr. and Mrs. Jones are waiting in the obstetrician's office for a routine prenatal check up. The couple is Roman Catholic and they do not believe in abortion. The obstetrician has recommended a screening test to rule out neural tube defects. Mrs. Jones does not see any benefit from this testing procedure and does not want to undergo the procedure.

24. Which one of the following factors is the LEAST important consideration during the assessment phase of this visit?
    A. The nurse is not Roman Catholic.
    B. The test is a venipuncture and carries little risk.
    C. Most couples receive normal results from prenatal tests.
    D. Results of the tests will be provided before the delivery date.

25. Which one of the following considerations should the nurse deal with FIRST?
    A. The couple believes that testing is used to identify anomalies in order to terminate pregnancies.
    B. The couple's clear-cut beliefs about pregnancy termination are very different from the reality of raising an abnormal child.
    C. The nurse believes that pregnancy termination for fetal abnormalities is often the best option.
    D. The nurse believes that raising a child with a terminal illness is extremely difficult.

26. Which one of the following goals would be MOST appropriate for the nurse in this situation?
    A. To provide nonjudgmental supportive counseling
    B. To help the couple make their decision
    C. To provide follow-up care to the couple
    D. To educate the couple about neural tube defects

27. Which of the following statements by Mrs. Jones indicates that the nurse's goal was met?
    A. "I had no idea what was involved in raising a disabled child."
    B. "Your ideas have been very helpful. I think one of them will work."
    C. "We will discuss this and call you tomorrow with our decision."
    D. "I had no idea what neural tube defects were."

CHAPTER 6
Communication and Health Assessment of the Child and Family

1. Match each term with it corresponding description.

   A. verbal communication
   B. nonverbal communication
   C. abstract communication
   D. paralanguage
   E. confirming behaviors
   F. disconfirming behaviors
   G. triage
   H. empathy
   I. sympathy
   J. family
   K. family structure
   L. sociogram
   M. family function
   N. anthropometry

   __D__ the pitch, pause, intonation, rate, volume, and stress apparent in speech

   __N__ an essential parameter of nutritional status; the measurement of height, weight, head circumference, proportions, skinfold thickness, and arm circumference

   __H__ the capacity to understand what another person is experiencing from within that person's frame of reference

   __C__ takes the form of play, artistic expression, symbols, photographs, and choice of clothing

   __K__ refers to the composition of the family

   __I__ involves having feelings or emotions in common with another person rather than merely understanding those feelings

   __B__ often called body language and includes gestures, movements, facial expressions, postures, and reactions

   __L__ a drawing that indicates the significant persons in an individual's life

   __J__ refers to all those individuals who are considered by the family member to be significant to the nuclear unit

   __A__ involves language and its expressions; vocalizations

   __M__ concerned with how the family members behave toward one another and with the quality of the relationship

   __E__ response behavior that includes nodding the head, requesting clarification

   __F__ response behavior that includes tapping finger, turning away from speaker

   __G__ assessing symptoms and forming clinical judgment for further medical care

2. Which nursing action would negatively affect the communication process between the nurse and the client?
   A. Messages delivered to the client are congruous.
   B. Communication includes the child as well as the parent.
   C. The nurse uses verbal and nonverbal communication to reflect approval of the client's statement.
   D. The nurse uses a slow, even, steady voice to convey instruction.

3. Mrs. Green has brought her daughter Karen to the clinic as a new patient. Karen, age 12 years, requires a physical exam so she can play volleyball. Which one of the following techniques used by the nurse to establish effective communication during the interview process is NOT correct?
   A. The nurse introduces himself/herself and asks the name of all family members present.
   B. After the introduction, the nurse is careful to direct questions about Karen to Mrs. Green since she is the best source of information.
   C. After the introduction and explanation of her role, the nurse begins the interview by saying to Karen, "Tell me about your volleyball team."
   D. The nurse chooses to conduct the interview in a quiet area with few distractions.

4. While conducting an assessment of the child, the nurse communicates with the child's family. Which one of the following does the nurse recognize as NOT productive in obtaining information?
   A. Obtaining input from the child, verbal and nonverbal
   B. Observing the relationship between parents and child
   C. Using broad open-ended questions
   D. Avoiding the use of guiding statements to direct the focus of the interview

5. The receptionist at the clinic where you are employed as a nurse has forwarded a call to you from Mrs. Garcia, mother of four-year-old Maria. Mrs. Garcia tells you that Maria has had a fever all morning of around 100° F. Maria has now started with diarrhea and vomiting. As you phone triage this call, which one of the following do you recognize as appropriate?
   A. Reassure Mrs. Garcia that Maria is not very sick and will be fine in a day or two
   B. Confer with the practitioner at once
   C. Wait to document in Maria's medical record until Maria comes in for a visit
   D. Offer advice for home care and instruct Mrs. Garcia to call or come to the clinic if symptoms are not improving

6. The capacity to understand what another person is feeling by experiencing from that person's frame of reference is described as:
   A. sympathy.
   B. empathy.
   C. reassurance.
   D. encouragement.

7. The nurse is conducting an interview with eight-year-old Jesus and his mother, Mrs. Lopez. Mrs. Lopez is worried because Jesus has been acting up at home and at school and disrupting everyone. An interpreter has been requested since the mother speaks very little English. When using an interpreter for communication with Mrs. Lopez, the nurse realizes that:
   A. the interpreter will have very little to do because Jesus can interpret for his mother.
   B. when the interpreter and Mrs. Lopez speak for a long period, it will be necessary to interrupt to refocus the interview.
   C. the nurse will need to communicate directly with Mrs. Lopez and ignore the interpreter.
   D. the nurse will need to pose questions to elicit only one answer at a time from Mrs. Lopez.

8. The nurse recognizes which of the following statements as TRUE or FALSE when planning how to communicate effectively with children?

   _F_ Nonverbal components of the communication process do not convey significant message.

   _T_ Children are alert to their surroundings and attach meaning to gestures.

   _T_ Active attempts to make friends with children before they have had an opportunity to evaluate unfamiliar person increases their anxiety.

   _T_ The nurse should assume a position that is at eye level with the child.

   _F_ Communication through transition objects such as dolls or stuffed animals delays the child's response to verbal communication offered by the nurse.

9. To effectively provide anticipatory guidance to the family, the nurse should:
   A. provide information to deal with each problem as it develops.
   B. provide teaching and interventions based on needs identified by the professional.
   C. be suspicious of the parent's ability to deal effectively with the child's needs.
   (D.) assist the parents in building competence in their parenting abilities.

10. Communication with children must reflect their developmental thought process. Match the development stage with the description of communication guidelines to be used. (Stages may be used more than once.)

    A. infancy
    B. early childhood
    C. school-age years
    D. adolescence

    _B_ focus communication on the child; experiences of others are of no interest to them

    _A_ primarily use and respond to nonverbal communication

    _B_ interpret words literally and are unable to separate fact from fantasy

    _B_ assign human attributes to inanimate objects

    _C_ require explanations and reasons why procedures are being done to them

    _C_ have a heightened concern about body integrity, being overly sensitive to any activity that constitutes a threat to it

    _D_ often willing to discuss their concern with an adult outside the family and often welcome the opportunity to interact with a nurse

11. Which one of the following BEST describes the appropriate use of play as a communication technique in children?
    A. Small infants have little response to activities that focus on repetitive actions like patting and stroking.
    B. Few clues about intellectual or social developmental progress is obtained from the observation of child's play behaviors.
    C. Therapeutic play has little value in reduction of trauma from illness or hospitalization.
    (D.) Play sessions serve as assessment tools for determining children's awareness and perception of illness.

12. Several creative communication techniques are often used with children. Identify which is being used in each of the following examples.

    A. ___Storytelling___ The nurse shows Tina a picture of a child having an intravenous infusion started and asks Tina to describe the scene.

    B. ___"I" Messages___ "I am concerned about how the medicine treatments are going because I want you to feel better."

    C. ___Bibliotherapy___ The nurse reads Tina a story from a book and asks her to retell the story.

    D. ___Drawing___ The nurse provides Tina with crayons and paper and asks her to draw a picture of her family.

    E. ___Directed Play___ The nurse gives Tina a doll and a stethoscope and allows Tina to listen to the doll's heart.

13. A complete pediatric health history includes ten expected components. List these components.

    _____   _____

    _____   _____

    _____   _____

    _____   _____

    _____   _____

14. In eliciting the chief complaint, the nurse identifies which one of the following techniques as NOT appropriate?
A. Limiting the chief complaint to a brief statement restricted to one or two symptoms
B. Use labeling-type questions such as, "How are you sick?" to facilitate information exchange
C. Record the chief complaint in the child's or parent's own words
D. Use open-ended neutral questions to elicit information

15. Which component of the pediatric health history is the following? "Nausea and vomiting for three days. Started with abdominal cramping past eating hamburger at home. No pain or cramping at present. Unable to keep any foods down but able to drink clear liquids without vomiting. No temperature elevation, no diarrhea."
A. Chief complaint
B. Past history
C. Present illness
D. Review of systems

16. The nurse recognizes which one of the following as NOT part of the past history included in a pediatric health history?
    A. Symptom analysis
    B. Allergies
    C. Birth history
    D. Current medications

17. What are the MOST important previous growth patterns to record when completing a child's history of growth and development?

    _____

    _____

18. What are the MOST important developmental milestones to record when completing the child's health history?

    _____

    _____

    _____

19. The nurse knows that the BEST description of the sexual history for a pediatric health history:
    A. includes a discussion of plans for future children.
    B. allows the client to introduce sexual activity history.
    C. includes a discussion of contraception methods only when the client discloses current sexual activity.
    D. alerts the nurse to the need for sexually transmitted disease screening.

20. The _genogram_ uses symbols to diagram data about the family structure.
    The _pedigree_ records the family medical history in chart form.
    The _ecomap_ is a visual presentation of the family's support system.

21. Indications for the nurse to conduct a comprehensive family assessment include which of the following?
    1. Children with developmental delays
    2. Children with history of repeated accidental injuries
    3. Children with behavioral problems
    4. Children receiving comprehensive well-child care

    A. 1, 2, 3, and 4
    B. 2, 3, and 4
    C. 1, 2, and 3
    D. 2 and 3

22. Assessment of family structure is best conducted:
    A. after the first meeting with the client.
    B. only when a problem is suspected within the family.
    C. towards the end of the interview when rapport has been established.
    D. by interviewing the client about other family members' roles within the family.

23. Assessment of family interactions and roles, decision making and problem solving, and communication is known as assessment of:
   A. family structure.
   B. family function.
   C. family composition.
   D. home and community environment.

24. Describe the four principal areas of concern the nurse should focus on when assessing family structure.

   _____

   _____

   _____

   _____

25. The dietary history of a pediatric client includes:
   A. a 12-hour dietary intake recall.
   B. a more specific, detailed history for the older child.
   C. financial and cultural factors that influence food selection.
   D. criticism of parents' allowance of non-essential foods.

Critical Thinking • Case Study

Mrs. Brown brings her 11-year-old son, Kenny, to the clinic for a physical. She is concerned because Kenny comes home from school "very tired and only wants to watch television." Kenny's bedtime has not changed, he performs well in school, and his mother denies stress or problems within the home. On physical exam, Kenny is above the 90th percentile for weight by 25 pounds.

26. To effectively establish a setting for communication, the nurse, upon entering the room with Mrs. Brown and Kenny, introduces herself/himself and explains her/his role and the purpose of the interview. Kenny is included in the interaction as the nurse asks his name and age and what he is expecting at his visit today. The nurse next informs Mrs. Brown and Kenny that Kenny is 25 pounds overweight and that his diet and exercise plan must be "terrible" for Kenny to be in "such bad shape." Which aspect of effective communication has the nurse forgotten that will MOST significantly impact the exchange of information during this interview?
   A. Assurance of privacy and confidentiality
   B. Preliminary acquaintance
   C. Directing the focus away from the complaint of fatigue to one of obesity
   D. Injected her/his own attitudes and feelings into the interview

27. Based on the information provided, the nurse can correctly record which of the following?
   A. Chief complaint
   B. Present illness
   C. Past medical history
   D. Symptom analysis

28. Mrs. Brown, Kenny and the nurse agree to the need to conduct a more intensive nutritional assessment. Which one of the following ways to record Kenny's dietary intake would the nurse suggest as MOST reliable in providing needed information to currently assess Kenny's dietary habits?

   A 12-hour recall
   B. 24-hour recall
   C. Food diary for 3-day period
   D. Food frequency questionnaire

29. During the physical exam which of the following physical findings by the nurse could be consistent with excess carbohydrate nutrition?

   A. Caries
   B. Skin elastic and firm
   C. Hair stringy, friable, dull and dry
   D. Enlarged thyroid

30. The physical exam has been completed to reflect that other than his obesity, Kenny is in excellent physical health with normal blood counts. The completed nutritional assessment reflects that Mrs. Brown has little knowledge about proper nutrition and that Kenny has a large intake of "junk" foods high in fat and calories but low in nutrients. Based on the data collected, which of the following nursing diagnoses would be MOST appropriate?

   1. altered family process related to parents' knowledge deficit
   2. altered family coping related to family's inability to purchase needed foods
   3. altered individual coping related to fatigue from poor dietary habits
   4. altered nutrition: more than body requirements related to eating practices
   5. altered nutrition: more than body requirements related to knowledge deficit of parent

   A. 1, 2, and 4
   B. 3 and 4
   C. 3, 4, and 5
   D. 4 and 5

31. Once the problem is defined, the nurse includes Mrs. Brown in the problem-solving process. Why is it important for the nurse to include the parent in the problem-solving process?

   _____

   _____

CHAPTER 7
Physical and Developmental Assessment of the Child

1. In examining pediatric clients, the normal sequence of head-to-toe direction is often altered to accommodate the client's developmental needs. The nurse identifies which of the following goals as LEAST likely to guide the examination process?
   A. Minimizing the stress and anxiety associated with the assessment of body parts
   B. Record the findings according to the normal sequence
   C. Fostering a trusting nurse-child relationship
   D. Preserving the essential security of the parent-child relationship

2. Mr. Alls brings his son, Keith, in for Keith's regular well infant exam. Keith is 12 months old. The nurse knows that the BEST approach to the physical examination for this client will be to:
   A. have the infant sit in the parent's lap to complete as much of the examination as possible.
   B. place the infant on the exam table with parents out of view.
   C. perform examination in head-to-toe direction.
   D. completely undress Keith and leave him undressed during the examination.

3. Behavior that signals the child's readiness to cooperate during the physical examination would NOT include:
   A. talking to the nurse.
   B. making eye contact with the nurse.
   C. allowing physical touching.
   D. sitting on parent's lap, playing with doll.

4. The National Center for Health Statistics has growth charts available for pediatric clients. A major difference between the age-related charts is that the chart for ages birth to 36 months records height as ___recumbant___ ___length___ while the chart for ages 2 to 18 years records height as ___stature___ _____ .

5. The assessment method that the nurse expects to provide the BEST information about the physical growth pattern of a preschool-age child is:
   A. recording height and weight measurements of the child.
   B. keeping a flow sheet for height, weight, and head circumference increases.
   C. obtaining a history of sibling growth patterns.
   D. measuring the height, weight, and circumference of the child.

6. Identify the following statements regarding the growth or development patterns of pediatric clients as TRUE or FALSE.

___T___ Comparing children's growth trends with those of their parents is essential in evaluating adequate growth.

___F___ Breast-fed infants grow faster than bottle-fed infants during the 6- to 18-month age period.

___T___ Growth is a continuous but uneven process, and the most reliable evaluation lies in comparison of growth measurements over a prolonged time.

___T___ Growth measurements during the physical examination should be age-specific and include length, height, weight, skinfold thickness, and arm and head circumference.

7. Which one of the following evaluations for growth should be followed closely?
   A. Height and weight falls above the 5th percentile on the growth chart
   B. Height and weight falls below the 5th percentile on the growth chart
   C. Height and weight falls below the 95th percentile on the growth chart
   D. Height and weight falls within the 50th percentile on the growth chart

8. Head circumference is:
   A. measured in all children up to the age of 24 months.
   B. equal to chest circumferences at about 1 to 2 years of age.
   C. about 8 to 9 cm smaller than chest circumference during childhood.
   D. measured slightly below the eyebrows and pinna of the ears.

9. In infants and young children, the __apical__ pulse should be taken because it is the most reliable. This pulse should be counted for __1 full minute__ because of the possibility of irregularities in rhythm. When counting respirations in infants, observe the __abdominal__ movements and count for __1 full minute__ because their movements are irregular.

10. The nurse should take the vital signs of an infant in what order?
    A. Measure temperature, then count the pulse, and then count respirations
    B. Count the pulse, then count respirations and then measure the temperature
    C. Count respirations, then count the pulse, and then measure the temperature
    D. Measure the temperature, then count respirations, and then count the pulse

11. Which one of the following findings would the nurse recognize as normal when measuring the vital signs of a 5-year-old child?
    A. Femoral pulses graded at +1
    B. Oral temperature of 100.9 degrees F
    C. Blood pressure of 101/61
    D. Respiratory rate of 28

12. The nurse knows to eliminate which of the following observations when recording the general appearance of the child?
    A. Impression of child's nutritional status
    B. Behavior, interactions with parents
    C. Hygiene, cleanliness
    D. Vital signs

13. Match the assessment finding or descriptions with the terminology. (A term may be used more than once.)

A.	cyanosis	F.	jaundice	K.	koilonychia
B.	pallor	G.	plethora	L.	wryneck or torticolles
C.	erythema	H.	tissue turgor	M.	opisthotomos
D.	ecchymosis	I.	edema	N.	genu valgum
E.	petechiae	J.	pitting edema	O.	genu varum

___A___ appears in dark-skinned clients as ashen-gray lips and tongue

___D___ appears in light-skinned clients as purplish to yellow-green areas

___B___ may be a sign of anemia, chronic disease, edema, or shock

___C___ redness of the skin which may be the result of infection, local inflammation, or increased temperature from climatic conditions

___D___ large, diffuse areas, usually blue or black in color and the result of injury

___E___ small distinct pinpoint hemorrhages

___F___ yellow staining of the skin usually caused by bile pigments

___K___ "spoon nails"; sometimes seen in iron deficiency anemia

___L___ injury to the sternocleidomastoid muscle with subsequent holding of the head to one side with the chin pointing toward the opposite side

___M___ hyperextension of the neck and spine

___I___ swelling or puffiness of skin

___J___ temporary indentation that occurs when the finger is pushed into the skin

___G___ intense redness of the lips or cheeks as a compensatory response to chronic hypoxia

___H___ amount of elasticity to the skin

___O___ lateral bowing of the tibia

___N___ knees are close together but feet are spread apart; knock-knee

14. The nurse is assessing skin turgor in 10-month-old Ryan. The nurse grasps the skin on the abdomen between the thumb and index finger, pulls it taut, and quickly releases it. The tissue remains suspended or tented for a few seconds then slowly falls back on the abdomen. Which of the following evaluations can the nurse correctly assume?
    A. The tissue shows normal elasticity.
    B. The child is properly hydrated.
    C. The assessment was done incorrectly.
    D. The child has poor skin turgor.

15. The nurse is assessing 7-year-old Mary's lymph nodes. The nurse uses the distal portions of his/her fingers and gently but firmly presses in a circular motion along the occipital and postauricular node areas. The nurse records the findings as "tender, enlarged, warm lymph nodes." The nurse knows that:
    A. findings are within normal limits for Mary's age.
    B. assessment technique was incorrect and should be repeated.
    C. findings suggest infection or inflammation in the scalp area or external ear canal.
    D. recording of the information is complete because it includes temperature and tenderness.

16. The nurse recognizes an assessment finding of the head and neck that does NOT need referral as:
    A. head lag before 6 months of age.
    B. hyperextension of the head with pain on flexion.
    C. palpable thyroid gland including isthmus and lobes.
    D. closure of the anterior fontanel at the age of 9 months.

17. Sinuses that are present soon after birth are the _maxillary_ and _ethmoid_ sinuses.

18. Normal findings on examination of the pupil may be recorded as PERRLA, which means

    _____ .

19. Match the term with the description.

    A. hypertelorism   _D_ rolling out of the eye lid
    B. ptosis   _E_ turning in of the eye lid
    C. sunset eyes   _H_ inflammation and blockage of lacrimal sac or duct
    D. ectropion   _I_ farsightedness
    E. entropion   _M_ granulomas or cyst of internal sebaccous glands
    F. hordeolum   _A_ large spacing between the eyes
    G. blepharitis   _C_ upper eye lid covers no part of the iris
    H. dacyocystitis   _N_ ability to focus on one visual field with both eyes at
    I. hyperopia   the same time
    J. myopia   _K_ one eye deviates from point of fixation
    K. strabismus   _G_ inflammation of edge of eye lid
    L. amblyopia   _F_ stye
    M. chalazion   _B_ upper eye lid covers part of the pupil or the lower
    N. binocularity   part of the iris
                                _J_ nearsightedness
                                _L_ type of blindness resulting from uncorrected
                                     "lazy" eye

20. Which one of the following assessments is an expected finding in the child's eye examination?
    A. Opaque red reflex of the eye
    B. Ophthalmoscopic exam reflects veins are darker in color and about one fourth larger in size than the arteries.
    C. Strabismus in the 12-month-old infant
    D. 5-year-old child who reads the Snellen Eye chart at the 20/40 level

21. When assessing the ear in the 2-year-old child, the nurse should:
    A. expect cerumen in the external ear canal.
    B. use the smallest speculum to prevent trauma to the ear.
    C. pull the pinna up and back to better visualize the canal.
    D. pull the pinna down and back to better visualize the canal.

22. The test that measures the compliance of the tympanic membrane and the middle ear pressure is:
    A. Rinne test.
    B. threshold acuity sweep test.
    C. vestibular testing.
    D. tympanometry.

23. Four-year-old Billy has been brought to the clinic by his parents because they have noticed a sudden foul odor in the mouth accompanied by a discharge from the right nares. The nurse knows that this is MOST likely to suggest:
    A. poor dental hygiene.
    B. foreign body in the nose.
    C. gingival disease.
    D. thumb-sucking.

24. The nurse is assessing the mouth and throat of 7-month-old Alex. Which of the following is recognized as a normal finding?
    A. Membranes are bright pink, smooth, glistening.
    B. White curdy plaques located on the tongue
    C. Redness and puffiness along the gum line
    D. Tip of the tongue extends to gum line.

25. When assessing 4-year-old Gail's chest, the nurse would expect:
    A. movement of the chest wall to be symmetric bilaterally and coordinated with breathing.
    B. respiratory movements to be chiefly thoracic.
    C. anteroposterior diameter to be equal to the transverse diameter.
    D. retraction of the muscles between the ribs on respiratory movement.

26. The nurse asks 12-year-old Susan to repeat the words "99" several times while the palmar surfaces of the nurse's hands are placed on the child's chest. The nurse is palpating for conduction of sound through the respiratory tract. What is this called?
    A. Pleural friction rub
    B. Crepitation
    C. Normal respiratory movements
    D. Vocal fremitus

27. On auscultation of 8-year-old Tammie's lung fields, the nurse hears inspiratory sounds that are louder, longer and higher-pitched than on expiration. These sounds are heard over the chest except over the scapula and sternum. These sounds are:
    A. bronchovesicular breath sounds.
    B. vesicular breath sounds.
    C. bronchial breath sounds.
    D. adventitious breath sounds.

28. When the nurse is palpating for cardiac thrills, the nurse knows that thrills are:
    A. vibrations caused by the flow of blood from one chamber to another through a narrowed opening.
    B. best felt with the dorsal surface of the hands.
    C. found at the point of maximum intensity.
    D. louder on inspiration than expiration.

29. A heart sound that is the result of vibrations produced during ventricular filling and normally heard in some children is:
   A. S1.
   B. S2.
   C. S3.
   D. S4.

30. When listening over the aortic area of the heart, the nurse should place the stethoscope where?
   A. 2nd right intercostal space close to sternum
   B. 2nd left intercostal space close to sternum
   C. 5th left intercostal space close to sternum
   D. 5th right intercostal space, left midclavicular line

31. Examination of the abdomen is performed correctly by the nurse in the following order:
   A. inspection, palpation, percussion, and auscultation.
   B. inspection, percussion, auscultation, and palpation.
   C. palpation, percussion, auscultation, and inspection.
   D. inspection, auscultation, percussion, and palpation.

32. While assessing the male genitalia of 4-year-old Ben, the nurse notes that the urethral meatus is opening on the ventral side of the glans or shaft. This finding is consistent with:
   A. a normal finding.
   B. hypospadias and needs referral.
   C. epispadias and needs referral.
   D. phimosis and needs referral

33. In performing an examination for scoliosis, the nurse understands that which one of the following is an INCORRECT method?
   A. The child should be examined only in his/her underpants (and bra if an older girl).
   B. The child should stand erect with the nurse observing from behind.
   C. The child should squat down with hands extended forward so the nurse can observe for asymmetry of the shoulder blades.
   D. The child should bend forward so that the back is parallel to the floor so that the nurse can observe from the side.

34. How would the nurse test for the Brudzinski sign and what would a positive sign in the presence of symptoms suggest?

   Child lies supine & flex child's head
   _____

35. The Denver Developmental Screening Test is limited by its inability to predict:
   A. developmental delays in children of cultural ethnic groups.
   B. gross motor delays.
   C. language delays.
   D. personal-social delays.

36. When discussing the results of an abnormal Denver Developmental Screening test with a parent, the nurse would:
    A. ask the parent if the child's performance was typical behavior.
    B. emphasize the failed items first, delayed items second, and then the passed items.
    C. explain that referral for the child should be immediate.
    D. explain the necessity for testing all items to the right of the child's age line to determine developmental delays.

Critical Thinking • Case Study

Mary, a 13-year-old, has come to the clinic with her mother with a complaint of right side abdominal pain of 24 hours' duration. She tells you, the nurse, that she has had some nausea and vomiting but no diarrhea. Her appetite is depressed and she feels hot and feverish. Mary has taken Tylenol for pain but with little relief. A complete blood count has been ordered and results are pending.

37. In preparing Mary for physical exam, you know that during the examination as an adolescent Mary will likely:
    A. prefer her parents to be present during the entire exam.
    B. desire to undress in private and will feel more comfortable when provided with a gown.
    C. prefer traumatic procedures such as ears and mouth exams last.
    D. need to have heart and lungs auscultated first.

38. The nurse completes the physical examination and evaluates which one of the following as an abnormal finding?
    A. Bowel sounds are stimulated by stroking the abdominal surface with the fingernail.
    B. Mary has no abdominal discomfort when she is supine with the legs flexed at the hips and knees.
    C. Mary's eyes are open during palpation of the abdomen.
    D. When the nurse presses firmly over the area distal to the right side of the abdomen and quickly releases this pressure, pain is intensified in the lower right side.

39. Which one of the following organs is located in the lower right quadrant of the abdomen?
    A. Bladder
    B. Liver
    C. Ovaries
    D. Appendix

40. Mary's parents are apprehensive about Mary and ask the nurse if "it is serious." Which one of the following is the BEST response?
    A. "Mary has appendicitis and will need to have surgery immediately."
    B. "You will have to ask the doctor about her condition."
    C. "Mary has some abdominal pain which is not normal. We are watching her very carefully and will be able to tell you more when the laboratory tests are completed."
    D. "Mary should be able to go home as soon as the doctor finishes with the examination and the laboratory tests are completed."

41. While inspecting the abdomen which one of the following does the nurse recognize as a normal finding?
    A. Peristaltic waves
    B. Silvery, whitish lines when the skin is stretched out
    C. Bulging at the umbilicus
    D. Protruding abdomen with skin pulled tight

CHAPTER 8
Health Promotion of the Newborn and Family

1. The chemical factors in the blood that stimulate the initiation of the first respiration in the neonate are ___low O2___, ___high CO2___ and ___low pH___.

2. The primary thermal stimulus that helps initiate the first respiration is ___sudden chilling___.

3. The nurse recognizes that tactile stimulation probably has some effect on initiation of respiration in the neonate. Which one of the following is of NO beneficial effect?
    A. Normal handling of the neonate
    B. Drying the skin of the neonate
    C. Slapping the neonate's heel or buttocks
    D. Placing the infant skin to skin with the mother

4. The nurse knows which one of these neonates will MOST likely need additional respiratory support at birth?
    A. The infant born by normal vaginal delivery
    B. The infant born by cesarean birth
    C. The infant born vaginally after 12 hours of labor
    D. The infant born with high levels of surfactant

5. During the transition from fetal to neonatal circulation, the newborn's cardiovascular system accomplishes which of the following anatomic and physiologic alterations?
    1. closure of the ductus venosus
    2. closure of the foramen ovale
    3. closure of the ductus arteriosis
    4. increased systemic pressure and decreased pulmonary artery pressure

    A. 1, 2, 3, and 4
    B. 1, 2, and 3
    C. 2, 3, and 4
    D. 1, 3, and 4

6. Identify the following statements about infant adjustments to extrauterine life as either TRUE or FALSE.
    ___T___ Factors that predispose the neonate to excessive heat loss are large surface area, thin layer of subcutaneous fat and the lack of shivering to produce heat.
    ___F___ Nonshivering thermogenesis is an effective method of heat production in the neonate since it is able to produce heat with little use of oxygen.
    ___T___ Brown fat or brown adipose tissue has a greater capacity to produce heat than does ordinary adipose tissue.
    ___F___ The longer the infant is attached to the placenta, the less blood volume will be received by the neonate.
    ___T___ Deficient production of pancreatic amylase impairs utilization of complex carbohydrates.

___F___ Deficiency of pancreatic lipase assists the neonate in the digestion of cow's milk.

___F___ Most salivary glands are functioning at birth even though most infants do not start drooling until teeth erupt.

___T___ The stomach capacity for most newborn infants is about 90 cc.

___F___ The newborn should be expected to void within the first 48 hours.

7. Match the term with the description.

   A. meconium   ___B___ pale yellow to golden; pasty consistency
   B. breast-fed infant stools ___A___ first stool dark green; pasty, sticky consistency
   C. formula-fed infant stools ___C___ pale yellow to light brown; firmer in consistency with more offensive odor

8. Newborns receive passive immunity in the form of IgG from the
   __maternal circulation__ and __breast milk__ .

9. The nurse recognizes that all of the following effects of maternal sex hormones in the newborn are normal EXCEPT:
   A. hypertrophied labia.
   B. secretion of witch's milk from the newborn breasts.
   C. pseudomenstruation.
   D. bleeding from the breast nipples.

10. Fill in the blanks in the following statements as they pertain to sensory functions in the normal newborn.
    A. The newborn can fixate on a bright object that is within __8 inches__ and in the midline of the visual field.
    B. Infants have visual preferences for the colors of __green__ , __pink__ , and __yellow__ and for designs such as __geometric__ __shapes__ and __checkerboards__
    C. The newborn's response to __low__ frequency sounds is one of decreased motor activity and crying while exposure to __high__ frequency sound elicits an alerting reaction.

11. The nurse is performing the 5-minute Apgar on a newborn. Which one of the following observations is included in the Apgar score?
    A. Blood pressure
    B. Temperature
    C. Muscle tone
    D. Weight

12. Match the period of reactivity with the observations the nurse is likely to observe during each period.

    A. first period of reactivity   ___A___ excellent bonding period and time to start breast feeding
    B. second stage of first period of reactivity   ___B___ period of infant sleep lasting two to four hours; heart rate and respiratory rates decrease
    C. second period of reactivity   ___C___ gastric and respiratory secretions are increased; passage of meconium commonly occurs

13. The nurse uses the Brazelton Neonatal Behavioral Assessment Scale to assess the newborn's behavioral responses. How would the nurse define *habituation*?
    A. Responsiveness of the newborn to auditory and visual stimuli
    B. Process whereby the newborn becomes accustomed to stimuli
    C. The infant is easily aroused from sleep state.
    D. The infant has a reactive Moro reflex with good muscle tone and coordination.

14. The nurse recognizes that one of the following is NOT correct about the relationship of newborn weight to gestational age:
    A. All infants below the weight of 2500g (5 1/2 pounds) are premature by gestational age.
    B. Gestational age is more closely related to fetal maturity than is birth weight.
    C. Classification of infants by both weight and gestational age can be beneficial for predicting mortality risks.
    D. Heredity influences are a normal part of assessment.

15. On assessment of a 24-hour newborn, the nurse makes several observations. Which is normal?
    A. Cyanotic color centrally and peripherally
    B. Axillary temperature of 96 degrees F
    C. Infant's posture is one of flexion of head and extremities, which rest on chest and abdomen.
    D. Respirations of 68

16. Match the following term with its description.

    A. milia   E. acrocyanosis   I. caput succedaneum
    B. erythema toxicum   F. cutis marmorata   J. cephalhematoma
    C. Harlequin color change   G. mongolian spots   K. vernix caseosa
    D. nevus flammeus   H. telangiectatic nevi L. lanugo

    __G__ irregular areas of deep blue pigmentation, usually in sacral and glutteal regions seen in the newborn

    __A__ distended sebaceous glands that appear as tiny white papules on the cheeks, chin and nose in the newborn

    __C__ lower half of body becomes pink and upper half is pale when newborn lies on side

    __I__ edema of the soft scalp tissue

    __B__ pink papular rash with vesicles superimposed on thorax, back, buttocks and abdomen in the newborn

    __D__ port-wine stain

    __J__ hematoma between periosteum and skull bone

    __E__ cyanosis of hands and feet

    __H__ "stork bites"; flat, deep pink, localized areas usually seen at back of neck

    __F__ transient mottling when infant is exposed to decreased temperature, stress, or overstimulation

    __L__ fine downy hair present on the newborn's skin

    __K__ cheese-like substance, mixture of sebum and desquamating cell covers the skin at birth

17. Newborns lose up to 10% of their birth weight by 3 to 4 days of age. The factor that does NOT contribute to this process is:
    A. limited fluid intake in breast-fed infants.
    B. incomplete digestion of complex carbohydrates.
    C. loss of excessive extracellular fluid.
    D. passage of meconium.

18. When assessing blood pressure in the newborn, the nurse knows which of the following is TRUE?
    A. A difference in systolic BP in which the BP in the calf is 10 mm Hg less than in the upper arm needs referral.
    B. Routine BP measurements of full-term neonates are an excellent predictor of hypertension.
    C. A normal BP reading for a 3-day-old infant would be approximately 90/60.
    D. BP should be measured routinely on all healthy newborns as recommended by the American Academy of Pediatrics.

19. A widened, tense, bulging fontanel can be a sign of ___↑___ intracranial pressure while a markedly sunken, depressed fontanel is a sign of _dehydration_.

20. Assessment of the newborn include which of the following?
    1. clinical gestational age assessment
    2. general measurements
    3. general appearance
    4. head-to-toe assessment
    5. parent-infant attachment

    A. 1, 2, 3, 4, and 5
    B. 1, 2, 3, and 4
    C. 2, 3, 4, and 5
    D. 2, 3, and 4

21. Which of the following observations from the eye assessment of a newborn are recognized as normal?
    A. Purulent discharge at age 48 hours
    B. Absence of the red reflex at age 24 hours
    C. No pupillary reflex at age 3 weeks
    D. Presence of strabismus at age 48 hours

22. It is important to assess for nasal patency in the newborn because newborns are usually _obligatory nose breathers_.

23. The nurse correctly identifies the need to notify the physician for which of the following neonates?
    A. The 24-hour-old neonate found to have Epstein pearls on the side of the hard palate
    B. The 2-day-old neonate with periodic breathing
    C. The 24-hour-old neonate who has nasal flaring
    D. The 2-hour-old neonate with a bluish, white, moist, umbilical cord with one vein and two arteries visible

24. Match the term with its description.

A. anal patency
B. Down syndrome
C. rooting reflex
D. Babinski
E. Moro reflex
F. tonic neck

__C__ Touching cheek along the side of the mouth causes infant to turn head toward that side and begin to suck.

__D__ fanning of the toes and dorsiflexion of the great toe; disappears after one year of age

__E__ symmetric abduction and extension of the arms, fingers fan out; thumb and index finger form a C

__A__ passage of meconium from rectum during first 48 hours of life

__B__ transverse palmar crease

__F__ infant in supine position turns head to one side with jaw over shoulder with extension of the arm and leg on the side to which the head is turned and flexion of the opposite side

25. Complete the following.
    A. The loss of heat to cooler solid objects in the environment that are not in direct contact with the infant is termed __radiation__.
    B. Heat loss from the body from direct contact of skin with a cooler solid object is termed __conduction__.
    C. Placing the infant in the direct flow of air from a fan causes rapid heat loss through __convection__.
    D. Loss of heat through skin moisture is termed __evaporation__.

26. The nurse implements all of the following actions to maintain a patent airway in a newborn. Which one will be LEAST effective?
    A. Maintaining the healthy infant in a supine or side-lying position during sleep
    B. Maintaining the infant with breathing problems in a prone position during sleep
    C. When suctioning the infant in the delivery room, suction the pharynx first, then the nasal passages
    D. Continuing oral feedings for the infant with nasal flaring and intercostal retractions

27. Identify the correct medication to be given to provide preventive care.
    A. __silver nitrate__ prophylactic eye treatment against ophthalmia neonatorum
    B. __Vit K__ administered by injection to prevent hemorrhagic disease of the newborn
    C. __Hep B shot__ first dose given between birth and 2 days of age to decrease incidence of HBV.

28. In screening for phenylketonuria (PKU) the nurse knows:
    A. blood samples should be taken after 24 hours of age and again at 2 weeks of age.
    B. blood should be drawn using a venous blood sample.
    C. preparation includes instructing parents to keep the infant NPO for 2 hours before the test.
    D. to completely saturate the filter paper by applying blood to both sides of the paper.

29. The nurse should involve the parents in the care of their newborn. Teaching is LEAST likely to include:
   A. the use of Ivory soap, oils, powder, and lotions with each bath.
   B. cleaning of the vulva by a front-to-back direction or cleaning of the foreskin by wiping around the glans. If the foreskin is retracted it must be by gentle retraction only as far as it will go with gentle return to normal position as necessary. The foreskin is not retracted in the newborn because it is normally tight.
   C. care of the umbilical stump, including placing the diaper below the cord to avoid irritation and wetness of the site.
   D. care of the circumcision site to include the fact that on the second day a yellowish white exudate forms normally as part of the granulating process.

30. Human milk is preferable to cow's milk because:
   A. human milk has a non-laxative effect.
   B. human milk has more calories per ounce.
   C. human milk has greater mineral content.
   D. human milk offers greater immunologic benefits.

31. The nurse is instructing new parents about proper feeding techniques for their newborns. Indicate which of the following statements are TRUE and which are FALSE.
   ___T___ Infants need at least two hours of sucking daily.
   ___T___ After feeding, infants should be placed on the right side to prevent regurgitation and distention.
   ___T___ Breast-fed infants tend to be hungry every two to three hours.
   ___T___ Supplemental feedings should not be offered to the breast-fed infant because they cause nipple confusion.
   ___T___ Supplemental water is not needed in breast-fed infants, even in hot climates.
   ___T___ Five behavioral stages occur during successful feeding. These are prefeeding, approach, attachment, consummatory and satiety behaviors.

32. Which one of the following actions by the nurse will LEAST likely promote the attachment process of the infant and parent?
   A. Recognizing individual differences present in the infant and explaining these normal characteristics to the parent
   B. Assisting the mother to assume the en face position when she is presented with her infant
   C. Explaining to the parents how to react to their infant with the use of reciprocal interacting
   D. Explaining to the parents the need for infants to have an organized schedule of daily activities which allows the infant to remain in his/her crib during awake periods

Michael was born by normal vaginal delivery to Marilyn and Doug Madison. Assessment at birth reflects a heart rate of 120, respiratory effort good with a strong cry, muscle tone, active movement, reflex irritability, turns head away when nose is suctioned, and color assessment of body pink with feet and hands blue. Michael's weight is 6 pounds and his length is 21 inches. Mrs. Madison is allowed to hold Michael and put him to breast in the delivery room. The Madisons do not plan on circumcision for Michael.

33. What is the Apgar score for Michael?
    A. 8
    B. 10
    C. 9
    D. 7

34. The nurse is conducting a gestational age assessment of Michael based on the six neuromuscular signs. What are these signs and what results would indicate a higher maturity rating?

    _____

    _____

    _____

    _____

    _____

    _____

35. Listed below are nursing actions that the nurse would perform during the transitional period. List these actions in order of priority.
    1. taking head and chest circumference measurements
    2. assessing for neonatal distress
    3. administering prophylactic medications
    4. scoring for gestational age
    5. assessing vital signs

    A. 2, 5, 1, 3, 4
    B. 1, 2, 5, 3, 4
    C. 2, 3, 1, 5, 4
    D. 2, 5, 4, 1, 3

36. Identify four nursing goals that are the basics for safe and effective care for the newborn by order of priority.

    _____

    _____

    _____

    _____

37. You are assigned to care for Michael in the newborn nursery. Michael is now 1 day old. List six daily assessments that the nurse recognizes should be conducted and documented.

_____

_____

_____

_____

_____

_____

38. Mrs. Madison and Michael are being discharged tomorrow. You are preparing to provide Mrs. Madison with the newborn discharge teaching plan. Michael is Mrs. Madison's first infant and on assessment you find that Mrs. Madison has several questions about her techniques of breast-feeding. You show Mrs. Madison how to hold Michael for feeding, how to properly position him to facilitate sucking, how to care for her breast and provide her with a video to reinforce your instruction. When you return later, Mrs. Madison asks you about the use of supplemental feedings. Which of the following is the best response?
    A. "It is okay to give Michael supplements but only after he is put to the breast."
    B. "Why would you think about that now? We'll discuss it tomorrow when you are ready to go home."
    C. "There is no need to give Michael supplemental feedings. Supplemental feeding may decrease your milk production."
    D. "You will need to give Michael supplemental feedings sometimes because you may not have enough milk."

39. The nurse correctly evaluates the teaching plan as effective when:
    A. Mrs. Madison is discharged to take Michael home.
    B. Mrs. Madison explains to the nurse how to successfully breast-feed Michael.
    C. Mrs. Madison is seen by the nurse to successfully breast-feed Michael. Additionally, Mrs. Madison discusses with the nurse the information that the nurse had previously shared with her on breast-feeding.
    D. Mrs. Madison verbalizes that she has no further questions about breast-feeding and is able to describe to the nurse the teaching that had been provided.

40. Mrs. Madison and Michael are being discharged just 24 hours after birth. What should the nurse include in the early discharge newborn home care instructions for each of the following areas?

    wet diapers ___6-10 / day_____

    stools ___2-3/day c̄ breastfeeding_____

    activity ___4-5 wakeful periods_____

    cord ___nonodorus, ↑ diaper line, apply drying solution___

    position of sleep ___side or back_____

CHAPTER 9
Health Problems of the Newborn

1. Match the term with the description.

   A. cephalopelvic disproportion

   B. crepitus

   C. moniliasis

   D. Staphylococcus aureus

   E. icterus

   F. hemolytic

   G. fiberoptic blanket

   H. bronze-baby syndrome

   I. heterozygous

   J. homozygous

   _____ causes impetigo

   _____ suited for home phototherapy

   _____ fetal head cannot pass through the maternal pelvis

   _____ rare reaction to phototherapy in which the serum, urine, and skin turn grayish brown

   _____ candidiasis

   _____ having dissimilar genes at a given position on a pair of chromosomes

   _____ coarse, crackling sensation can be produced by rubbing together of fractured bone fragments

   _____ having the same genes at a given point on a pair of chromosomes

   _____ related to destruction of red blood cells

   _____ jaundice

2. Birth injuries may occur during the delivery of the infant. Birth injuries are NOT usually the result of:
   A. forceful extraction deliveries.
   B. dystocia.
   C. excess amniotic fluid.
   D. breech presentations.

3. Which one of the following soft tissue birth injuries is most likely to need further evaluation?
   A. Subcutaneous fat necrosis
   B. Ecchymoses
   C. Petechiae appearing in areas other than the presenting part
   D. Petechiae appearing on the areas of the presenting part

4. Nursing care for soft tissue injury is NOT usually directed toward:
   A. assessing the injury.
   B. preventing breakdown and infection.
   C. providing explanations and reassurance to the parents.
   D. explaining the need for careful follow-up of injury after the infant's discharge.

5. Match the following types of extracranial hemorrhagic injury to the correct description.

   A. caput succedaneum

   B. subgaleal hemorrhage

   C. cephalhematoma

   _____ bleeding into the area between the periosteum and bone; does not cross the suture line

   _____ bleeding into the potential space that contains loosely arranged connective tissue

   _____ edematous tissue above the bone; extends across sutures

6. Fracture of the clavicle is the most frequent birth injury. Which one of the following would the nurse expect to observe on the physical examination of this infant?
   A. Crepitus felt over the affected area
   B. Symmetrical moro reflex
   C. Complete fracture with overriding fragments
   D. Positive scarf sign

7. Match the following types of paralyses with the correct description. (Types of paralyses may be used more than once.)

   A. facial paralysis   B. brachial palsy   C. phrenic nerve paralysis

   _____ arm hangs limp with the shoulder and arm adducted and internally rotated
   _____ inability to close the eye completely on the affected side with drooping of the corner of the mouth and absence of forehead wrinkling; injury to cranial nerve VII
   _____ usually spontaneously disappears in a few days but may take several months
   _____ causes diaphragmatic paralysis with respiratory distress the most common sign of injury; usually unilateral injury with affected side lung not expanding
   _____ nursing care includes maintaining proper positioning and preventing contractures
   _____ nursing care is aimed at aiding the infant in sucking and the mother with feeding techniques
   _____ undressing begins with the unaffected side while dressing begins with the affected side
   _____ artificial tears are instilled to prevent drying

8. Which one of the following does the nurse recognize as NOT being correct in describing erythema toxicum neonatorium?
   A. It is a benign, self-limiting rash that appears within the first 2 days of life.
   B. The rash is most obvious during crying episodes.
   C. The rash may be located on all areas of the body including the soles of the feet and the palms of the hands.
   D. Lesions appear as 1- to 3-mm, white or pale yellow pustules with an erythematous base. Smears of the pustules show increased numbers of eosinophils and lowered numbers of neutophils.

9. The nurse is preparing to teach a class to new parents about candidiasis. In organizing the presentation, which of the following statements does the nurse recognize as TRUE or FALSE?
   A. _____ Candidiasis is a yeast-like fungus that can be transmitted by maternal vaginal infection during delivery, person-to-person contact, and from contaminated articles.
   B. _____ In the neonate, candidiasis is usually found in the oral and diaper areas.
   C. _____ It is difficult to distinguish between oral candidiasis and coagulated milk in the infant's mouth because both are easily removed by simple wiping.
   D. _____ Thrush appears when the oral flora are altered as a result of antibiotic therapy or poor handwashing by the infant's caregiver.
   E. _____ Oral candidiasis is treated with the administration of oral nystatin four times a day before feedings and at night.
   F. _____ The infant can spread candidial dermatitis into the mouth with contaminated hands; therefore, the parents should be taught to place clothes over the diaper to break this cycle.
   G. _____ It is not necessary to boil bottles or nipples for infants with oral candidiasis because the fungus is heat resistant.
   H. _____ Oral nystatin should be placed in the far back of the throat to allow the infant to swallow it easily.

10. Which one of the following is NOT a correct description of impetigo and should be omitted by the nurse from the teaching plan?
    A. Impetigo is caused by Staphylococcus aureus.
    B. Impetigo is an eruption of vesicular lesions that occur on skin that has not been traumatized.
    C. Distribution of the lesions usually occurs on the perineum, trunk, face and buttocks.
    D. Impetigo requires the infected child or infant be isolated from others until all lesions have healed.

11. Label the following statements with the correct birthmark identification.
    A. _____ These lesions are pink, red, or purple and often thicken, darken, and proportionately enlarge as the child grows.
    B. _____ These are red, rubbery nodules with a rough surface which are recognized as tumors that involve only capillaries.
    C. _____ These are multiple flat, light brown and often characterize the autosomal-dominant hereditary disorder neurofibromatosis.

12. Treatment for port-wine stain includes laser therapy. The teaching plan for treatment expectations includes:
    A. The lesion will have a bright pink appearance for 10 days after treatment.
    B. Expose the infant to sunlight for 15 minutes daily after treatments.
    C. Administer salicylates before each treatment for pain.
    D. After treatment, gently wash the area daily with soap and dab it dry.

13. _____ is an excessive accumulation of bilirubin in the blood and is characterized by _____ , a yellow discoloration of the skin.

14. In discussing the pathophysiology of bilirubin, the nurse knows that red blood cell destruction results in _____ and _____.
    _____ _____ is an insoluble substance bound to albumin. In the liver this is changed to a soluble substance, _____ _____.

15. What is the term used to describe the yellow staining of the brain cells that can result in bilirubin encephalopathy?
    A. Jaundice
    B. Physiologic jaundice
    C. Kernicterus
    D. Icterus neonatorum

16. Which one of the following statements about bilirubin encephalopathy is TRUE?
    A. Development may be enhanced by metabolic acidosis, lowered albumin levels, intracranial infections, and increases in the metabolic demands for oxygen or glucose.
    B. It produces no permanent neurologic damage.
    C. Serum bilirubin levels alone can predict the risk of brain injury.
    D. It produces permanent liver damage by deposits of conjugated bilirubin within the cell.

17. A newborn developed jaundice at 48 hours' age that peaked at 72 hours and declined at about age 7 days. The MOST likely cause of this hyperbilirubinemia is:
    A. physiologic jaundice.
    B. pathologic jaundice.
    C. hemolytic disease of the newborn.
    D. breast milk jaundice.

18. Of the four infants listed below, which one would the nurse recognize as being LEAST likely to develop jaundice?
    A. An infant with subgaleal hemorrhage which is now resolving
    B. An infant with cephalhematoma which is now resolving
    C. The infant who has feedings started early, which will stimulate peristalsis and rapid passage of meconium
    D. The infant who is of Native American descent

19. Which one of the following therapies would the nurse expect to implement for breast-feeding-associated jaundice?
    A. Increase frequency of breast-feedings
    B. Permanent discontinuation of breast-feedings
    C. Discontinuation of breast-feedings for 24 hours with the use of home phototherapy
    D. Increase frequency of breast-feedings and addition of caloric supplements

20. Newborns are more prone to produce higher levels of bilirubin because they:
    1. have a higher concentration of circulating erythrocytes.
    2. have red blood cells with a shorter life span.
    3. have reduced albumin concentrations.
    4. have an anatomically underdeveloped liver.

    A. 1, 2, 3, and 4
    B. 1, 2, and 3
    C. 2, 3, and 4
    D. 3 and 4

21. Which one of the following is TRUE regarding diagnostic evaluations for bilirubin?
    A. Newborn levels of unconjugated bilirubin must exceed 5 mg/dl before jaundice is observable.
    B. Hyperbilirubinemia is defined as a serum bilirubin value of above 8 mg/dl in full-term infants.
    C. When jaundice occurs before the infant is 24 hours of age, bilirubin level assessment is unnecessary.
    D. Transcutaneous bilirubinometry is an effective cutaneous measurement of bilirubin in full-term infants being treated with phototherapy.

22. Implementation of phototherapy for an infant with jaundice does NOT include:
    A. shielding the infant's eyes by an opaque mask to prevent exposure to the light.
    B. recognizing that once phototherapy has been started, visual assessment of jaundice increases in validity; therefore, fewer serum bilirubin levels will be necessary.
    C. charting of the phototherapy including the time it was started and stopped, the manufacturer of the fluorescent lamp, the number of lamps, and the photometer measurement of light intensity.
    D. assessing the infant for side effects including loose, greenish stools, skin rashes, hyperthermia, dehydration, and increased metabolic rates.

23. Complete the following:

A. Erythroblastosis fetalis is caused by _____ _____.

B. The nurse is reviewing maternal laboratory results. The nurse knows that the

_____ _____ is the test that monitors anti-Rh antibody titers.

The test performed postnatally to detect antibodies attached to the circulating erythrocytes of affected infants is called _____ _____ .

C. In order to be effective in preventing maternal sensitization to the Rh factor, the nurse must administer Rho immune globulin (RhoGam) to the Rh negative mother within

_____ _____ after the first delivery or abortion and with each subsequent pregnancy. To further decrease the risk of Rh immunization RhoGam is administered at _____ weeks of gestation. RhoGam is administered by the _____ route.

24. Explain how the nurse is expected to assist the practitioner with a blood exchange transfusion in the newborn?

_____

_____

25. In the full-term neonate, which one of the following fits the definition of hypoglycemia? Plasma glucose concentrations of:
   A. 46 mg/dl at birth.
   B. 60 mg/dl at 72 hours of age.
   C. 48 mg/dl at 36 hours of age.
   D. 45 mg/dl at 12 hours of age.

26. What assessment finding is the nurse MOST likely to see in the infant as a result of hypoglycemia?
   A. Forceful, low pitched cry
   B. Tachypnea
   C. Jitteriness, tremors, twitching
   D. Vomiting, refusal to eat

27. Which of the following nursing interventions are recognized as appropriate for the infant with hypoglycemia?
   1. Early institution of bottle-feeding or breast-feeding
   2. Increase environmental stimulants
   3. Protect from cold stress and respiratory difficulty that predispose the infant to decreased blood glucose levels
   4. Force early oral glucose feedings

   A. 1, 2, 3, and 4
   B. 1 and 3
   C. 3 and 4
   D. 1, 2, and 3

28. Full-term infants at risk for hypoglycemia shortly after birth include:
    1. those born to diabetic mothers.
    2. those that are small for gestational age.
    3. those that are large for gestational age.

    A. 1, 2, and 3
    B. 1 and 2
    C. 2 and 3
    D. 1 and 3

29. Hyperglycemia in the newborn is defined as a blood glucose concentration greater than
    _____ in the full-term infant and greater than _____ in the pre-term infant.

30. Infants at risk for early-onset hypocalcemia are:
    A. postterm infants.
    B. infants that develop jaundice.
    C. infants born to hypertensive mothers.
    D. small-for-gestational-age infants who experience perinatal hypoxia.

31. The nurse caring for the infant with hypocalcemia and receiving intravenous calcium
    gluconate recognizes that which one of the following is included in the care plan?
    A. Scalp veins are the preferred site for intravenous administration of calcium gluconate.
    B. Observe for signs of hypercalcemia including vomiting and bradycardia.
    C. Stimuli should be increased until calcium levels rise.
    D. Calcium gluconate is compatible with sodium bicarbonate.

32. The nurse is assessing Sarah, a neonate born at home, and observes slight blood oozing from
    the umbilicus. What is the MOST likely cause of Sarah's hemorrhagic disease?
    A. The neonate was born with an anatomically immature liver.
    B. Coagulation factors (II, VII, IX, X) are deactivated in the neonate.
    C. Vitamin K was administered to the neonate shortly after birth.
    D. The newborn was born with a sterile intestine and was unable to synthesize vitamin K until
       feedings began.

33. The goal is to prevent hemorrhagic disease in the newborn by prophylactic administration of
    vitamin K (AquaMEPHYTON). How does the nurse correctly administer this drug?

    _____

    _____

34. When teaching the parents of the newborn about testing for PKU, the nurse should include
    which one of the following key points?
    A. The test is performed only on infants expected to have the disorder.
    B. The test is performed on cord blood.
    C. The test is not reliable if the blood sample is taken after the infant has ingested a source of
       protein.
    D. The test should be performed on all newborns before they leave the hospital, and a repeat
       blood specimen should be obtained by 2 weeks of age if the first test was taken within the
       first 24 hours of life.

35. Dietary instructions for the parents of a child with phenylketonuria include:
    1. maintaining a low-phenylalanine diet through adolescence.
    2. increasing intake of high-protein foods such as meat and dairy products.
    3. measuring vegetables, fruits, juices, breads, and starches.
    4. avoiding aspartame.
    5. introduction of solid foods as cereal, fruits and vegetables during infancy as usual.
    6. utilization of soy formula during infancy.

    A. 1, 2, 3, and 4
    B. 1, 3, 4, 5, and 6
    C. 3, 4, and 5
    D. 1, 3, 4, and 5

36. In educating the parents of a newborn with galactosemia, the nurse includes which one of the following in the plan?
    A. All food labels should be read carefully for the presence of lactose.
    B. Once the diagnosis is made and the diet is altered, little follow-up of these infants is necessary.
    C. Breast milk is acceptable for infants with galactosemia.
    D. Signs of visual impairment are unlikely in children with this disorder.

37. Diagnostic evaluation testing for congenital hypothyroidism in the newborn includes:
    1. a low level of T4.
    2. a high level of TSH.
    3. mandatory testing of all newborns within the first 24 to 48 hours or before discharge.
    4. venous blood samples taken on two separate occasions.

    A. 1 and 3
    B. 1, 2, and 3
    C. 1, 2, and 4
    D. 2 and 4

Critical Thinking • Case Study

Mrs. Becker had a normal pregnancy and delivery without complications at 39 weeks gestation. She is breast-feeding her 2-day-old neonate, Ben, when she notices that Ben's skin looks yellow. The total serum bilirubin level is 13 mg/dl.

38. Mrs. Becker asks the nurse about Ben's condition and the seriousness of his illness. Which one of the following is the BEST response?
    A. "Ben has pathologic jaundice, a serious condition."
    B. "Ben has breast milk jaundice and you will need to stop breast-feeding."
    C. "Ben probably has physiologic jaundice, a normal finding at his age."
    D. "Infants with serum bilirubin levels of 13 mg/dl will develop bilirubin encephalopathy and severe brain damage."

39. The physician orders that Mrs. Becker increase her frequency of breast-feeding to every two hours and to avoid supplementation. The rationale for this management is being discussed by the nurse with Mrs. Becker. Which one of the following does the nurse recognize as the basis for the ordered treatment?
    A. The jaundice is related to the process of breast-feeding, probably from decreased caloric and fluid intake by breast-fed infants.
    B. The jaundice is caused by a factor in the breast milk that breaks down bilirubin to a lipid-soluble form, which is reabsorbed in the gut.
    C. The jaundice is caused by the mother's hemolytic disease.
    D. The jaundice is increased because the infant was put to breast early, which increases the amount of time meconium is kept in the gut before excretion.

40. The serum bilirubin level has not decreased as the physician desired and phototherapy has been ordered. The priority goal at this time is:
    A. the family will be prepared for home phototherapy.
    B. the infant will receive adequate intravenous hydration.
    C. the infant will experience no complications from phototherapy.
    D. the infant will have hourly bilirubin level testing completed.

41. When caring for Ben the nurse should take all but which of the following actions to prevent complications?
    A. Make certain that eyelids are closed before applying eye shields. Check eyes at least every shift for discharge or irritation.
    B. Monitor axillary temperature closely to detect hyperthermia and/or hypothermia.
    C. Maintain 18 inches' distance between infant and light.
    D. Apply oil daily to skin to avoid breakdown.

42. The BEST expected patient outcome for Ben while on phototherapy is:
    A. newborn begins feeding soon after birth.
    B. family demonstrates an understanding of therapy and prognosis.
    C. newborn displays no evidence of infection.
    D. newborn displays no evidence of eye irritation, dehydration, temperature instability, or skin breakdown.

CHAPTER 10
The High-Risk Newborn and Family

1. Identify the following.

   _____ An infant whose birth weight is less than 2500 g. regardless of gestational age.

   _____ An infant whose birth weight is less than 1000 g.

   _____ An infant whose birth weight falls below the 10th percentile on intrauterine growth curves.

   _____ An infant whose birth weight falls above the 90th percentile on intrauterine growth charts.

   _____ An infant born before completion of 37 weeks of gestation.

   _____ An infant born between the 38th week and completion of the 42nd week of gestation.

   _____ An infant born after 42 weeks gestation.

   _____ Death of a fetus after 20 weeks of gestation.

   _____ Death that occurs in the first 27 days of life.

   _____ Describes the total number of fetal and early neonatal deaths per 1000 live births.

   _____ The capacity to balance heat production and conservation and heat dissipation.

   _____ An environment that permits the infant to maintain a normal core temperature with minimum oxygen consumption and caloric expenditure.

   _____ Heat loss that occurs when infants are exposed to drafts, increased air flow.

   _____ Use of double-walled incubators can effectively reduce this heat loss in high risk newborn.

   _____ This type of heat loss can be reduced by warming all items that come into direct contact with the newborn.

2. _____ _____ _____ and _____ _____ continue to be identified as leading causes of infant mortality.

3. List ways in which the nurse working with women of child-bearing age can reduce infant mortality and morbidity within the community.

   _____

   _____

   _____

4. Which one of the following is NOT used in the classification of high-risk newborns?
   A. According to birth size
   B. According to gestational age
   C. According to mortality
   D. According to birth age

5. A neonatal intensive care facility that provides a full range of maternal newborn services and that has the capacity to provide care for the most complex neonatal complications with at least one full-time neonatologist on staff is known as:
   A. Level I facility.
   B. Level II facility.
   C. Level III facility.
   D. Level IV facility.

6. When the high-risk neonate needs transportation to a facility that can provide intensive care, the nurse recognizes that priority care for this neonate must include:
   A. transfer of both the mother and infant.
   B. immediate transport often before stabilization of the neonate.
   C. delay of transport until the neonate has sufficiently stabilized for transport.
   D. a transport team composed of at least a neonatologist, a respiratory therapist, and one neonatal nurse.

7. A thorough systematic physical assessment is a must in the care of the high-risk neonate. Subtle changes in _____ _____ , _____ , _____ or _____ _____ often indicate an underlying problem.

8. At birth the newborn is immediately assessed to determine any apparent problems and to identify those that demand immediate attention. The assessment NOT usually conducted at birth or immediately after birth is:
   A. assignment of a gestational age score.
   B. assignment of an Apgar score.
   C. evaluation for obvious congenital anomalies.
   D. evaluation for neonatal distress.

9. Identify the following statements about high-risk care of the neonate as either TRUE or FALSE.
   A. _____ Neonates under intensive observation are placed in a controlled environment and monitored for heart rate, respiratory activity, and temperature.
   B. _____ Sophisticated monitoring and life-support systems can replace the observations of the infant by nursing personnel.
   C. _____ Electrodes for cardiac monitors should not be applied to the back or upper arms of the neonate.
   D. _____ Infants who are mechanically ventilated and have low Apgar scores can have lower blood pressures.
   E. _____ An accurate output can be obtained in the neonate by use of a urine collecting bag or by weighing the infant's diaper. Regardless of the method utilized, 40 gram weight of urine would be recorded as 40 ml of urine.
   F. _____ The nurse is preparing the infant for a heel stick. This preparation is done to create adequate vasodilation and is accomplished by placing a heating pad on the infant's heel.
   G. _____ Nurses are allowed to turn off alarm systems for electronic monitoring devices when their sounds disturb the infant's parents.

10. The major source of increased production of heat during cold stress in the high-risk neonate is _____ .

11. Low-birth-weight infants are at a disadvantage for heat production when compared to full-term infants because they have:
    1. small muscle mass.
    2. fewer deposits of brown fat.
    3. less insulating subcutaneous fat.
    4. poor reflex control of skin capillaries.

    A. 1, 2, 3, and 4
    B. 2, 3, and 4
    C. 1, 2, and 3
    D. 1, 3, and 4

12. Cold stress produces three major consequences that add additional hazards to the neonate. These are:

    _____

    _____

    _____

13. The nurse recognizes an intervention LEAST likely to be effective for high-risk neonates as which one of the following?
    A. Maintaining a neutral thermal environment
    B. Placing the heat-sensing probe on the infant's abdomen when the infant is in the prone position
    C. Keeping oxygen that is supplied to the infant via a hood around the head warmed and humidified
    D. Warming all items that come in direct contact with the infant including the hands of caregivers

14. A primary objective in the care of high-risk infants is to maintain respiration. Describe how the nurse should complete the respiratory assessment.

    _____

    _____

15. The best way to prevent infection in the high-risk neonate begins with:
    A. meticulous and frequent hand washing of all persons coming in contact with the infant.
    B. observing continually for signs of infection.
    C. requiring everyone working in the NICU to put on fresh scrub clothes before entering the unit.
    D. performing epidemiologic studies at least monthly.

16. Baby girl Miller has been admitted to the NICU with low-birth-weight and possible infection. Parenteral fluids have been ordered for hydration and antibiotic administration.

    A. What are the preferred sites for peripheral IV infusions in this infant?

    _____

    B. In many neonatal centers a specially inserted catheter is used for IV hydration and medication administration because it is less expensive and decreases trauma to the neonate. What is the catheter called? _____

    C. The nurse starts a peripheral line and places the neonate on an infusion pump to regulate the rate of IV administration. Ten minutes later the nurse observes for signs of infiltration. What signs would the nurse be looking for?

    _____

17. A complication that develops with the use of the umbilical catheter is thrombi. The nurse best recognizes this complication because of the appearance of:
    A. increased warmth in lower extremities.
    B. bluish discoloration seen in the toes, called "cath toes".
    C. bounding pedal pulses.
    D. hemorrhage from the umbilical catheter area.

18. What is the BEST indication that the preterm infant can tolerate nipple feedings?
    A. The infant requires approximately 40 minutes to complete a feeding.
    B. The infant has a sustained respiratory rate of 68.
    C. Infant is able to suck on a pacifier.
    D. Infant has a coordinated suck-swallow reflex.

19. A 1500g. infant appears to be ready for enteral feedings. Which one of the following would the nurse include in the implementation of gavage feedings?
    A. Insert the tube into the unobstructed nares.
    B. Perform the procedure with the infant in a supine position with the head elevated 45 degrees.
    C. Aspirate the contents of the stomach, measure these contents and replace the residual before beginning the feeding. The amount of residual is subtracted from the total feeding to prevent over-distending the stomach.
    D. Allow the feeding to flow by gravity, then push a small amount of the feeding into the stomach, then allow the remainder of the feeding to flow by gravity.

20. _____ increases oxygenation during tube feeding and has been shown to increase readiness in low-birth-weight infants for bottle-feeding.

21. One of the major goals of care for the high-risk neonate is conservation of energy. This is LEAST likely accomplished by which of the following actions?
    A. Organizing nursing care activities so the infant is not over stimulated and not over disturbed
    B. Maintaining a neutral thermal environment
    C. Keeping the infant in the supine position as much as possible to decrease expenditure of energy by unnecessary movement
    D. Employing gavage feeding

22. In caring for preterm infants' skin, the nurse knows to:
   A. use scissors to remove dressings or tape from the infant's extremities.
   B. use solvents to remove tape from the neonate's skin.
   C. use alkaline-based soaps in removal of stool.
   D. use transparent elastic film dressings to secure and protect central lines.

23. Manifestations of acute pain in the neonate include:
   A. increased transcutaneous oxygen saturation.
   B. increased heart rate and rapid, shallow respirations.
   C. hypoglycemia.
   D. all of the above.

24. Describe interventions that can be used to promote developmental care for preterm infants.

   _____

   _____

25. _____ is the most widely used narcotic analgesic for
   pharmacologic management of neonatal pain.

26. Promoting a healthy parent-child relationship for the family with a high-risk neonate is BEST
   accomplished by the nurse:
   A. reinforcing parents during their caregiving activities and interactions with their infant.
   B. discouraging them from talking about the baby.
   C. reassuring them that the infant is doing well.
   D. encouraging the mother to stay by the infant's bedside to promote bonding.

27. The term _____ is applied to physically healthy children
   who are perceived by the parents to be at high risk for medical or developmental problems.

28. Discharge instructions for the parents of the preterm infant should NOT include:
   A. warning parents that their infant may still be in danger and will need constant attention.
   B. providing information to the parents on how to contact personnel for later questions.
   C. instructions about car safety seats including how these seats can be adapted for smaller
      children with the placement of blanket rolls on each side of the infant to support the head
      and trunk.
   D. providing adequate information about immunization needs.

29. To help parents deal with neonatal death, the nurse does which of the following?
   A. Discourages the parent from staying with the infant before death to prevent over
      attachment
   B. Explains to the parents that the infant would have had many developmental problems and
      it is better that the infant did not suffer
   C. Gives the parents the opportunity to hold and talk with the infant before and after death
   D. Forces the parents to see the infant after death because closure is necessary

30. A physical characteristic usually observed in the preterm infant and NOT observed in the full-term infant is:
   A. proportionately equal head in relation to the body.
   B. skin is often translucent, smooth, shiny with small blood vessels clearly visible underneath the epidermis.
   C. soles of feet and palms of hand have distinct creases extending across the entire palms and down the complete soles of the feet.
   D. absence of lanugo and little vernix caseosa.

31. Apnea in the preterm infant is defined as a lapse of spontaneous breathing lasting for how many seconds?
   A. 5
   B. 10
   C. 15
   D. 20

32. Bryan is a 2 day old preterm infant being cared for in the NICU. He had some apnea periods but in report the nurse was told he had had no episodes today. His apnea monitor alarm has just sounded. What is the FIRST action of the nurse?
   A. Use tactile stimulation, rubbing on the back to stop the apneic spell
   B. Suction the nose and oropharynx
   C. Assess the infant for color and for presence of respiration
   D. Place the infant on the abdomen

33. The preterm infant is having regular respirations for up to 20 seconds with subsequent apneic periods that last no longer than 10 seconds and occur three times in succession. What is this called?
   A. Obstructive apnea
   B. Periodic breathing
   C. Central apnea
   D. Mixed apnea

34. A late and serious sign of respiratory distress in the neonate is:
   A. central cyanosis.
   B. respiratory rate of 90 breaths/minute.
   C. substernal retractions.
   D. nasal flaring.

35. When nasopharyngeal passages, the trachea, or the ET tube is being suctioned in the newborn, which one of the following is a correct procedure?
   A. Pulse oximeter is observed before, during, and after suctioning to provide an ongoing assessment of oxygenation status.
   B. Continuous suction is applied as the catheter is withdrawn.
   C. The catheter is inserted gently and slowly and suction is conducted to a point where the catheter meets resistance before the catheter is withdrawn.
   D. The time the airway is obstructed by the catheter is limited to no more than 10 seconds.

36. Discuss the importance of surfactant to the preterm infant's lungs.

   _____

   _____

37. Match the following.

A. pulmonary interstitial emphysema

B. lung compliance

C. continuous positive airway pressure (CPAP)

D. intermittent mandatory ventilation (IMV)

E. positive end-expiratory pressure (PEEP)

F. nasal flaring

G. grunting

H. synchronized intermittent mandatory ventilation (SIMV)

_____ method that infuses air or oxygen under a preset pressure by means of nasal prongs, a face mask, or an endotracheal tube

_____ method the allows infant to breathe spontaneously at own rate but provides mechanical cycled respirations and pressure at regular preset intervals by means of a endotracheal tube and ventilator

_____ develops in the preterm infant with RDS and immature lungs as a result of overdistention of distal airways

_____ method that provides increased end-expiratory pressure during expiration and between mandatory breaths, preventing alveolar collapse

_____ lung distensibility

_____ abnormal sounds made upon respiration as a result of increased effort required to fill the lungs; associated with atelectasis

_____ widening of the nostril during inspiration, signals respiratory distress

_____ infant triggered ventilator with signal detector and assist/control mode

38. Susie, a 20 minute old neonate, was observed at birth to have meconium staining. If Susie has meconium in the lungs, this MOST likely will:
A. prevent air from entering the lungs.
B. trap inspired air in the lungs.
C. cause no problems with breathing.
D. lead to respiratory alkalosis.

39. An important nursing function is close observation of neonates at risk for developing air leaks. These infants include:
A. infants with respiratory distress syndrome (RDS).
B. infants with meconium stained amniotic fluid.
C. infants receiving CPAP or positive-pressure ventilation.
D. all of the above.

40. Infants diagnosed with bronchopulmonary dyplasia have special care needs. These needs include:
A. opportunities for adequate rest.
B. increases in environmental stimuli.
C. decreases in caloric intake.
D. rapid weaning from ventilators.

41. The laboratory evaluation for the diagnosis of sepsis is LEAST likely to include:
A. blood cultures.
B. spinal fluid culture.
C. urine culture.
D. gastric secretions culture.

42. Clinical signs seen in necrotizing enterocolitis are:
    A. increased abdominal girth.
    B. increased gastric residual.
    C. positive stool hematest.
    D. all of the above.

43. Preterm infants can develop patent ductus arteriosus (PDA). Therapy often includes the administration of:
    A. theophyllin.
    B. indomethacin.
    C. digoxin.
    D. heparin.

44. Why does the nurse carefully monitor and record amounts of all blood drawn for tests in the preterm infant?
    A. Early prevention of anemia
    B. Prevention of infection
    C. Prevention of polycythemia
    D. Detection of factors that contribute to hypothermia

45. A preterm infant is in danger of developing retinopathy of prematurity (ROP). Of the following nursing actions, which one is LEAST likely to be effective in the prevention of ROP?
    A. Correct oxygen administration
    B. Decreasing environmental stimuli, direct light
    C. Observing for clinical signs of metabolic acidosis
    D. Monitoring of oxygenation status

46. The nurse recognizes that which of the following interventions is CONTRAINDICATED in the preterm infant with increased intracranial pressure?
    A. Avoiding interventions that produce crying
    B. Administration of hyperosmolar solutions
    C. Administering analgesics to reduce discomfort
    D. Turning the head to the right without body alignment

47. The nurse is able to distinguish between seizures and jitteriness in the neonate. Identify which one of the following is NOT a description of seizures.
    A. Seizures are not accompanied by ocular movement.
    B. Seizures have their dominant movement as tremor.
    C. In seizures the dominant movement cannot be stopped by flexion of the affected limb.
    D. Seizures are highly sensitive to light manual stimulation.

48. John is a newborn just delivered of a diabetic mother. The nurse will watch John for signs that he is rapidly developing what?
    A. Hyperglycemia
    B. Hypoglycemia
    C. Failure of the pancreas
    D. Dehydration

49. Infants born to narcotic-addicted mothers may exhibit all of the following clinical manifestations EXCEPT:
   A. tremors and restlessness.
   B. frequent sneezing.
   C. coordinated suck and swallow reflex.
   D. high-pitched, shrill cry.

Critical Thinking • Case Study

Baby Mark was born at 36 weeks gestation and weighed 2300 g at birth. Apgar score at 1 minute was 5. Baby Mark was suctioned and oxygen administration started. He responded with spontaneous respirations. You are the nurse who has been assigned to care for him in the special care nursery. Mark's admission vital signs are pulse 150, respirations 56, and axillary temperature of 96.4 degrees F. Mark is placed in a radiant warmer and oxygen continued by oxygen hood.

50. You would classify Baby Mark as:
   1. full-term infant.
   2. preterm infant.
   3. low-birth-weight.
   4. small for gestational age.

   A. 1 and 4
   B. 2 and 4
   C. 2 and 3
   D. 1 and 3

51. You identify Mark as being at risk for developing respiratory distress syndrome. Why?
   1. gestational age
   2. low Apgar score
   3. hypothermia
   4. respiratory rate of 56

   A. 1, 2, 3, and 4
   B. 1, 2, and 3
   C. 2, 3, and 4
   D. 2 and 3

52. The nurse's plan for oxygen administration includes:
   A. frequent suctioning.
   B. frequent assessment to include unobstructed nares.
   C. nipple feeding with respiratory rates of 70 and below.
   D. turning off monitor alarms to allow the neonate to rest.

53. Baby Mark's parents are visiting him for the first time. How can the nurse assist the parents in feeling more comfortable in the NICU atmosphere?
   A. Discourage questions of a technical nature.
   B. Tell the parents that Mark is going to be fine.
   C. Explain what is happening with Mark and why he is receiving this type of care.
   D. Leave the parents alone with the infant.

54. The nurse will develop a plan of care for Mark that recognizes which of the following as the BEST expected outcome?
    A. Oxygen is administered correctly, and arterial blood gases are within normal limits.
    B. Monitor for thermal environment changes.
    C. Record oxygen delivery rates every two hours.
    D. Assess respiratory status every hour.

55. Mark has had an apneic episode. What should the nurse include in the documentation of this episode?

    _____

    _____

56. As a nurse in the NICU you are assigned to care for a 4 pound preterm infant named Maria. In report you learn that Maria is still on gavage feedings and that tomorrow she is scheduled to begin bottle feeding. If Maria tolerates her bottle feedings well, she is scheduled to go home in a few days. The nurse caring for a preterm infant closely observes for behaviors that indicate readiness for bottle-feedings. Name these behaviors.

    _____

    _____

57. The nurse in the special care nursery should position the preterm infant in the _____ position to improve oxygenation. On discharge from the nursery to home the nurse instructs the parents to place the infant in the _____ position while sleeping.

CHAPTER 11
Conditions Caused by Defects in Physical Development

1. Match the following.

   A. growth
   B. hyperplasia
   C. hypertrophy
   D. differentiation
   E. organogenesis
   F. teratogenesis
   G. sensitive or critical periods

   _____ prenatal growth process disturbed to produce a structural or functional defect

   _____ Major impact of environmental factors coincides with this period.

   _____ beginning of all major organ systems

   _____ Cells divide and synthesize new proteins.

   _____ increase in cell number

   _____ increase in cell size

   _____ Early cells are modified and specialized to form the individual.

2. Parental responses to the birth of an infant with a physical disability are BEST described as:
   A. hostility and bitterness.
   B. disbelief and denial.
   C. strengthening of the psychologic attachment the mother has formed during pregnancy with the unborn child.
   D. establishment of realistic goals.

3. The nurse can independently implement which one of the following actions in the preoperative neonate?
   A. Start a peripheral intravenous line
   B. Begin administration of prophylactic antibiotics
   C. Provide accurate information to the newborn's parents regarding what to expect postoperatively
   D. Begin pain management control

4. Primary roles of the nurse in the care of an infant born with a physical defect are:
   A. to discourage the parents from talking about the infant.
   B. to show the parents photographs of other infants with similar defects and assure them the defect can be corrected.
   C. to supply only information as requested by the parents.
   D. to support and encourage the parents in their caregiving tasks.

5. Identify the following statements about postoperative care of the neonate as TRUE or FALSE.

_____ The newborn's poor chest wall stability, along with smaller and more reactive airways, contributes to postoperative respiratory compromise.

_____ Most postoperative neonates require mechanical ventilation.

_____ Neonates are highly subject to acidosis and hypoxia and require continuous monitoring of acid-base balance and oxygen status.

_____ The preterm infant is at high risk for developing respiratory complications from general anesthesia.

_____ The neonate is particularly sensitive to vagal stimulation which can be induced by postoperative nasogastric tubes, endotracheal tubes and suctioning.

_____ The neonate's risk for rapid fluid shifts can be intensified by stress and loss of fluid during surgical procedures.

6. Critical guidelines for neonatal postoperative care include continuous monitoring of oxygen and acid-base status. What actions would the nurse expect to take to achieve this goal?
   A. Monitor neonatal weight postoperatively and keep accurate intake and output record
   B. Monitor axillary temperature, blood pressure, and heart rate every 15 minutes x 4, every 30 minutes x 2, every 1 hour x 6, then every 2 hours for 24 hours
   C. Monitor surgical site/skin status for drainage, bleeding and amount of output from tubes
   D. Monitor pulse oximetry and arterial blood gases

7. The nurse has completed the physical assessment of Baby Boy Andrews and has noticed a cutaneous dimple with dark tufts of hair between L5 and S1. Which of the following medical conditions should the nurse suspect?
   A. Spina bifida occulta
   B. Spina bifida cystica
   C. Meningocele
   D. Cranioschisis

8. Research has shown that supplemental folic acid can reduce the recurrence rates of spina bifida, anencephaly, or encephalocele. How should this supplement be administered?
   A. Daily folic acid dose to 4.0 mg beginning 1 month before conception and during the first trimester
   B. Daily folic acid dose of 0.4 mg as soon as pregnancy is confirmed
   C. Daily folic acid dose of 4.0 mg given through the use of multivitamin preparations beginning 1 month before conception and throughout the first trimester
   D. Daily folic acid dose of 4.0 mg beginning with the confirmation of pregnancy and continuing throughout pregnancy

9. Match the medical condition with its description.

   A.   anencephaly   _____ failure of neural tube to close and fuse
   B.   myelodysplasia   _____ results from disturbances in the dynamics of CSF absorption and flow
   C.   myelomeningocele
   D.   hydrocephalus   _____ congenital malformation where both cerebral hemispheres are absent
                               _____ any malformation of the spinal canal and cord

10. The major complications of myelomeningocele are _____ _____
    _____ and _____.

11. Therapeutic management that provides the most favorable (morbidity and mortality) outcome for the child born with myelomeningocele is:
    A. early physical therapy.
    B. closure of the defect within first 24 hours.
    C. vigorous antibiotic therapy.
    D. splint application to lower extremities.

12. Management goal for genitourinary function in the infant with myelomeningocele is _____ while the goal for the older child is _____.

13. Myelomeningocele may be associated with hydrocephalus. What should the nurse assess to identify an infant with hydrocephalus?
    A. Upward eye slanting
    B. Strabismus
    C. Wide or bulging fontanels
    D. Decreased head circumference

14. Upon delivery of an infant with myelomeningocele, which one of the following nursing actions may be CONTRAINDICATED?
    A. Examination of the membranous cyst for intactness
    B. Diapering the infant
    C. Keep moist sterile normal saline dressings on defect
    D. Keep infant in the prone position

15. An infant born with spina bifida who needs intermittent urinary catheterization has developed sneezing, wheezing, and a rash over his lower pelvic and genital area. The nurse would suspect this infant has developed:
    A. asthma.
    B. emphysema.
    C. latex allergy.
    D. anaphylaxis.

16. Hydrocephalus that is a result of maldevelopment or an intrauterine infection is called _____. Hydrocephalus that is caused by infection, neoplasm, or hemorrhage is called _____.

17. Surgical shunts are often required to provide drainage in the treatment of hydrocephalus. What is the preferred shunt for infants?
    A. Ventriculoperitoneal shunt
    B. Ventriculoatrial shunt
    C. Ventricular bypass
    D. Ventriculopleural shunt

18. The nurse recognizes that which one of the following would be included in the postoperative care of a client with a shunt?
    A. Positioning the patient in a head-down position
    B. Continuous pumping of the shunt to assess function
    C. Monitoring for abdominal or peritoneal distention
    D. Positioning the child on the side of the operative site to facilitate drainage

19. The major complications of VP shunts are _____ and _____.

20. Posterior fontanel is closed by age _____.
    Anterior fontanel is closed by age _____.
    Sutures are unable to be separated by ICP by age _____.

21. Identify the following statements about microcephaly as TRUE or FALSE.

    _____ Microcephaly is defined as a head circumference greater than 5 standard deviations below the mean.

    _____ Primary microcephaly can be caused by irradiation between 4 to 20 weeks of gestation.

    _____ Secondary microcephaly can be caused by infection during the third trimester, the perinatal period, or early infancy.

    _____ All children with microcephaly are mentally retarded.

    _____ There is no treatment for microcephaly.

    _____ Nursing care is supportive and directed toward helping parents adjust to a child with cognitive impairment.

22. Therapeutic management for craniosynostosis is:
    A. placement of ventriculoperitoneal shunt.
    B. removal of neoplasm.
    C. release of fused sutures.
    D. supportive assistance for parents.

23. The nurse, in preparing the nursing care plan for the infant born with craniofacial abnormalities, recognizes which of the following as TRUE?
    A. Children with this deformity face erroneous assumptions of mental retardation.
    B. Abnormalities include deformities involving the skull and facial bones.
    C. A helmet is often required after surgery to protect the operative site and bone grafts for 6 months to 2 years.
    D. All of the above are true.

24. Positional plagiocephaly may be resolved by instructing the parents to position the infant how?

    _____

    _____

25. Match the degree of developmental hip dysplasia with its description.

    A. acetabular dysplasia

    B. subluxation

    C. dislocation

    _____ Femoral head remains in contact with the acetabulum, but the head of the femur is partially displaced.

    _____ Femoral head remains in the acetabulum (mildest form).

    _____ Femoral head loses contact with the acetabulm.

26. The nurse observes which of the following signs in the infant with developmental dysplasia?
    A. Negative Ortolani test
    B. Asymmetrical folds in skin of legs
    C. Lengthening of the limb on the affected side
    D. Limitation in adduction of the leg

27. Match the expected therapeutic management for developmental hip dysplasia with the age group.

    A. newborn to 6 months   _____ more difficult; includes operative reduction and
    B. 6 to 18 months   innominate osteotomy procedures designed to
    C. older child   construct an acetabular roof

                                     _____ abduction devices as Pavlik harness; can also
                                                  include skin traction, hip spica cast

                                     _____ gradual reduction by traction and individualized
                                                  home traction program followed by a attempted
                                                  closed reduction of the hip

28. Why is the practice of double or triple diapering the infant with developmental dysplasia of the hip no longer recommended?

    _____

    _____

29. Match the congenital clubfoot conditions with its description.

    A. talipes varus   _____ eversion or bending outward
    B. talipes valgus   _____ inversion or bending inward
    C. talipes equinus   _____ plantar flexion, in which the toes are lower than the
    D. talipes calcaneus   heel

                              _____ dorsiflexion, in which the toes are higher than the
                                       heel

30. Treatment of clubfoot includes:
    A. correction of the deformity.
    B. maintenance of the correction until normal muscle is gained, often accomplished by casts or orthoses.
    C. follow-up observation to detect possible recurrence of the deformity.
    D. all of the above

31. Match the following.

    A. metatarsus varus   _____ seal limbs, deficiency of long bones with
    B. amelia   development of hands and feet attached at or near
    C. meromelia   the shoulders
    D. phocomelia   _____ absence of complete extremity
    E. atresia   _____ medial adduction of the toes and forefoot

                              _____ partial absence of extremity

                              _____ absence of a normal opening

32. An important assessment for identifying cleft palate is for the nurse to:
    A. assess sucking ability of infant.
    B. assess color of lips.
    C. palpate the palate with the gloved finger.
    D. all of the above.

33. Which of the following feeding practices should be used when feeding the infant with a cleft of the lip or palate?
    A. Use a large, hard nipple with a large hole
    B. Use a normal nipple
    C. Use ESSR feeding technique
    D. Hold breast feeding until after surgical correction of the defect

34. In providing postoperative care for the infant with a cleft lip or palate, which one of the following is acceptable?
    A. Use of tongue depressor in the mouth to assess surgical site
    B. Continuous elbow restraints to prevent injury
    C. Placement of infant in the prone position after cleft lip repair
    D. Placement of the infant in the prone position after cleft palate repair

35. In preparing the parents of a child with cleft palate, the nurse includes which of the following in the long term family teaching plan?
    A. Tooth development will be delayed.
    B. Guideline use for speech development
    C. Use of decongestants and tylenol to care for frequent upper respiratory symptoms
    D. All of the above

36. The priority nursing intervention in the immediate care of a postoperative infant after repair of a cleft lip or cleft palate is to:
    A. keep the infant well hydrated.
    B. prevent vomiting.
    C. maintain an open airway.
    D. administer medications to prevent drooling.

37. The nurse observes frothy saliva in the mouth and nose of the neonate and frequent drooling. When fed, the infant swallows normally but suddenly the fluid returns through the nose and mouth of the infant. The nurse would suspect what medical condition?
    A. Esophageal atresia
    B. Cleft palate
    C. Anorectal malformation
    D. Biliary atresia

38. In assessment for anorectal malformation the nurse inspects for patency of the anus and rectum and meconium passage. Why is the passage of meconium not always an indicator of anal patency in females?

_____

_____

39. The best definition of biliary atresia is:
    A. jaundice persisting beyond 2 weeks of age with elevated direct bilirubin levels.
    B. progressive inflammatory process causing intrahepatic and extrahepatic bile duct fibrosis.
    C. absence of bile pigment.
    D. hepatomegaly and palpable liver.

40. The term used to describe a hernia that is constricted and cannot be reduced manually is

    _____ .

41. Identify the following statements about umbilical hernia as either TRUE or FALSE.
    _____ The disorder affects blacks more than whites.
    _____ It affects preterm infants more than full-term infants.
    _____ It may be present in association with Down syndrome.
    _____ It is most prominent when the infant is crying.
    _____ It usually spontaneously resolves by 3 to 4 years of age.

42. Which one of the following is CONTRAINDICATED as part of the therapeutic management for the neonate with congenital diaphragmatic hernia?
    A. Endotracheal intubation
    B. Gastrointestinal decompression
    C. Positioning the infant with the head and chest elevated above the abdomen
    D. Bag and mask ventilation

43. Match the following.

    A. gastroschisis
    B. omphalocele
    C. phimosis
    D. inguinal hernia
    E. femoral hernia
    F. cryptorchidism
    G. hypospadias
    H. epispadias
    I. hydrocele
    J. bladder exstrophy
    K. hydronephrosis

    _____ prevents retraction of the foreskin
    _____ herniation of the abdominal contents through the umbilical ring
    _____ Herniation is lateral to the umbilical ring.
    _____ externalization of the bladder
    _____ painless inguinal swelling
    _____ swelling in the groin area associated with severe pain (most common in females)
    _____ fluid in the processus vaginalis
    _____ One or both of the testes do not descend.
    _____ Urethral opening is located below the glans penis or along the ventral surface of penile shaft.
    _____ opening of urethra on dorsum of penis
    _____ renal pelvis and calyces become dilated

44. Identify the primary criterion used when assigning gender sex to an infant born with doubtful sex.

    _____

    _____

45. TORCH complex is a group of microbial agents that cause similar manifestations in the neonate. List what each letter stands for.

T _____

O _____

R _____

C _____

H _____

46. The nurse can expect the infant with fetal alcohol syndrome on assessment to exhibit which of the following?
   A. Normal prenatal growth patterns
   B. Normal feeding patterns
   C. Thicker upper lip and longer palpebral fissures
   D. Irritability

Critical Thinking • Case Study

Jane Williams is a newborn diagnosed with myelomeningocele. She has been admitted to the NICU.

47. Which one of the following is the primary nursing goal for Jane before surgical correction of the myelomeningocele?
   A. Observe for increasing paralysis
   B. Prevent infection
   C. Prevent skin breakdown
   D. Limit environmental stimulus

48. Thirty-six hours after birth, the nurse notes that Jane has developed an elevated temperature, is irritable, and is lethargic. What would the nurse suspect?
   A. Hydrocephalus
   B. Infection
   C. Latex allergy
   D. Urinary retention

49. Which one the following nursing diagnoses is MOST relevant to Jane's care?
   A. Altered bowel elimination related to neurological deficits
   B. High risk for infection related to the presence of infectious organisms
   C. Altered nutrition related to immobility
   D. Altered self-concept related to physical disability

50. Develop goals related to Jane's care in the NICU.

_____

_____

_____

51. Which one of the following is the BEST way to have Jane's tactile stimulation needs met before repair of the myelomeningocele?
   A. By frequent cuddling and being held in parent's arms
   B. By having black and white drawings placed within the infant's view
   C. By frequent caressing and stroking while the infant is placed on a pillow across the parent's lap
   D. By frequent changing of the infant's diaper and dressing

52. Jane has corrective surgery and is 6 hours postoperative. The nurse must observe the abdomen closely for the development of _____.

53. After closure of the meningomyelocele, Jane's nursing care should include which one of the following?
   A. Measuring the head circumference daily
   B. Keeping external stimulus at a minimum
   C. Strict limitation of leg movement
   D. Withholding breast or bottle feedings

CHAPTER 12
Health Promotion of the Infant and Family

1. Terms—Biologic Development

   A. binocularity
   B. depth perception
   C. visual preference
   D. respiratory rate
   E. heart rate
   F. sinus arrhythmia
   G. hemopoietic changes
   H. physiologic anemia
   I. digestive process
   J. ptyalin

   K. amylase
   L. lipase
   M. trypsin
   N. suckling
   O. sucking
   P. swallowing
   Q. infantile swallow reflex
   R. mature swallow reflex
   S. Santmyer swallow

   T. immunologic system
   U. thermoregulation
   V. thermogenesis
   W. total body fluid
   X. renal structures
   Y. endocrine system
   Z. righting reflexes
   AA. crawling
   BB. creeping

   ___I___ immature at birth; do not begin functioning until age 3 months

   ___B___ stereiopsis; begins to develop by age 7 to 9 months

   ___T___ receives a significant amount of maternal protection for this system until about 3 months of age

   ___D___ begins to slow in infants and is relatively stable

   ___F___ heart rate that increases with inspiration and decreases with expiration

   ___A___ the fixation of two ocular images into one cerebral picture (fusion); begins to develop by 6 weeks of age and should be well established by age 4 months

   ___G___ fetal hemoglobin is present for the first 5 months

   ___C___ looking at the human face is the choice for infants

   ___H___ caused by high levels of fetal hemoglobin which is thought to depress the production of erythropoietin

   ___E___ slows and is often in sinus arrhythmia

   ___J___ amylase; present in small amounts in the newborn but usually has little effect

   ___P___ deglutition; the ability to collect the food and propel it into the esophagus

   ___N___ first seen at birth; denotes extension and a pulling-in pattern of tongue movements, as in licking

   ___BB___ propelling forward on hands and knees with belly off floor

   ___L___ infants do not achieve adult levels of fat absorption because of the limited secretion of this enzyme

   ___K___ pancreatic enzyme needed for digestion of complex carbohydrates

   ___M___ secreted in sufficient quantities to catabolize protein into polypeptides and some amino acids in infants

   ___O___ the action used in the bottle fed infant; infants control the stream of milk by pushing the tongue against the rubber nipple holes

   ___R___ somatic reflex; tongue remains behind the central incisors and the mandible no longer thrusts forward; tongue pressure and movement against the hard palate pushes the food back in to the pharynx

   ___Z___ elicit postural responses of flexion or extension and are responsible for motor activities such as rolling over, assuming the crawl position and maintaining normal head-trunk-limb alignment during activities

infantile swallow reflex

✓ ___Q___ visceral reflex; food lies in a shallow groove on the top of the tongue; the fluid flows by gravity down the tongue and along the sides of the mouth. The process is efficient for fluids but not for solids.

___X___ complete maturity of this system occurs during the latter half of the second year

___V___ shivering

___S___ a special reflex exhibited by infants; when a puff of air is directed at the face; the infant will exhibit a reflex swallow.

___W___ comprises 75% of the body weight at birth

___AA___ propelling forward with belly on floor

___U___ more efficient during infancy than in the newborn stage

___Y___ adequately developed at birth but functions are immature

2. Terms—Psychosocial development

A. acquiring a sense of trust/overcoming a sense of mistrust
B. narcissism
C. grasping
D. biting
E. cognition
F. sensorimotor phase
G. separation

H. object permanence
I. symbols
J. use of reflexes
K. primary circular reactions
L. secondary circular reactions
M. imitation
N. play

O. affect
P. secondary schemas
Q. reactive attachment disorder (RAD)
R. solitary play
S. Infant Temperament Questionnaire (ITQ)
T. spoiled child syndrome
U. graduated extinction

___L___ the third stage of the sensorimotor period; lasts until 8 months of age; reactions are repeated and prolonged for the response that results; grasping becomes pulling

x ___A___ the phase according to Erikson that the infant is concerned with

___C___ reaching out to others; initially reflexive; has powerful social meaning for the parents

___B___ total concern for oneself; at its height in the newborn

___E___ the ability to know; most commonly explained by Piaget's theory of development

___I___ mental representations; a major intellectual achievement of the sensorimotor period

___D___ occurs in the second stage of infancy; a more aggressive and active way that infants use to hold onto what is their own and how they attempt to more fully control their environment

___G___ a crucial event in the sensorimotor phase in which infants learn to detach themselves from other objects in the environment

x ___F___ the term used by Piaget to describe the period from birth to 24 months

___K___ marks the beginning of the replacement of reflexive behavior with voluntary acts in the sensorimotor period; occurs from 1 to 4 months; sucking and grasping become deliberate acts to elicit certain responses

x ___H___ a major accomplishment for the infant in the sensorimotor phase; the realization that objects that leave the visual field still exist

___J___ identifies the first stage of the sensorimotor period; the experience of perceiving patterns or ordering; provides a foundation of the subsequent stages

___P___ occurs during the fourth sensorimotor stage of Piaget; infants use previous behavior achievements as the foundation of adding new skills

___M___ infants in the second half of the first year develop this ability that requires the differentiation of selected acts from several events

___R___ the type of play that infants engage in; denotes one-sided play

___N___ infants take pleasure in performing acts after they have mastered them; consumes most of the infant's waking hours

_____T_____ excessive self centered and immature behavior resulting from the failure of parents to enforce consistent age appropriate limits

_____O_____ outward manifestation of emotion and feeling; seen as infants begin to develop a sense of permanency

_____Q_____ a psychologic and developmental problem that stems from maladaptive or absent attachment between the infant and parent

_____u_____ approach to dealing with night crying; to let the child cry for progressively longer times between brief parental interventions that consist only of reassurance

_____S_____ a screening tool that focuses on nine temperament variables

3. Terms—Child Care

A. in home child care   C. center based child care   E. sick child care
B. family daycare home   D. work based group child care

_____E_____ available for times when the child is ill and often located in community hospitals

_____C_____ usually refers to a licensed daycare facility that provides care for six or more children, for six or more hours in a 24 hour day

_____A_____ may consist of a full time baby sitter who lives in the home or comes to the home

_____D_____ an option that is becoming increasingly popular to provide quality and convenient child care to employees

_____B_____ typically provides child care and protection for up to five children for part of a 24 hour day

4. Terms—Promoting Optimum Health

A. fluoride
B. whole-cell pertussis vaccine
C. acellular pertussis vaccine
D. inactivated polio virus vaccine (IPV)

E. oral polio virus vaccine (OPV)
F. ComVax
G. Hib conjugate vaccines
H. varicella zoster immune globulin (VZIG)

I. Vaccine Adverse Event Reporting System (VAERS)
J. National Childhood Vaccine Injury Act (NCVIA) of 1986/ Vaccine Compensation Amendments of 1987

_____C_____ contains one or more immunogens derived from the Bordetella pertussis organism; highly purified; associated with fewer local and system reactions

_____E_____ currently licensed for use in the United States; carries a rare risk of vaccine associated polio paralysis (VAPP)

_____A_____ an essential mineral for building caries resistant teeth; needed beginning at 6 months of age if the infant does not receive water with an adequate fluoride content

_____D_____ currently licensed for use in the United States; administered at 2 and 4 months; when used exclusively eliminates the risk of vaccine associated polio paralysis (VAPP)

_____F_____ combines Hib and hepatitis B in one vaccine

X___H___ cell-free live-attenuated vaccine for varicella; recommended for healthy children 12–18 months of age

_____G_____ provide protection against serious infections caused by Haemophilus Influenza Type b; especially bacterial meningitis, epiglottitis, bacterial pneumonia, septic arthritis, and sepsis

_____J_____ a law to provide compensation for children who are inadvertently injured by vaccines and provide greater protection from liability for vaccine manufacturers

_____I_____ Any adverse reactions after administration of any vaccine are reported to this agency.

_____B_____ prepared from inactivated cells of Bordetella pertussis; contains multiple antigens

5. Terms—Injury Prevention

A.	clothing closures, food items, pacifiers	D.	baby powder
B.	syringe cap	E.	Latex balloons
C.	easy open tear down strips	F.	bed/crib safety hazards

G. plastic bags
H. cords
I. changing table

___G___ a cause of suffocation because it is light weight and can be easily become wrapped around the head of an active infant

___E___ the leading cause of pediatric choking deaths from children's products

___A___ common causes of aspiration in infants, because they are often small, cylindrical, and/or pliable

___C___ a safety device used to prevent tampering that can be aspirated and is very difficult to locate because it is clear

___B___ a potential aspiration hazard when using a syringe to accurately measure and dispense oral liquid medication to young children

___I___ a danger area for falling; usually high and narrow

___D___ a mixture of talc and other silicates that is hazardous if aspirated

___H___ should be less than 30 cm 12 inches to decrease the risk of strangulation

___F___ pose a number of hazards from suffocation to strangulation

6. If the infant weighs 7.5 kg at age 5 months, about how many kilograms was his/her probable birth weight?
   A. 7.0
   B. 4.0
   C. 3.3
   D. 15.4

   $$\frac{3.4}{2\overline{)7.5}}$$
   $$\frac{6}{15}$$

7. If the infant's head circumference is 46 cm at 6 months, how many centimeters would you expect his/her head circumference to be at 8 months?
   A. 46.5
   B. 47
   C. 47.5
   D. 49

   1 cm / 2 months

8. The infant's posterior fontanel usually closes by:
   A. 6 to 8 weeks.
   B. 3 to 6 months.
   C. 12 to 18 months.
   D. 9 to 12 months.

   2-3 months
   bute

9. Match the neurologic reflex with its expected behavioral response AND the age of its appearance in infancy (one selection from Column 2 and one selection from Column 3).

A. labyrinth righting

B. neck righting

C. body righting

D. Otolith righting

E. Landau

F. parachute

___F___ When infant is suspended in a horizontal prone position and suddenly thrust downward, hand and fingers extent forward as if to protect against falling.

___D___ When body of an erect infant is tilted, head is returned to upright erect position.

___C___ This is a modification of the neck righting reflex in which turning hips and shoulders to one side causes all other body parts to follow.

___E___ When infant is suspended in a horizontal prone position, the head is raised and legs and spine are extended

___B___ While infant is supine, head is turned to one side. Shoulder, trunk, and finally pelvis will turn toward that side.

___A___ Infant in prone or supine position is able to raise head.

___D___ 7 to 12 months; persists indefinitely

___C___ 6 months until 24 to 26 months

___A___ 2 months; strongest at 10 months

___E___ 6 to 8 months until 12 to 24 months

___F___ 7 to 9 months; persists indefinitely

___B___ 3 months until 24 to 36 months

10. Which one of the following statements is TRUE about the proportion of the chest at the end of the first year?
    A. The contour of the chest is more like a neonate's than an adult's.
    B. The anteroposterior diameter is larger than the lateral diameter.
    C. The chest is small in relation to the size of the heart.
    D. The chest circumference is about equal to the head circumference.

11. Which one of the following characteristics of vision is developed at the earliest age?
    A. Binocularity
    B. Stereopsis
    C. Corneal reflex
    D. Convergence

12. Which characteristic of the infant's respiratory system predisposes him/her to middle ear infection?
    A. A short, angled eustachian tube
    B. A short, straight eustachian tube
    C. The close proximity of the trachea to the bronchi
    D. The size of the lumen of the eustachian tube

13. The nurse can expect that an infant will respond to his/her own name by about:
    A. 3 months of age.
    B. 4 months of age.
    C. 6 months of age.
    D. 10 months of age.

14. Which one of the following hemopoietic changes would be considered abnormal in the first 5 months of life?
    A. Low iron levels
    B. Physiologic anemia
    C. Fetal hemoglobin present
    D. Low hemoglobin

15. All of the following digestive processes are deficient in an infant until about 3 months except:
    A. amylase.
    B. lipase.
    C. saliva.
    D. trypsin.

16. The _____liver_____ is the most immature of all of the gastrointestinal organs throughout infancy.

17. Which one of the following suckling actions is characteristic of the breast-fed infant?
    A. The tongue moves rhythmically forward to the gums and lips and backward.
    B. The infant controls the stream of milk by pushing his/her tongue against the nipple.
    C. The sucking action causes a rapid flow of milk.
    D. The tongue moves from the soft palate to the front of the mouth.

18. Which one of the following is a characteristic of the somatic swallow reflex?
    A. The mandible does not thrust forward.
    B. The tongue is more concave.
    C. It prepares the infant for solids.
    D. It develops before the age of 6 months.

19. After birth, normal levels of immunoglobulin in humans are:
    A. reached by 1 year of age.
    B. reached in early childhood.
    C. transferred from the mother.
    D. reached by 9 months of age.

20. Which of the following mechanisms decreases the newborn's thermoregulation efficiency?
    A. Shivering
    B. Limited adipose tissue
    C. Dilation of the capillaries
    D. Constriction of the capillaries

21. The infant is predisposed to a more rapid loss of total body fluid and dehydration because:
    A. of a high proportion of extracellular fluid.
    B. of a high proportion of intracellular fluid.
    C. total body water is at about 40%.
    D. extracellular fluid is 20% of the total.

22. Complete maturity of the kidney occurs:
    A. at birth.
    B. by 6 months.
    C. by 1 year.
    D. by 24 months.

23. Until the renal structures mature, the range of specific gravity for the infant ranges from 1._0_ _0_ _0_ to 1._0_ _1_ _0_ .

24. The expected immaturity of the infant's functioning endocrine system will be demonstrated in the infant's:
   A. growth patterns.
   B. thyroid levels.
   C. stress response.
   D. immunoglobulin levels.

25. Fine motor development is evaluated by observing the 10-month-old infant of the:
   A. ability to stack blocks.
   B. pincer grasp.
   C. righting reflexes
   D. tonic neck reflex.

26. Which one of the following characteristics disappears by about 3 months?
   A. Ability to stack blocks
   B. Pincer grasp
   C. Righting reflexes
   D. Tonic neck reflex

27. Which one of the following assessment findings would be considered MOST abnormal?
   A. The infant who displays head lag at 3 months of age
   B. The infant who starts to walk at 18 months of age
   C. The infant who begins to sit unsupported at 9 months of age
   D. The infant who begins to roll from front to back at 5 months of age

28. If parents are concerned about the fact that their 14-month-old infant is not walking, the nurse would particularly want to evaluate whether the infant:
   A. pulls up on the furniture.
   B. uses a pincer grasp.
   C. transfers objects.
   D. has developed object permanence.

29. Which one of the following factors determines the quality of the infant's formulation of trust?
   A. The quality of the interpersonal relationship
   B. The degree of mothering skill
   C. The quantity of the mother's breast milk
   D. The length of suckling time

30. Piaget's theory of cognitive development as it pertains to the infant involves which three crucial events?
   A. Trust, readjustment, and the regulation of frustration
   B. Separation, object permanence, and mental representation
   C. Imitation, personality development, and temperament
   D. Ordering, comfort, and satisfaction with his/her body

31. The development of the sexual identity begins:
    A. after the first year.
    B. during the phallic stage.
    C. at birth.
    D. at puberty.

32. Parenting:
    A. is an instinctual ability.
    B. is a learned acquired process.
    C. begins shortly after birth.
    D. shapes the infant's environment positively.

33. Separation anxiety and stranger fear normally begin to appear by:
    A. 4 weeks.
    B. 6 months.
    C. 14 months.
    D. 4 years.

34. A maltreated child who manifests behaviors such as limited eye contact and poor impulse control may be suffering from:
    A. separation anxiety.
    B. stranger fear.
    C. reactive attachment disorder.
    D. spoiled child syndrome.

35. Which one of the following play activities would be LEAST appropriate to suggest to parents for their 3-month-old infant?
    A. Playing music and singing along
    B. Using rattles
    C. Using an infant swing
    D. Placing toys a bit out of reach

36. Knowledge of the infant's temperament should NOT be used to help parents to:
    A. see an organized view of the child's behavior.
    B. choose childrearing techniques.
    C. identify a difficult child.
    D. see their child in a better perspective.

37. If parents are concerned about "spoiling" their child, the nurse should encourage them to respond to the newborn's crying episodes with:
    A. a delayed response of holding the infant.
    B. a prompt response of holding the infant.
    C. letting the infant cry a little.
    D. maintaining a feeding schedule.

38. Which one of the following data could be considered evidence that the child is being spoiled by the parents?
    A. The child who has a difficult temperament and a short attention span
    B. The toddler who has a temper tantrum
    C. The infant who has colic
    D. The child who always cries if he/she doesn't get his/her way

39. Limit setting and discipline should begin in:
    A. middle childhood or adolescence.
    B. infancy with voice tone and eye contact.
    C. early childhood with voice tone and eye contact.
    D. infancy with time out in a chair for misbehavior.

40. In guiding parents who are choosing a day care center, the nurse should stress that state licensure represents a program that maintains:
    A. optimal care.
    B. health features.
    C. minimum requirements.
    D. safety features.

41. A 12-month-old infant would be likely to have:
    A. 2 teeth.
    B. 4 teeth.
    C. 6 teeth.
    D. 12 teeth.

42. Which one of the following reasons to put shoes on an infant is CORRECT?
    A. To protect foot from injury
    B. To support foot muscles
    C. To support the ankle
    D. To protect the arch

43. When the infant reaches 6 months of age, the breast-feeding mother should supplement the breast milk with:
    A. formula.
    B. nothing.
    C. water.
    D. iron.

44. The greatest threat to successful breast-feeding for the employed mother is:
    A. lack of feeding options.
    B. danger of bacterial contamination.
    C. fatigue.
    D. inefficient breast pumping.

45. Which one of the following formula feeding patterns would warrant further evaluation for a 1-year-old infant?
    A. Four feedings of 5 oz. each
    B. Five feedings of 8 oz. each
    C. Three feedings of 6 oz. each
    D. Four feedings of 6 oz. each

46. The primary reason for introducing solid food to infants is to:
    A. supply nutrients not found in formula or breast milk.
    B. replace nutrients found in breast milk.
    C. socialize them to the culturally acceptable food.
    D. promote the disappearance of the extrusion reflex.

47. If sweetening of the infant's home-prepared foods is performed, the risk of botulism can be avoided by:
    A. honey.
    B. corn syrup.
    C. refined sugar.
    D. none of the above.

48. Studies have shown that excessive fruit juice consumption increases the likelihood of:
    A. short stature.
    B. scurvy.
    C. rickets.
    D. nursing caries.

49. When introducing new food, the parents should NOT:
    A. decrease the quantity of the infant's milk.
    B. mix food with formula to feed through a nipple.
    C. introduce new foods in small amounts.
    D. offer the new food by itself at first.

50. Which one of the following techniques is recommended to assist in weaning the infant?
    A. Eliminate the night time feeding first.
    B. Always wean to a bottle first.
    C. Always wean directly to a cup.
    D. Gradually replace one bottle or breast-feeding at a time.

51. Describe the considerations that should be included in a culturally sensitive approach to weaning.

    _____

    _____

52. Cosleeping with the parents is commonly associated with:
    A. Sudden Infant Death Syndrome.
    B. colic.
    C. single parenting.
    D. breast-fed infants.

53. Match the sleep disturbance with the technique for management.

    A. nighttime feeding   _C_ Check at progressively longer intervals each night.
    B. developmental night   _E_ Keep a night light on.
       crying   _B_ Reassure parents that this is a temporary phase.
    C. trained night crying   _D_ Establish a consistent before-bedtime routine.
    D. refusal to go to sleep   _A_ Put infant to bed awake.
    E. nighttime fear

54. Which one of the following side effects of immunization would MOST likely be considered severe?
   A. Febrile episode
   B. Malaise
   C. Encephalitis
   D. Behavioral changes

55. The nurse should withhold immunization with the oral polio vaccine if which one of the following situations exists?
   A. The child had a temperature of 104° after the last immunization.
   B. The child has a cold with a temperature of 100°.
   C. The child has had a kidney transplant.
   D. The child had a seizure the day after the last immunization.

56. Which one of the following techniques has been demonstrated by research to minimize local reactions when administering immunizations to infants?
   A. Select a 1-inch needle to deposit vaccine deep into the thigh muscle mass.
   B. Use an air bubble to clear the needle after the injection.
   C. Change the needle in the syringe after drawing up the vaccine.
   D. Apply a topical anaesthetic to the site for a minimum of one hour.

57. To prevent aspiration in the infant, the nurse should avoid using:
   A. baby powder made from cornstarch.
   B. pacifiers made from a padded nipple.
   C. syringes to dispense oral medication.
   D. pacifiers with one-piece construction.

58. Which one of the following hazards causes the majority of deaths in young children?
   A. Plastic garment bags
   B. Ill-fitting crib slats
   C. Latex balloons
   D. Ill-fitting crib mattresses

59. Which one of the following situations involving cords would be considered LEAST hazardous?
   A. A bib that is not removed at bedtime
   B. A pacifier that is hung around the infant's neck with a 10 inch string
   C. A play telephone with a 10-inch cord
   D. A toy tied to the playpen with a 15-inch ribbon

60. The BEST place in the car for the infant car restraint is in the:
   A. back seat facing back.
   B. back seat facing front.
   C. passenger seat with an air bag, facing front.
   D. passenger seat without an air bag, facing back.

61. To prevent falls, the parents should take any of the following precautions EXCEPT:
   A. never leave the child on a changing table unattended.
   B. keep necessary articles within easy reach.
   C. change the infant's diaper on the floor.
   D. use a walker to strengthen walking muscles.

62. One way to distract an infant while changing his/her diaper that is NOT recommended is to:
   A. give the infant the bottle of talc baby powder to hold.
   B. sing and play with the infant.
   C. play the same game each time.
   D. none of the above ideas are recommended.

Critical Thinking • Case Study

Jennifer Klein, a 6-month-old infant, is admitted to the Pediatric Unit with bronchiolitis. Both of her parents work and the baby attends day care. Jennifer is the first child, and the parents seem anxious about the admission as well as her care at home and her normal development. It is clear that the parents need information about general health promotion for their infant.

63. Which areas should be assessed to determine the status of the parents' current health promotion practices? (Check all that apply.)

   _____ respiratory status (lung sounds)

   ___✓___ nutrition

   _____ fever patterns

   ___✓___ sleep and activity

   ___✓___ number and condition of teeth

   _____ fluid and hydration status

   _____ condition of the mucous membranes of the mouth

   ___✓___ immunization status

   ___✓___ safety precautions used in the home

64. Which one of the following nursing diagnoses would be used MOST often for health promotion related to development in an infant Jennifer's age?
   A. Activity intolerance
   B. Ineffective thermoregulation
   C. High risk for injury
   D. Altered parenting

65. Which one of the following strategies is used MOST often to help new parents like Jennifer's adjust to the parenting role?
   A. Parenting classes
   B. Anticipatory guidance
   C. First aid courses
   D. Cardiopulmonary resuscitation courses

66. By the time Jennifer is ready for discharge, the nurse evaluates that her parents have achieved improved parenting skills. Which one of the following methods would BEST measure the plan's success?
   A. Jennifer is afebrile.
   B. Reports from the other staff are positive.
   C. Verbalizations from the parents indicate that they understand.
   D. A home visit demonstrates that positive changes have occurred.

CHAPTER 13
Health Problems During Infancy

1. Nutritional Disturbances and Feeding Difficulties

A. coenzymes
B. apoenenzyme
C. holoenzyme
D. microminerals
E. lacto-ovovegetarians
F. vegans
G. Zen macrobiotics
H. Recommended Dietary Allowances (RDAs)
I. Dietary Reference Intake (DRIs)

J. Dietary Guidelines for Americans
K. Food Guide Pyramid
L. diarrhea
M. aflatoxin
N. food allergy
O. food intolerance
P. allergens
Q. sensitization

R. atopy
S. lactase
T. congenital lactose intolerance
U. late onset lactose intolerance
V. La Leche League
W. regurgitation
X. spitting up
Y. Feeding Checklist

___G___ more restrictive than pure vegetarians in that cereals, especially brown rice, are the mainstay of the diet

___C___ forms when vitamin coenzymes enter the body and combine with a protein apoenzyme

___F___ pure vegetarians who eliminate any food of animal origin, including milk and eggs

___A___ substances that regulate specific metabolic activity; vitamins act in this way

___D___ trace elements; have daily requirements of less than 100 mg

___B___ a protein enzyme that has been synthesized with the cell

___K___ dietary advice for the public that replaces the basic four food groups; used to convey nutrition information to the public and applies to children as young as 2 years of age

___M___ a mycotoxin mold that has been implicated in the etiology of kwashiorkor; present in large numbers in the intestines of children with the disease

___H___ The standard developed by the National Academy of Sciences, Food and Nutrition Board; the most widely used standard that identifies areas of nutritional concern.

___E___ exclude meat from their diet but eat milk and eggs and sometimes fish

___I___ guidelines for nutritional intake that encompass the RDAs yet extend their scope to include additional parameters related to nutritional intake; include estimated average nutrient requirements for age and gender categories, tolerable upper-limit nutrient intakes that are associated with a low risk of adverse effects and the standard RDAs

___L___ a major factor in malnutrition in many developing and underdeveloped nations

___J___ dietary advice for the public that encourages eating a variety of foods, maintaining ideal body weight, consuming adequate starch and fiber and limiting intake of fat, cholesterol, sugar, salt, and alcohol

___R___ allergy with a hereditary tendency

___N___ hypersensitivity; refers to those reactions to food that involve immunologic mechanisms, usually immunoglobulin E

___V___ an agency with local groups to provide reassurance and support for the breast feeding mother

___O___ refers to those reactions to food that involve known or unknown nonimmunologic mechanisms; such as lactose intolerance

___S___ an enzyme that is needed for the digestion of lactose

___W___ return of undigested food from the stomach, usually accompanied by burping

___P___ usually proteins that are capable of inducing IgE antibody formation

___X___ dribbling of unswallowed formula from the infant's mouth immediately after a feeding

___Q___ the initial exposure of an individual to an allergen resulting in an immune response; subsequent exposure than induces a much stronger response that is clinically apparent

___T___ a rare disorder that appears soon whether the infant receives infant formula or human milk

___Y___ a 25 item observational scale developed specifically for the purpose of observing mother infant dyads with nonorganic failure to thrive

___U___ manifested later in life; more common in Orientals, Southern Europeans, Arabs, Jews and Blacks. Manifested by diarrhea, abdominal pain, distention and flatus shortly after ingesting mill products

2. Disorders

A.   example/demonstration   C.   positional plagiocephaly E.   SHARE
B.   apparent life-   D.   Autism Society of
     threatening events   America
     (ALTEs)

___C___ flattening of the skull that occurs when the infant's head position is not varied

___E___ a siblings' group for the support of people with autism

___A___ teaching technique to use with parents of infants with nonorganic failure to thrive who are learning infant care

___D___ provides information about education treatment programs and techniques and facilities related to autism

___B___ associated with only a minority of Sudden Infant Death Syndrome victims; previously referred to inaccurately as "near miss SIDS"; includes a combination of apnea, color change and change in muscle tone that is frightening to the observer

3. In the United States, which of the following populations is at risk for developing a vitamin D deficiency?
   A. Lower socioeconomic groups
   B. Those that consume raw cow's milk
   C. Children with measles
   D. Children with rheumatoid arthritis

4. The most common vegetable consumed by children and adolescents is
   ____french fries_____.

5. The children at risk for vitamin C deficiency are those:
   A. with low fruit intake.
   B. living below the poverty level.
   C. receiving high doses of salicylates.
   D. receiving inadequate calcium.

6. The greatest concern with minerals is:
   A. deficiency.
   B. excess causing toxicity.
   C. nervous system disturbances from excess.
   D. hemochromatosis.

7. Match the type of vegetarianism with its description.

A. Lacto-ovovegeterians

B. Lactovegetarians

C. Pure vegetarians (vegans)

D. Zen macrobiotics

___C___ This group eliminates any food of animal origin including milk and eggs.

___D___ This group is most restrictive of all. Brown rice is the mainstay of the diet.

___A___ This group excludes meat from their diet but eats milk, eggs, and sometimes fish.

___B___ This group excludes meat and eggs, but drinks milk.

8. On what nutrient should the nutritional assessment focus for any family who is vegetarian?

_____protein_____

9. To increase iron absorption the nurse should recommend that the parents mix the iron with:
A. formula.
B. cereal.
C. sweet potatoes.
D. apple juice.

10. Which one of the following is the source that applies to children that should be used to convey nutrition information to the public?
A. Recommended Dietary Allowances (RDAs)
B. The basic four food groups
C. Food Guide Pyramid
D. Dietary Guidelines for Americans

11. Which of the following combinations of foods would ensure the most complete protein for a strictly vegetarian family if eaten together at the same meal?
A. Milk and chicken
B. Sunflower seeds and rice
C. Rice and red beans
D. Eggs and cheese

12. In the United States, protein and energy malnutrition (PEM) occurs where:
A. the food supply is inadequate.
B. the food supply may be adequate.
C. the adults eat first, leaving insufficient food.
D. the diet consists mainly of starch grains.

13. Kwashiorkor occurs in populations where:
A. the food supply is inadequate.
B. the food supply is adequate for protein.
C. the adults eat first, leaving insufficient food.
D. the diet consists mainly of starch grains.

14. Childhood nutritional marasmus usually results in populations where:
A. the food supply is inadequate.
B. the food supply is adequate for protein.
C. the adults eat first, leaving insufficient food.
D. the diet consists mainly of starch grains.

15. Which one of the following therapeutic management treatments would be considered INAPPROPRIATE for PEM, kwashiorkor or marasmus?
    A. Provide high-protein, high-carbohydrate diet.
    B. Replace fluids and electrolytes.
    C. Provide a high fiber diet, high fat diet.
    D. Provide a structured play program.

16. The rate for obesity in children according to the Nutritional Health and Nutritious Examination Survey had _____↑_____ by ____21____%.

17. Obesity in adults has been shown to be linked to:
    A. adolescent obesity.
    B. infant obesity.
    C. breast feeding.
    D. bottle feeding.

18. The primary goal in regard to obesity in infants is:
    A. safe weight loss.
    B. prevention.
    C. decrease the fat content in the milk.
    D. decrease the total quantity of food.

19. Recently there has been additional evidence that poor nutrition in the United States may be the result of:
    A. availability of food.
    B. nutritional habits.
    C. access to food markets.
    D. farming techniques.

20. If the infant seems unsatisfied when solid foods are added, the parents should NOT:
    A. substitute water for a bottle of formula.
    B. add 4 to 5 ounces of fruit juice to each meal.
    C. use a nipple with a smaller hole.
    D. decrease the quantity of milk at each meal.

21. Which one of the following foods is NOT generally considered allergenic?
    A. Orange juice
    B. Eggs
    C. Bread
    D. Rice

22. Which one of the following clinical manifestations may indicate that an infant has an allergy to cow's milk?
    A. Sleeplessness
    B. Colic
    C. Vomiting and diarrhea
    D. All of the above

23. Which one of the following diagnostic strategies is the MOST definitive for identifying a milk allergy?
   A. Stool analysis for blood
   B. Serum IgE levels
   C. A challenge of milk after elimination
   D. Skin testing

24. To avoid atopy, parents should consider:
   A. soy formula.
   B. breast feeding.
   C. starting solid foods at 4 months.
   D. goat's milk.

25. Treatment of cow's milk allergy in infants involves changing the formula to:
   A. soy-based formula.
   B. goat's milk.
   C. casein/whey hydrolysate milk.
   D. milk pretreated with microbial derived lactase.

26. Congenital lactose intolerance refers to:
   A. a rare form of lactose intolerance.
   B. the form of lactose intolerance associated with giardiasis.
   C. an intolerance that is manifested later in life.
   D. all of the above.

27. Indicate whether statement is TRUE or FALSE.

   ___F___ Breast milk lacks fat for adequate growth.

   ___F___ Standard growth charts reflect normal growth patterns of the breast-fed infant.

   ___F___ Breast-fed infants grow slower in the first few months of life as a result of protein deficiency.

   ___F___ Head circumference of breast-fed infants is greater than the head circumference of formula-fed infants.

   ___T___ Breast-fed infants demonstrate self-regulation in regard to energy intake.

   ___F___ Breast-fed infants have more episodes of otitis media and diarrhea than bottle fed infants.

   ___F___ Breast-fed infants are usually growth deficient during the first year of life.

28. Match the common breast-feeding problem with the strategy for it.

   A. engorgement   ___A___ Prevent this problem with frequent feedings.
   B. painful nipples   ___B___ Have infant nurse on the unaffected side first.
   C. let down reflex   ___C___ May need to use oxytocin nasal spray.
   D. inadequate milk supply ___D___ Avoid use of supplemental feedings.
   E. plugged ducts   ___E___ Position infant's chin toward affected area.
   F. mastitis   ___F___ May need antibiotics to treat this problem.

29. If a sensitivity to cow's milk is suspected as the cause of an infant's colic the parents should:
    A. try substituting casein hydrolysate formula.
    B. try substituting soy formula.
    C. be reassured that the symptoms will disappear spontaneously at about 3 months of age.
    D. be assessed for areas of improper feeding techniques.

30. The etiology for colic that is commonly accepted is:
    A. carbohydrate malabsorption.
    B. excessive air swallowing.
    C. colonic fermentation.
    D. infant temperament.

31. Which of the following phrases BEST defines rumination?
    A. It is the involuntary return of undigested food from the stomach, usually accompanied by burping.
    B. It is the dribbling of unswallowed formula from the infant's mouth immediately after a feeding.
    C. It is the active, voluntary return of swallowed food into the mouth.
    D. It is the same as vomiting.

32. Match the category of failure to thrive and the description

    A. Organic failure to thrive (OFTT)   __B__ has a definable cause that is unrelated to any physiologic disease process, such as disturbance in maternal-child attachment

    B. Nonorganic failure to thrive (NFTT)   __A__ result of a physical cause, such as a congenital heart defect

    C. idiopathic failure to thrive   __C__ unexplained by the usual organic and environmental etiologies and may be classified as NFTT

33. List five factors other than parent-child interaction that can lead to inadequate feeding of the infant.

    _____

    _____

    _____

    _____

    _____

34. A term that health care workers may use to avoid the social stigma of nonorganic failure to thrive is ___growth delay / failure___ .

35. If failure to thrive has been a long standing problem, the infant will have evidence of:
    A. weight and height depression.
    B. weight depression only.
    C. height depression only.
    D. neither height nor weight depression.

36. Which one of the following characteristics in an infant with failure to thrive is MOST significant?
    A. Difficult feeding pattern with vomiting and aversion behavior
    B. Crying, excessive irritability and sleep pattern disturbances
    C. Lack of fit between the child's temperament and that of the parents
    D. Irregularity in activities of daily living and difficult temperament pattern

37. Which one of the following strategies might be recommended for an infant with failure to thrive to increase caloric intake?
    A. Utilize developmental stimulation by a specialist during feedings.
    B. Avoid solids until after the bottle is well accepted.
    C. Be persistent through 10 to 15 minutes of food refusal.
    D. Vary the schedule for routine activities on a daily basis.

38. The incidence of diaper dermatitis is generally reported as greater in bottle-fed infants than in breast-fed infants, because in breast-fed infants there is a lower:
    A. ammonia content in the urine.
    B. pH content of the feces.
    C. microbial content of the feces.
    D. number of stools per day.

39. Which one of the following strategies should the nurse recommend to the parents of an infant with diaper dermatitis?
    A. Apply fluorinated hydrocortisone sparingly.
    B. Avoid cornstarch because it promotes yeast growth.
    C. Use a hand held dryer on the open lesions.
    D. Use diapers with super absorbent gel.

40. Which one of the following disorders is NOT a manifestation of seborrhagic dermatitis?
    A. Eczema
    B. Cradle cap
    C. Blepharitis
    D. Otitis externa

41. Which one of the following recommendations for the care of atopic dermatitis is controversial?
    A. Use the wet method of skin care.
    B. Use the dry method of skin care.
    C. Limit the infant's exposure to allergens.
    D. Avoid exposure of the infant to skin irritants.

42. Identify the following statements as either TRUE or FALSE.
    ___F___ The incidence of Sudden Infant Death Syndrome (SIDS) is associated with diphtheria, tetanus and pertussis vaccines.
    ___T___ Maternal smoking during and after pregnancy has been implicated as a contributor to SIDS.
    ___F___ Parents should be advised to position their infants on their abdomen to prevent SIDS.
    ___F___ The nurse should encourage the parents to sleep in the same bed as the infant who is being monitored for apnea of infancy in order to detect subtle clinical changes.
    ___T___ The psychogenic theory of autism which is unsupported by current findings depicts the parents of the autistic child as detached individuals.

Six-month-old Jason Fitch has come to the office today for his routine immunizations. His mother says she thinks everything is just fine, except that Jason seems to have a lot of food intolerances.

The nurse continues the assessment and finds that Jason is eating many of the food items the rest of the family eats including milk products in very small amounts. There is no particular pattern to the way the new foods are being introduced.

Jason exhibits a variety of symptoms related to skin irritations. He is developing rashes around his mouth, rectum and elsewhere on his body when he eats certain foods.

43. Based on the prevalence of the common health problems of infancy what areas should the nurse include in an initial assessment of a 6 month old?
    A. Nutrition
    B. Temperament
    C. Sleep patterns
    D. All of the above

44. Based on the data from the assessment interview, which one of the following goals is BEST for the nurse to establish?
    A. To prevent outbreaks of food allergy
    B. To prevent death from anaphylaxis
    C. To prevent genetic transmission
    D. All of the above

45. Which one of the following recommendations would be MOST appropriate for Jason's mother?
    A. Reconsider breast feeding.
    B. Eliminate cow's milk.
    C. Add only one new food at each 5 day interval.
    D. Eliminate solids until 9 months of age.

46. At an earlier visit, the nurse had determined that there was altered parenting related to lack of knowledge in Jason's family. Which one of the following outcome criteria would help the nurse to evaluate the mother's ability provide a constructive environment for Jason? Jason's mother is able to:
    A. identify eating patterns that contribute to symptoms.
    B. share her feelings regarding her parenting skills.
    C. practice appropriate precautions to prevent infection.
    D. identify the rationale for prevention of the skin rashes.

CHAPTER 14
Health Promotion of the Toddler and Family

1. Promoting Optimum Growth and Development

A.	terrible twos	K.	superego	U.	operations
B.	weight	L.	tertiary circular reactions	V.	punishment and obedience orientation
C.	height				
D.	head circumference	M.	new means through mental combinations	W.	separation
E.	chest circumference			X.	individuation
F.	autonomy vs. doubt and shame	N.	domestic mimicry	Y.	parallel play
		O.	egocentrism	Z.	Toddler Temperament Scale/ TBAQ
G.	negativism	P.	preoperational phase		
H.	ritualism	Q.	egocentric speech	AA.	sibling rivalry
I.	ego	R.	collective monologue	BB.	regression
J.	id	S.	socialized speech	CC.	fears
		T.	preoperational thinking		

__N__ imitation of household activity

__C__ The average at 2 years of age is 86.6 cm (34 inches).

__A__ term often used to describe the toddler years; period from 12 to 36 months of age

__E__ increases in size during the toddler years; shape also changes

__G__ the persistent negative response to requests; characteristic of the toddler's behavior

__B__ The average at 2 years of age is 12 kg (27 pounds).

__F__ the developmental task of the toddler years

__H__ the toddler's need to maintain sameness and reliability; provides a sense of comfort

__J__ the impulsive part of the psyche

__L__ the fifth stage of the senorimotor phase of development where the child uses active experimentation to achieve previously unattainable goals; object permanence is one of the most dramatic achievements of this stage

__I__ may be thought of as reason or common sense during the toddler phase of psychosocial development

__K__ the conscience

__D__ Growth slows somewhat at the end of infancy; total increase during the second year is 2.5 cm.

__M__ the final sensorimotor stage that occurs during ages 19 to 24 months

__O__ the ability to envision situations from perspectives other than one's own

__Q__ consists of repeating words and sounds for the pleasure of hearing oneself and is not intended to communicate

__U__ the ability to manipulate objects in relation to each other in a logical fashion

__P__ spans ages 2 to 7 years; bridges the self-satisfying behavior of infancy and social behavior of latency; uses egocentric language dependent of perception

__X__ those achievements that mark children's assumption of their individual characteristics in the environment

__W__ the child's emergence from a symbiotic fusion with the mother

__Y__ playing alongside, not with, other children

_R___ egocentric speech that reflects the child's lingering self centeredness

_AA__ the natural jealousy and resentment of children to a new child in the family

_CC__ common during the toddler stage, includes problems with sleep, animals, engines, strangers and separation

_T___ implies that children think primarily based on their own perception of an event; problem solving is based on what they see or hear directly, rather than on what they recall about objects and events

_BB__ a retreat from a present pattern of functioning to past levels of behavior; usually occurs in instances of stress, when the toddler attempts to cope by reverting to patterns of behavior that were successful in earlier stages of development; common in toddlers

_S___ one of the two types of speech used by children in the toddler years; used for communication; egocentric in that children communicate about themselves to others

_Z___ tools that assist in identifying temperamental characteristics; reliable instruments used to assess toddler temperament and other behaviors

_V___ the most basic level of moral judgment; whether an action is good or bad depends on whether it results in reward or punishment

2. Promoting Optimum Health

A. pedodontist
B. plaque
C. dental caries
D. periodontal disease
E. scrub method
F. gingivitis
G. swish and sallow method
H. fluorosis
I. nursing caries
J. convertible restraint
K. five-point harness
L. padded shield
M. T-shield
N. boosters
O. low shield model
P. belt positioning model

_P___ a booster that uses a lap/shoulder belt; the preferred type of booster

_M___ a harness system that consists of retracting shoulder straps attached to a flat chest shield with a rigid stalk that attaches to a restraint between the legs

_O___ a booster that primarily uses a lap belt

_N___ depend on the vehicle belts to hold the child in place

_I___ nursing bottle caries; bottle mouth caries; occurs when the child is placed in the crib or bed with a bottle of milk, juice, soda pop, or sweetened water at nap or bedtime or uses the bottle as a pacifier while awake

_K___ a harness system that consists of a strap over each shoulder, one on each side of the pelvis and one between the legs

_G___ may be used to clean teeth when brushing is impractical

_J___ a car seat that is suitable for infants in the rearward-facing position and for toddlers in the forward-facing position

_H___ a condition characterized by an increase in the degree and extent of the enamel's porosity as a result of excessive fluoride ingestion by young children

_E___ a brushing technique that is suitable for cleaning primary teeth where the tips of the bristles are place firmly at a 45-degree angle against the teeth and gums and are moved back and forth in a vibratory motion

_L___ a harness system that uses shoulder straps attached to a shield that is held in place by a crotch strap

_C___ decay

_F___ inflammation of the gums

_D___ gum disease

_A___ a pediatric dentist; toddlers should have the first appointment soon after the first teeth erupt usually around 1 year of age

_B___ soft bacterial deposits that adhere to the teeth and cause decay

3. If the chest circumference of a toddler is 50 cm, how many cm would you expect the head circumference to be?
   A. 25
   B. 35
   C. 50
   D. 60

4. Which one of the following factors is MOST important in predisposing toddlers to frequent infections?
   A. Short straight internal ear canal and large lymph tissue
   B. Pulse and respiratory rate slower and blood pressure increases
   C. Abdominal respirations
   D. Less efficient defense mechanisms

5. One of the MOST important digestive system changes that is completed during the toddler period is the:
   A. increased acidity of the gastric contents.
   B. voluntary control of the sphincters.
   C. protective function of the gastric contents.
   D. increased capacity of the stomach.

6. Which one of the following statements is MOST characteristic of the behaviors of a 24-month-old?
   A. Motor skills are fully developed, but occur in isolation from the environment.
   B. The toddler walks alone, but falls easily.
   C. The toddler's activities begin to produce purposeful results.
   D. The toddler is able to grasp small objects, but cannot release them at will.

7. Using Erikson's theory as a foundation, the primary developmental task of the toddler period is to:
   A. satisfy the need for basic trust.
   B. achieve a sense of accomplishment.
   C. learn to give up dependence for independence.
   D. acquire language or mental symbolism.

8. Piaget's theory of cognitive development depicts the toddler as a child who:
   A. continuously explores the same object each time it appears in a new place.
   B. is able to transfer information from one situation to another.
   C. has a persistent negative response to any request.
   D. has a rudimentary beginning of a superego.

9. The principle characteristics of Piaget's preoperational phase are:
   1. dependence on perception in problem solving.
   2. egocentric use of language.
   3. the ability to manipulate objects in relation to each other in a logical way.
   4. the ability to problem solve based on what they recall about objects and events.

   A. 1, 2, 3
   B. 1 and 2
   C. 2 and 3
   D. 2, 3, and 4

10. Match the characteristic of preoperational thought with its description.

A. egocentrism   D. centration   G. magical thinking
B. transductive reasoning   E. animism   H. inability to conserve
C. global organization   F. irreversibility

   D   focusing on one aspect rather than considering all possible alternatives

   A   inability to envision situations from perspectives other than one's own

   F   inability to undo or reverse the actions initiated physically

   E   attributing lifelike qualities to inanimate objects

   B   thinking from the particular to the particular

   H   not able to understand the idea that a mass can be changed in size shape, volume, or length without losing or adding to the original mass

   G   believing that thoughts are all powerful and can cause events

   C   changing any one part of the whole changes the entire whole

11. According to Kohlberg, the BEST way to discipline children is to:
    A. use a punishment and obedience orientation.
    B. withhold privileges.
    C. use power to control behavior.
    D. give explanations and help the child to change.

12. By the age of 2, the toddler generally:
    A. has clear body boundaries.
    B. participates willingly in most procedures.
    C. recognizes sexual differences.
    D. is unable to learn correct terms for body parts.

13. Which of the following skills is NOT necessary for the toddler to acquire before separation and individuation can be achieved?
    A. Object permanence
    B. Lack of anxiety during separations from parents
    C. Delayed gratification
    D. Ability to tolerate a moderate amount of frustration

14. The usual number of words acquired by the age of 2 years is about:
    A. 50
    B. 100
    C. 300
    D. 500

15. The two-year-old child living in a bilingual environment will generally have:
    A. advanced speaking ability without adequate comprehension.
    B. advanced speaking ability along with advanced comprehension.
    C. delayed speaking ability with adequate comprehension.
    D. delayed speaking without adequate comprehension.

16. Which one of the following types of play decreases in frequency as the child moves through the toddler period?
    (A.) Solitary play
    B. Imitative play
    C. Tactile play
    D. Parallel play

17. List at least 5 characteristics of an 18 to 24-month-old child that would indicate readiness for toilet training.

    _____

    _____

    _____

    _____

    _____

18. Which one of the following techniques would be BEST to use when toilet training a toddler?
    (A.) Limit sessions to 5 or 10 minutes of practice
    B. Remove child from the bathroom to flush the toilet
    C. Assure the toddler's privacy during the sessions
    D. Place potty chair near a television to help distract the child during the sessions

19. Which one of the following statements is FALSE in regard to toilet training?
    (A.) Bowel training is usually accomplished after bladder training.
    B. Night time bladder training is usually accomplished after bowel training.
    C. The toddler who is impatient with soiled diapers is demonstrating readiness for toilet training.
    D. Fewer wet diapers signals that the toddler is physically ready for toilet training.

20. Which one of the following strategies is appropriate for parents to use to prepare a toddler for the birth of a sibling?
    A. Explain the upcoming birth as early in the pregnancy as possible.
    B. Move the toddler to his/her own new room.
    (C.) Provide a doll for the toddler to imitate parenting.
    D. Tell the toddler that a new playmate will come home soon.

21. The BEST approach for extinguishing a toddler's attention-seeking behavior of a tantrum with head banging is to:
    A. ignore the behavior.
    B. provide time out.
    C. offer a toy to calm the child.
    (D.) protect the child from injury.

22. Which one of the following techniques is BEST to deal with the negativism of the toddler?
    A. Quietly and calmly ask the child to comply.
    B. Provide few or no choices for the child.
    (C.) Challenge the child with a game.
    D. Remain serious and intent.

23. Which of the following statements about stress in toddlers is TRUE?
    A. Toddlers are rarely exposed to stress or the results of stress.
    B. Any stress is destructive because toddlers have a limited ability to cope.
    C. Most children are exposed to a stress free environment.
    D. Small amounts of stress help toddlers develop effective coping skills.

24. List 3 signs of increased stress in toddlers.

    _____thumb sucking_____

    _____pulling hair_____

    _____biting_____

25. Regression in toddlers occurs when there is:
    A. stress.
    B. a threat to their autonomy.
    C. a need to revert to dependency.
    D. all the above.

26. Which of the following statements is TRUE in regard to nutritional changes from the infant to the toddler years?
    A. Caloric requirements increase from 102 kcal/kg to 108 kcal/kg.
    B. Caloric requirements decrease from 108 kcal/kg to 102 kcal/kg.
    C. Protein requirements decrease from 2.2 kcal/kg to 1.5 kcal/kg.
    D. Protein requirements increase from 1.2 kcal/kg to 2.2 kcal/kg.

27. Reduced fluid requirement in toddlers represents a decrease in total body fluid with:
    A. an increase in intracellular fluid.
    B. an increase in extracellular fluid.
    C. a decrease in intracellular fluid.
    D. a decrease in extracellular fluid.

28. Which one of the following nutritional requirements increases during the toddler years?
    A. Calories
    B. Proteins
    C. Minerals
    D. Fluids

29. Physiologic anorexia in toddlers is characterized by:
    A. strong taste preferences.
    B. extreme changes in appetite from day to day.
    C. heightened awareness of social aspects of meals.
    D. all of the above.

30. Healthy ways of serving food to toddlers include:
    A. establishing a pattern of sitting at a table for meals.
    B. permitting nutritious nibbling in lieu of meals.
    C. discouraging between meal snacking.
    D. all of the above.

31. Developmentally, most children at 12 months:
    A. use a spoon adeptly.
    B. relinquish the bottle voluntarily.
    C. eat the same food as the rest of the family.
    D. reject all solid food in preference for the bottle.

32. The BEST approach to use for the toddler who prefers the bottle to all solid food is to:
    A. require the toddler to eat something.
    B. dilute the milk with water.
    C. withhold all food and water until the child takes solids.
    D. puree the solids and feed them through the bottle.

33. For a toddler with sleep problems, the nurse should suggest:
    A. using a transitional object.
    B. varying the bedtime ritual.
    C. restricting stimulating activities.
    D. all of the above.

34. Which one of the following strategies is INAPPROPRIATE for the parent to use to help the toddler adjust to the initial dental visit?
    A. Explain to the child that a check up won't hurt.
    B. Have the child observe his/her brother's examination.
    C. Have the child perform a check up on a doll.
    D. Ask the dentist to reserve a thorough exam for the another visit.

35. The MOST effective way to clean a toddler's teeth is:
    A. for the child to brush regularly with a toothpaste of his/her choice.
    B. for the parent to stabilize the chin with one hand and brush with the other.
    C. for the parent to brush the mandibular occlusive surfaces leaving the rest for the child.
    D. for the child to brush all except the mandibular occlusive surfaces.

36. Flossing is necessary:
    A. only after the permanent teeth erupt.
    B. to prevent fluorosis.
    C. for the toddler to learn.
    D. even if teeth are widely spaced.

37. Adequate fluoride ingestion:
    A. prevents gingivitis.
    B. prevents fluorosis.
    C. alters the anatomy of the tooth.
    D. reduces the amount of plaque.

38. Recommendations for toddlers to meet fluoride requirements include all of the following EXCEPT:
    A. supervise the use of toothpaste.
    B. prepare soy formula with fluoridated water.
    C. store fluoride products out of reach.
    D. administer fluoride supplements if water fluoride content is low.

39. One example of a treat that may actually damage the teeth is:
    A. aged cheese.
    B. celery sticks.
    C. sugarless gum.
    D. a handful of raisins.

40. Which of the following practices contributes to nursing bottle caries?
    A. Using a pacifier
    B. Feeding the last bottle before bedtime
    C. Long frequent nocturnal breast feeding
    D. All of the above

41. Match the major developmental achievement of the young child with its associated safety precaution that could be used to prevent injury.

    A. depth perception   _D_ Do not allow child to play near curb or parked cars.
        undefined   _E_ Choose large toys without sharp edges.
    B. able to open most   _C_ Supervise closely at all times.
        containers   _F_ Do not allow lollipop or similar objects when
    C. unaware of most dangers   walking or running.
    D. walks, runs, and moves   _A_ Remove unsecured or scatter rugs.
        quickly   _B_ Know the number of poison control center.
    E. puts things in mouth
    F. easily distracted

42. ___car___ injuries cause more accidental deaths in all pediatric age groups.

43. Children should use convertible car restraints until they:
    A. weigh 40 pounds.
    B. reach the age of one year.
    C. reach the age of eight years.
    D. weigh 60 pounds.

44. Which car safety device can be lethal to young children? ___airbags___

45. One of the BEST ways to prevent drowning in the toddler group is for parents to:
    A. learn cardiopulmonary resuscitation (CPR).
    B. supervise children whenever they are near any source of water.
    C. enroll the toddler in a swimming program.
    D. all of the above.

46. Prevention strategies have helped to decrease near drowning as one of the leading cause of "vegetative state" in children.
    TRUE or FALSE

47. The MOST common cause of burns in the toddler age group is the:
    A. flame burn from playing with matches.
    B. scald burn from high temperature tap water or hot liquids.
    C. hot object burn from cigarettes or irons.
    D. electric burn from electrical outlets.

48. The MOST fatal type of burn in the toddler age group is:
    A. flame burn from playing with matches.
    B. scald burn from high temperature tap water or hot liquids.
    C. hot object burn from cigarettes or irons.
    D. electric burn from electrical outlets.

49. Poisonings in toddlers can be BEST prevented by:
    A. consistently using safety caps.
    B. storing poisonous substances in a locked cabinet.
    C. keeping ipecac syrup in the home.
    D. storing poisonous substances out of reach.

50. The parents should consider moving the toddler from the crib to a bed after the toddler:
    A. reaches the age of 2 years.
    B. will stay in the bed all night.
    C. reaches a height of 35 inches.
    D. is able to sleep through the night.

51. Give an example of an item that could cause aspiration or suffocation next to each category that is hazardous to the toddler (e.g., Food: Hard candy)

    Foods: _____

    Play objects: _____

    Common household objects: _____

    Electrical items: _____

Critical Thinking • Case Study

Tasha Jackson is a 12-month-old infant who is visiting the clinic for her well baby check up. Tasha's mother Dora is expecting her second child in 3 months. Dora works full time and will be home for six weeks with the new baby. Tasha has been in day care since she was a baby. Mr. Jackson also works full time during the day.

52. List four areas that should by assessed by the nurse to obtain the information necessary to adequately give anticipatory guidance for a toddler at Tasha's age.

    _____

    _____

    _____

    _____

53. Which one of the following nursing interventions would be MOST appropriate to establish?
    A. Allow Mrs. Jackson to express her feelings.
    B. Give Mrs. Jackson advice about day care.
    C. Give Mrs. Jackson advice about sibling rivalry.
    D. All of the above

54. Dora Jackson shares with the nurse that she is concerned about her day care and is thinking about keeping Tasha at home for the six weeks after the baby is born. Which intervention has the highest priority in this situation?

A. Stress the importance of preparing Tasha for the new sibling.

B. Recommend that Ms. Jackson begin making plans to keep Tasha at home for the six weeks.

C. Recommend that any change in day care should take place well before the new baby's arrival.

D. Explore Ms. Jackson's concerns about her day care arrangements.

55. Which evaluation method would BEST delineate whether Ms. Jackson's concerns were warranted?

A. A home visit after the baby is born

B. A visit to the day care center

C. A return demonstration of baby care

D. Verbalization from Ms. Jackson that she is comfortable with her postpartum arrangements

CHAPTER 15
Health Promotion of the Preschooler and Family

1. Biologic and Psychologic

A. preschool period
B. placement stage
C. shape stage
D. design stage
E. combine
F. aggregate

G. pictorial stage
H. initiative
I. guilt
J. superego
K. Oedipal stage
L. castration complex

M. Electra complex
N. penis envy
O. preoperational phase
P. preconceptual phase
Q. intuitive thought phase

___M___ guilt that develops regarding a daughter's wish to marry her father and kill her mother

___I___ occurs in the preschool years; conflict arises when children overstep the limits of their ability and inquiry

___A___ the term used to describe the time during which the child is 3 to 5 years of age

___K___ phallic stage

___C___ the second stage of drawing development; the 3 year old draws a single-line outline form such as a rectangle, circle, oval, cross, or other odd shape

___Q___ occurs from age 4 to 7; the child begins to shift from totally egocentric thought to social awareness and ability to consider other viewpoints

___J___ conscience

___B___ the first stage of drawing development; a pattern of placing scribbles on paper that appears by age 2 years, and once developed, is never lost

___E___ when two diagrams are united in a drawing design

___N___ the desire to have a penis

___F___ when three or more united diagrams occur in a drawing

___L___ guilt that develops regarding a son's feelings toward his father that makes him fear the punishment of mutilation

___G___ the fourth stage of drawing development in which designs are recognizable as familiar objects

___P___ occurs from age 2 to 4 years; the first phase of Piaget's preoperational phase

___H___ the chief psychosocial task of the preschool period

___O___ spans the age from 2 to 7 years; the stage of Piaget's cognitive theory that involves the preschooler

___D___ the third stage of drawing development in which simple forms are drawn together to make structured designs

2. Social Development

A.	play	J.	telegraphic speech	T.	modeling
B.	right and left concepts	K.	associative play	U.	reinforcement
C.	causality	L.	imitative play	V.	quantity
D.	time concepts	M.	imaginary playmates	W.	severity
E.	magical thinking	N.	Behavioral Style Questionnaire	X.	distribution
F.	punishment and obedience orientation	O.	sexuality	Y.	onset
G.	naive instrumental orientation	P.	masturbation	Z.	duration
H.	sex typing	Q.	gifted/talented	AA.	stuttering
I.	individuation-separation process	R.	aggression	BB.	animism
		S.	frustration	CC.	desensitization

__H__ the process by which an individual develops the behavior, personality, attitudes, and beliefs appropriate for his or her culture and sex

__x__ different manifestations of the behaviors

__K__ group play in similar or identical activities but without rigid organization or rules

__G__ Actions are directed toward satisfying the child's own needs and less commonly the needs of others.

__C__ resembles logical thought superficially; the ability of preschoolers to explain a concept as they have heard it described by others, but their understanding is limited

__E__ the preschooler's belief that their own thoughts are all-powerful

__A__ the child's way of understanding, adjusting to, and working out life's experiences

__F__ the way that children from age 2 to 4 years judge whether an action is good or bad; judgement is based on whether it results in reward or punishment

__B__ A preschooler does not have the ability to understand these concepts.

__I__ complete by the preschool years; preschoolers are now able to relate to unfamiliar people easily and tolerate brief separations from parents with little or no protest

__L__ imaginative play; dramatic play; self expression

__D__ preschooler has incomplete understanding of this concept; interprets it according to his or her own frame of reference

__R__ behavior that attempts to hurt a person or destroy property

__U__ can shape aggressive behavior; closely associated with modeling

__M__ usually occurs between the ages of 2 and 3 years; more intelligent children tend to have the most vivid and complex experiences

__V__ the number of occurrences

__N__ used to identify temperamental characteristics in children who are in the age range of 3 to 7 years

__CC__ a type of condition that exposes the child to a feared object in a safe situation

__P__ self stimulation of the genitals

__Y__ the time the behavior started; sudden changes in behavior are most significant

__W__ the degree that behavior is interfering with social or cognitive functioning

__AA__ stammering; a normal speech pattern in the preschooler

__O__ a broad concept; two people unite intimately because of the special relationship they have together

__J__ formation of sentences of about three to four words; includes only the most essential words to convey meaning

__S__ the continual thwarting of self satisfaction by parental disapproval, humiliation, punishment and insults

_____ the amount of time the behavior has lasted; behaviors lasting greater than 4 weeks are significant

__BB__ ascribing lifelike qualities to inanimate objects

__Q__ specific academic aptitude, creative or productive thinking, leadership ability, ability in the visual or performing arts and psychomotor ability either singly or in combination

__T__ imitating behavior of significant others; a powerful influencing force in preschoolers

3. The approximate age range for preschool period begins at age __3__ years and ends at age __5__ years.

4. The average annual weight gain during the preschool years is __5__ pounds.

5. Which one the following statements about the preschooler's physical proportions is TRUE?
   A. Preschoolers have a squat and potbellied frame.
   B. Preschoolers have a slender, but sturdy frame.
   C. The muscle and bones of the preschooler have matured.
   D. Sexual characteristics can be differentiated in the preschooler.

6. Uninhibited scribbling and drawing can help to develop:
   A. symbolic language.
   B. fine muscle skills.
   C. eye hand coordination.
   D. all of the above.

7. To prevent injuries in preschoolers, parents should be able to:
   A. supervise them constantly.
   B. keep them within sight.
   C. enforce limits verbally.
   D. all of the above.

8. The resolution of the Oedipus/Electra complex occurs when the child:
   A. identifies with the same sex parent.
   B. realizes that the same sex parent is more powerful.
   C. wishes that the same sex parent were dead.
   D. notices physical sexual differences.

9. Because of the preschoolers egocentric thought, the BEST approach for effective communication is through:
   A. speech.
   B. play.
   C. drawing.
   D. actions.

10. Magical thinking according to Piaget is the belief that:
    A. events have cause and effect.
    B. God is like an imaginary friend.
    C. thoughts are all powerful.
    D. if the skin is broken, their insides will come out.

11. The moral and spiritual development of the preschooler is characterized by:
    A. concern for why something is wrong.
    B. actions that are directed toward satisfying the needs of others.
    C. thoughts of loyalty and gratitude.
    D. a very concrete sense of justice.

12. The preschooler's body image has developed to include:
    A. a well defined body boundary.
    B. knowledge about his/her internal anatomy.
    C. fear of intrusive experiences.
    D. anxiety and fear of separation.

13. Sex typing involves the process by which the preschooler:
    A. forms a strong attachment to the same-sex parent.
    B. identifies with the opposite-sex parent.
    C. develops sexual identification.
    D. all of the above.

14. Language during the preschool years:
    A. includes telegraphic speech.
    B. is simple and concrete.
    C. uses phrases not sentences.
    D. includes the ability to follow complex commands.

15. Bilingual children:
    A. experience adverse affects to their receptive language development.
    B. experience adverse affects to performance in the majority language.
    C. may experience superior improvement in the majority language.
    D. experience adverse affects to areas in addition to just language.

16. Which one of the following statements about social development of the preschooler is FALSE?
    A. Imaginary playmates are a normal part of the preschooler's play.
    B. Preschoolers have overcome much of their anxiety regarding strangers.
    C. Preschoolers use telegraphic speech between the ages of 3 and 4 years.
    D. Preschoolers particularly enjoy parallel play.

17. Television and videotapes:
    A. hinder the preschooler's development.
    B. should only be a part of the preschooler's social and recreational activities.
    C. are not an interactive activity.
    D. do not provide learning for the preschooler.

18. In regard to the development of temperament in the preschool years:
    A. temperamental characteristics change considerably during the preschool years.
    B. the effect of temperament on adjustment in a group becomes important during the preschool years.
    C. children need to be treated the same regardless of differences in temperament.
    D. there really is no tool that will adequately identify temperamental characteristics during the preschool years.

19. List at least 2 strategies parents may use to help their child prepare for the preschool or Kindergarten experience.

_____

_____

20. The BEST way for parents to respond to questions about sexuality is to give the child:
    A. an honest answer and find out what the child thinks.
    B. one or two sentences that answer the specific question only.
    C. an honest, short and to the point answer.
    D. an honest answer and a little less information than the child expects.

21. Which one of the following characteristics are NOT typically seen in a gifted/talented child?
    A. Constant questioning
    B. Play with imaginary friend
    C. Extremely mature social skills
    D. Temperamental

22. Which one of the following factors influences aggressive behavior?
    A. Frustration
    B. Modeling
    C. Gender
    D. All of the above

23. Which one of the following dysfunctional speech patterns is a normal characteristic of the language development of a preschool-aged child?
    A. Lisp
    B. Stammering
    C. Nystagmus
    D. Echolalia

24. Which one of the following sources of stress in the preschool-aged child is typical of a three year old?
    A. Insecurity
    B. Masturbation
    C. Jealousy
    D. Sexuality

25. Which one of the following approaches is recommended to help prevent stress in children?
    A. Allow time for rest.
    B. Prepare the child for changes.
    C. Monitor the amount of stress.
    D. All of the above.

26. Which one of the following examples would BEST help a preschool child dispel his/her fear of the water when learning to swim?
   A. Fear of the water is a healthy fear. It should not be dispelled.
   B. Allow the child to sit by the water with other children, play with water toys and get splashed lightly with the water.
   C. Reassure the child as he/she is brought slowly into the water with an adult who knows how to swim.
   D. Throw the child in the water and have an adult keep the child's head above water.

27. Preschool children with reported sleep problems may sleep (circle one) MORE or LESS than those children without sleep difficulties.

28. Identify the following statements as either TRUE or FALSE.
   ___F___ Sleep terrors can be described as a partial arousal from a very deep non-dreaming sleep.
   ___T___ Nightmares usually occur in the second half of the night.
   ___F___ With sleep terrors, crying and fright persist even after the child is awake.
   ___F___ With nightmares the child is not very aware of another's presence.

29. When educating the preschool child about injury prevention, the parents should:
   A. set a good example.
   B. help children establish good habits.
   C. be aware that pedestrian/motor vehicle injuries increase in this age group.
   D. all of the above.

Critical Thinking • Case Study

Sheila Roth arrives at the office for a routine preschool physical. Her son Jacob, who is not quite 3 years old, will attend the 3-year-old preschool program at a local private school this year. He has attended a home day care program since he was a baby, while his mother tends to her own interior decorating business.

The day care is run by an older woman who treats the twelve children in her program as if they are family. The helper at the day care is also very loving. The program is very structured in regard to schedule and usual routines.

Ms. Roth tells the nurse that she is looking forward to Jacob's new environment. His teacher is very creative and approaches the classroom from the perspective of the child's development. There will be a lot of choices for activities during the day.

30. Based on the information above, which one of the following is the BEST analysis of the data presented?
   A. Jacob needs some preparation for this new preschool experience.
   B. Jacob will have less trouble adjusting than a child who has never attended day care.
   C. Jacob is too young for such a drastic change.
   D. Jacob needs the individual attention he is getting at the day care.

31. Which one of the following expected outcomes would be MOST reasonable to establish?
    A. The nurse will help Ms. Roth assess Jacob's readiness for preschool.
    B. Jacob will attend preschool without any behavioral indications of stress.
    C. Ms. Roth will verbalize at least five strategies that can be used to help prepare Jacob for his preschool experience.
    D. Jacob will demonstrate behavior that indicates that he is adjusting to his preschool experience.

32. Which one of the following interventions would be INAPPROPRIATE for the nurse to suggest?
    A. Introduce Jacob to the teacher.
    B. Leave quickly the first day.
    C. Talk about the new school as exciting.
    D. Be confident the first day.

33. Which one of the following of Jacob's characteristics would indicate that he is ready for preschool?
    A. Social maturity
    B. Good attention span
    C. Academically ready
    D. All of the above

CHAPTER 16

Health Problems of Early Childhood

1. Match the term with its definition.

   A.   communicable disease   E.   reservoir   I.   direct
   B.   epidemic   F.   host   J.   vehicle
   C.   endemic   G.   carrier   K.   incubation period
   D.   infectious agent   H.   contact   L.   period of communicability

   __F__ provides subsistence or lodging to infectious agent

   __G__ harbors infectious agent without apparent disease

   __H__ person or animal that has been in association with source that could provide the infected agent

   __A__ illness caused by specific infectious agent through some transmission of agent

   __C__ disease occurring regularly within a geographic location

   __B__ disease occurring in greater than expected numbers within a community

   __E__ environment in which infectious agent lives and multiplies

   __D__ organism that is capable of producing infection

   __I__ contact and immediate transfer of infectious agent by kissing

   __J__ an object serving as intermediate means for transportation of infectious agent

   __L__ time period where infection may be directly or indirectly transported

   __K__ time between exposure to appearance of symptoms

2. Match the communicable disease with its description.

   A.   varicella   E.   rubeola   H.   rubella
   B.   diphtheria   F.   mumps   I.   scarlet fever
   C.   fifth disease   G.   pertussis   J.   poliomyelitis
   D.   roseola

   __C__ rash appears in three stages; stage I is erthema on face, chiefly on cheeks

   __A__ begins as macule rash, rapidly progresses to papule rash, then vesicles, and then breaks and forms crusts

   __B__ tonsillar pharyngeal areas are covered with white or gray membrane; complications include myocarditis and neuritis

   __D__ rash is rose-pink macules or maculopapules appearing first on trunk, then to neck, face, and extremities; is a nonpruritic rash

   __G__ cough occurs at night, and inspirations sound like crowing

   __F__ earache that is aggravated by chewing

   __E__ rash appears 3-4 days after onset and maculopapular eruption on face with gradual spread downward; koplik spots present before rash

   __H__ discrete pinkish red maculopapular rash appears on face and then downward to neck, arms, trunk, and legs; greatest danger is teratogenic effect on fetus

   __J__ can have permanent paralysis

   __I__ tonsils enlarged, edematous, reddened, and covered with patches of exudate; rash is absent on face; desquamation occurs.

3. Assessment of which of the following is NOT helpful in identifying potentially communicable diseases?
   A. Recent travel to foreign country
   B. Immunization history
   C. Past medical history
   D. Family history

4. Primary prevention of communicable disease is BEST accomplished by:
   A. immunization.
   B. control of the disease spread.
   C. adequate water supply.
   D. implementing good handwashing among hospital personnel.

5. Certain groups of children are at risk for serious complications from communicable diseases. These children do NOT include which of the following groups?
   A. Children with an immunodeficiency or immunologic disorder
   B. Children receiving steroid therapy
   C. Children with leukemia
   D. Children having recently undergone a surgical procedure

6. What antiviral agent is used to treat varicella infections in children at increased risk for complications associated with varicella?
   A. Varicella-zoster immune globulin
   B. Acyclovir
   C. Salicylates
   D. Steroids

7. Name the two diseases causes by the varicella zoster virus.

   _____chicken pox_____

   _____shingles_____

8. A major responsibility of the school nurse working with children at high-risk for communicable diseases is _____.

9. The American Academy of Pediatrics has recommended vitamin A supplements for certain pediatric patients with measles. Correct dosage of vitamin A and instruction to parents of these children include:
   1. single oral dose of 200,000 IU in children 1 year old.
   2. single oral dose of 100,000 IU in children 6-12 months old.
   3. dosage may be associated with vomiting and headache for a few hours.
   4. safe storage of the drug to prevent accidental overdose.

   A. 1, 2, 3, and 4
   B. 1, 2, and 4
   C. 1, 3, and 4
   D. 2 and 4

10. The nurse is conducting an educational session for the parents of a child diagnosed with varicella. Which one of the following is NOT an appropriate comfort measure to include in this session?
    A. Use Aveeno bath or oatmeal in bath water for added skin comfort.
    B. Use Caladryl lotion on rash to decrease itching.
    C. Use hot bath water to promote skin rash healing.
    D. Keep nails short and smooth to decrease infection from scratching.

11. Which one of the following does the nurse recognize as CONTRAINDICATED in providing comfort measures to children with communicable diseases?
    A. Use of acetaminophen for control of elevated temperature in child with varicella
    B. Use of imposed bed rest in child with pertussis
    C. Use of aspirin to control elevated temperature and/or symptoms in child with varicella
    D. Use of lozenges, saline rinses in child 8 years old with sore throat

12. Clinical manifestations differentiate bacterial conjunctivitis from viral conjunctivitis. Which one of the following is present with bacterial conjunctivitis but NOT usually found with viral conjunctivitis?
    A. Child awakens with crusting of eyelids.
    B. Child has increase in watery drainage from eyes.
    C. Child has inflamed conjunctiva.
    D. Child has swollen eyelids.

13. When instructing the parents caring for an infant with conjunctivitis, the nurse will include which one of the following in the plan?
    A. Accumulated secretions are removed by wiping from outer canthus inward.
    B. Hydrogen peroxide placed on Q-tips is helpful in removing crusts from eyelids.
    C. Compresses of warm tap water are kept in place on the eye to prevent formation of crusting.
    D. Washcloth and towel used by the infant are kept separate and not used by others.

14. Identify the following statements about stomatitis as TRUE or FALSE.

    A. __T__   Aphthous stomatitis may be associated with mild traumatic injury, allergy, and emotional stress.

    B. __T__   Aphthous stomatitis is painful, small, whitish ulcerations which will heal without complication in 4 to 12 days.

    C. __T__   Herpetic gingivostomatitis is caused by herpes simplex virus, usually type 1.

    D. __T__   Herpetic gingivostomatitis is commonly called "cold sores" or "fever blisters" and may appear in groups or singly.

    E. __F__   Treatment for stomatitis is aimed at relief of complications.

    F. __F__   When examining herpetic lesions, the nurse uses her uncovered index finger to check for cracks in the skin surface.

15. Anne, an 8 year old, has been diagnosed with giardiasis. The nurse would expect Anne to have MOST likely presented with which of these signs and symptoms?
    A. Diarrhea with blood in the stools
    B. Nausea and vomiting with a mild fever
    C. Abdominal cramps with intermittent loose stools
    D. Weight loss of 5 lbs over the last month

16. The nurse is instructing parents on the test tape diagnostic procedure for enterobiasis. Which one of the following is included in the explanation?
    A. Use a flashlight to inspect the anal area while the child sleeps.
    B. Perform the test 2 days after the child has received the first dose of mebendazole.
    C. Test all members of the family at the same time using frosted tape.
    D. Collect the tape in the morning before the child has a bowel movement or bath.

17. Children with pinworm infections present with the principal symptom of:
    A. perianal itching.
    B. diarrhea with blood.
    C. evidence of small rice-like worms in their stool and urine.
    D. abdominal pain.

18. The nurse has an order to administer mebendazole (Vermox) 100 mg to 5-year-old Megan for a positive pinworm test. The nurse recognizes which one of the following as an appropriate action when administering this medication?
    A. Vermox should be withheld in all children under 6 years of age.
    B. Advise the parents that Vermox will stain stools and vomitus bright red.
    C. Vermox will also effectively treat giardiasis.
    D. Vermox can be chewed, crushed or mixed with food.

19. Reduction of poisonings in children and infants can be accomplished by:
    A. use of child-resistant containers.
    B. educating parents and grandparents to place products out of reach of small children.
    C. educating parents to relocate plants out of reach of infants, toddlers, and small children.
    D. all of the above.

20. The most common accidentally ingested medications in children under 6 years of age are:
    A. cold and cough preparations.
    B. analgesics such as acetaminophen and ibuprofen.
    C. hormones such as oral contraception.
    D. antibiotics.

21. The first action parents should be taught to initiate in a poisoning is:
    A. induce vomiting.
    B. take the child to the family physician's office or emergency center.
    C. call the Poison Control Center.
    D. follow the instructions of the label of the household product.

22. Each toxic ingestion is treated individually. Gastric decontamination is aimed at removing the ingested toxic product by what five measures?

    _____

    _____

    _____

    _____

    _____

23. The major principles of emergency treatment for poisoning are _____,
_____, _____, _____, and
_____.

24. The nurse provides proper administration instructions to parents for ipecac syrup, including which one of the following?
A. Having 2 doses of emetic in the household for each child
B. Administering the emetic within 3 hours of toxic ingestion
C. Never administering out-of-date emetic
D. Forcing fluids and encouraging activity after the emetic is administered to facilitate its effectiveness

25. The nurse does NOT expect to assist in gastric lavage for the treatment of poisoning in which one of the following pediatric patients?
A. The 8-month-old child admitted to the emergency center who has eaten 8-10 holly berries
B. The 8-year-old child who took 3 of his Mom's birth control pills
C. The 6-year-old child who has an overdose of a noncorrosive substance and is convulsing
D. The 13-year-old girl who has an overdose of valium and is comatose

26. Potential causes of heavy metal poisoning in children include __lead__,
__mercury__, and __iron__.

27. Identify the following statements as TRUE or FALSE.

A. __T__   The neurologic system is of most concern when young children are exposed to lead because the developing brain is very vulnerable.

B. __T__   Young children will absorb more of the lead to which they are exposed than will adults.

C. __T__   Lead-based paint from old housing built before 1950 remains the most frequent source of lead poisoning in children.

D. __F__   Lead-containing pottery or leaded dishes do not contribute to lead poisoning because food does not absorb lead.

E. __T__   If the venous blood value is below 10 ug/dl of lead the child is considered to have a safe blood lead value.

F. __F__   The exposure risk is lower for children living in leaded environments whose diet is deficient in iron and calcium and high in fats because the diet slows the absorption of lead.

G. __T__   Pica is the habitual, purposeful, and compulsive ingestion of nonfood substances.

28. The nurse is to give a second injection of the chelation drug calcium disodium edetate. Which one of the following does the nurse recognize as being MOST helpful in preparing the young patient for the injection?
A. Inspect intake and output records before administration to verify kidney function.
B. Mix the drug with procain to lessen the pain associated with the injection.
C. Maintain seizure precautions at the bedside.
D. Use play therapy and aggressive play to provide the child with an outlet for frustration.

29. Diagnostic evaluations for lead poisoning include:
    A. blood levels for lead concentration including screening done on finger and heel sticks with blood collected by venipuncture to confirm diagnosis.
    B. recommended universal screening for all children, with children ages 6 years or older given priority.
    C. identifying children at high risk for anemia, since these children will most likely have higher lead levels.
    D. all of the above.

30. Therapeutic interventions for lead poisoning do NOT include:
    A. removal of the source of lead.
    B. improving nutrition.
    C. using chelation therapy.
    D. administration of dimercaprol intravenously.

31. Match the term with its description.

    A. child neglect   __D__ deliberate attempt to destroy a child's self-esteem
    B. physical neglect   __C__ failure to meet the child's needs for affection
    C. emotional neglect   __B__ deprivation of necessities such as food, clothing
    D. emotional abuse   __A__ failure to provide for the child's basic needs and adequate level of care
    E. physical abuse   __E__ deliberate infliction of physical injury on a child
    F. Munchausen syndrome   __F__ an illness that one person fabricates or induces in another person

32. Which one of the following parental characteristics does NOT describe abusive parent families?
    A. Teenage mothers are less likely to release frustration by striking out at their child.
    B. Abusive parents have difficulty controlling aggressive impulses.
    C. Free expression of violence is a consistent quality of abusive families.
    D. Abusive families are often more socially isolated and have fewer supportive relationships than nonabusive.

33. Which one of the following statements is FALSE?
    A. The position of the child in the family has little effect on the abusive situation.
    B. One child is usually the victim in an abusive family, and removal of this child often places the other sibling at risk.
    C. The abusive family environment is one of chronic stress, including problems of divorce, poverty, unemployment and poor housing.
    D. Child abuse is a problem of all social groups.

34. Match the term with its description.

A. incest

B. molestation

C. exhibitionism

D. pedophilia

E. sexual abuse

F. shaken baby syndrome

___E___ the use, persuasion, or coercion of any child to engage in sexually explicit conduct

___D___ preference of a prepubertal child by an adult as a means of achieving sexual excitement

___A___ any physical sexual activity between family members

___B___ "indecent liberties" as touching, fondling

___F___ violent shaking of infant can cause fatal intracranial trauma

___C___ indecent exposure

35. The nurse is talking with 13-year-old Amy, who has revealed that she is being sexually abused. Which one of the following is a CORRECT guideline for the nurse to utilize?
   A. Promise Amy not to tell what she tells you.
   B. Assure Amy that she will not need to report the abuse.
   C. Avoid using leading statements that can distort Amy's reporting of the problem.
   D. It is okay for the nurse to express anger, shock and to criticize Amy's family.

36. In identification of the abused child, the nurse knows:
   A. incompatibility between the history and the injury is probably the most important criterion on which to base the decision to report suspected abuse.
   B. it is necessary to exam for observable evidence of abuse.
   C. maltreated children rarely betray their parents by admitting to the abuse they received.
   D. all of the above.

Critical Thinking • Case Study

Jimmy is a 4 year old pre-kinder student who is brought to the school nurse's office by his teacher. She is concerned because Jimmy has purulent discharge in the corner of both eyes with the conjunctiva appearing inflamed. Jimmy is observed by the school nurse to be wiping his eyes frequently with his hands.

37. Based on the information provided, the nurse suspects the condition that Jimmy has is:
   A. bacterial conjunctivitis.
   B. viral conjunctivitis.
   C. allergic conjunctivitis.
   D. conjunctivitis caused by foreign body.

38. Based on knowledge of communicable disease, the nurse would prioritize which one of the following goals for Jimmy's plan of care?
   A. Will not become infected
   B. Will not spread disease
   C. Will experience minimal discomfort
   D. Will maintain skin integrity

39. The nurse calls Jimmy's parents to request that they come and pick Jimmy up from school. What is the BEST rationale for this action?

   A. Jimmy is tired and needs additional rest because of the infection.
   B. Jimmy is at high-risk for spreading the disease because of his age and his inability to wash hands after touching his eyes.
   C. Jimmy needs immediate medical attention to prevent complications.
   D. The nurse needs to discuss causes of this disease with Jimmy's mother so that its recurrence can be prevented.

40. It is important to include what information in the teaching plan for Jimmy's parents?

   A. Jimmy needs to have his own face cloth and towel.
   B. Eye medication will need to be administered before the eyes are cleaned.
   C. Jimmy cannot return to school until all symptoms have stopped.
   D. Jimmy will need his own eating utensils.

41. The nurse can expect treatment for this disease to include:

   A. use of continuous warm compresses held in place on each infected eye.
   B. application of broad-spectrum topical ophthalmic agents.
   C. oral broad-spectrum antibiotics.
   D. all of the above.

42. The effectiveness of nursing interventions for Jimmy's condition is BEST demonstrated by which one of the following evaluations?

   A. There is no spread of the disease within the school and family.
   B. Parents are able to demonstrate appropriate eye care.
   C. Jimmy reports no eye discomfort.
   D. Child engages in normal activities.

43. Albert, age 7, has been diagnosed with pinworms and Vermox has been ordered. The nurse knows that this drug should probably also be administered to:

   A. only Albert's siblings.
   B. only family members who test positive.
   C. all family members who are not pregnant or under 2 years of age.
   D. everyone who uses the same toilet facilities as Albert.

CHAPTER 17

Health Promotion of the School-Age Child and Family

1. The middle childhood is also referred to as school-age or the school years. What ages does this period represent?
   A. Ages 5 to 13 years
   B. Ages 4 to 14 years
   C. Ages 6 to 12 years
   D. Ages 6 to 16 years

2. Physiologically the middle years begin with _____ _____ and end at _____.

3. Which finding should the nurse expect when assessing physical growth in the school-age child?
   A. Increase of 2 to 3 kg per year
   B. Increase of 3 cm per year
   C. Little change in refined coordination
   D. Decrease in body fat and muscle tissue

4. Identify the following statements about the school-age child as either TRUE or FALSE.
   ___T___ In middle childhood there are fewer stomach upsets, better maintenance of blood sugar levels and an increased stomach capacity.
   ___F___ Caloric needs are higher in relation to stomach size when compared to the needs of preschool years.
   ___T___ The heart is smaller in relation to the rest of the body during the middle years.
   ___F___ During the middle years, the immune system develops little immunity to pathogenic microorganisms.
   ___T___ Back packs are preferred to other book totes during middle years.
   ___F___ Physical maturity correlates well with emotional and social maturity during the middle years.

5. What is the period that begins toward the end of middle childhood and ends with the thirteenth birthday?
   A. Puberty
   B. Preadolescence
   C. Early maturation
   D. All of the above

6. According to Freud, middle childhood is described as which one of the following periods?
   A. Anal
   B. Latency
   C. Oral
   D. Oedipal

7. According to Erikson, what is the developmental goal of middle childhood?
   A. Autonomy
   B. Trust
   C. Initiative
   D. Industry

8. Accord to Piaget, what is the stage of development for middle childhood?
   A. Concrete operational
   B. Preoperational
   C. Formal operational
   D. Sensorimotor

9. Early appearance of secondary sex characteristics of girls during preadolescence may be associated with which of the following feelings?
   A. Satisfaction with physical appearance and higher self-esteem
   B. Increase in self-confidence and a more outgoing personality
   C. Dissatisfaction with physical appearance and lower self-esteem
   D. Increased substance use and reckless vehicle use

10. Generally, the earliest age at which puberty begins in girls is age ____10____ and in boys age ___12___ .

11. Middle childhood is the time when children:
    1. learn the value of doing things with others.
    2. learn the benefits derived from division of labor in accomplishing goals.
    3. achieve a sense of industry and accomplishment.
    4. expand interests and engage in tasks that can be carried to completion.

    A. 1, 2, 3, and 4
    B. 1, 3, and 4
    C. 1 and 4
    D. 2 and 3

12. Dillon is a 6-year-old starting in a new neighborhood school. The first day of school he complains of a headache and tearfully tells his mother he does not want to go to school. Dillon's mother takes him to school and the nurse is consulted. The nurse recognizes that Dillon is a slow-to-warm-up child and suggests which one of the following?
    A. Put Dillon in the classroom with the other children and leave him alone.
    B. Insist that Dillon join and lead the class song.
    C. Include Dillon in activities without assigning him tasks until he willingly participates in activities.
    D. Send Dillon home with his mom since he has a headache.

13. During the concrete-operational period of middle childhood, which one of the following is the expected cognitive development?
    A. Are able to follow directions but unable to verbalize the actions involved in the process
    B. Are able to use their thought processes to experience events and actions and make judgments based on what they reason
    C. Are able to view from an egocentric outlook that is rigidly developed around the action to be completed
    D. Progress from conceptual thinking to perceptual thinking when making judgments

14. Match the following terms as they relate to the accomplishment of cognitive tasks of middle childhood.

A. conservation

B. identity

C. reversibility

D. reciprocity

E. classification skills

F. serialize

G. combinational skills

H. metalinguistic awareness

___F___ arrange objects according to some ordinal scale

___G___ ability to manipulate numbers and to learn the skills of addition, subtraction, multiplication and division

___E___ ability to group objects according to the attributes they share in common

___C___ ability to think through an action sequence, anticipate the consequences, and return and rethink the action in a different direction

___D___ ability to deal with two dimensions at one time and to comprehend that a change in one dimension compensates for a change in another

___B___ able to distinguish a shape change when nothing has been added or subtracted

___A___ ability to comprehend that physical matter does not appear and disappear by magic

___H___ ability to think about language and to comment on its properties

15. A major difference in moral development between young school-age children and older school-age children is BEST described by which one of the following?
   A. Younger children believe that standards of behavior come from within themselves.
   B. Children 6 to 7 years of age know the rules and understand the reasons behind the rules.
   C. Older school-age children are able to judge an act by the intentions that prompted it and not only by the consequences.
   D. All of the above

16. Which one of the following BEST identifies the spiritual development of school-age children?
   A. They have little fear of going to hell for misbehavior.
   B. They begin to learn the difference between the natural and the supernatural.
   C. They petition to God for less tangible rewards.
   D. They view God as a deity with few human traits.

17. Which one of the following would the nurse NOT expect to observe as a characteristic of peer group relationships in 8-year-old Mark?
   A. Mark demonstrates loyalty to the group by adhering to the secret code rules.
   B. Mark demonstrates a greater individual egocentric outlook as compared to other peer group members.
   C. Mark is willing to conform to the group's rule of "not talking to girls."
   D. Mark has a best friend within the peer group with whom he shares his secrets.

18. During the school-age years, children learn valuable lessons from age-mates. How is this accomplished?
   A. The child learns to appreciate the varied points of view that are within the peer group.
   B. The child becomes sensitive to the social norms and pressures of the group.
   C. The child's interactions among peers leads to the formation of intimate friendships between same-sex peers.
   D. All of the above

19. With school-age children, the relationship with the family can be observed in which one of the following statements?
    A. Children desire to spend equal time with family and peers.
    B. Children are prepared to reject parental controls.
    C. The group replaces the family as the primary influence in setting standards of behavior and rules.
    D. Children need and want restrictions placed on their behavior by the family.

20. Ms. Jones is a single mother caring for her 10-year-old son James. At an office appointment for James, his mother asks the nurse how to prevent James from becoming involved in gang violence. The BEST response is which one of the following?
    A. Try to be more of a "pal" to James so he will not seek outside approval.
    B. Relax restrictions on James because he needs to increase his independence and this will show that you trust him.
    C. Become aware of any gang-related activities in the community.
    D. Do not allow James to join "boys only" groups.

21. List three components of children's self-concepts.

    _____

    _____

    _____

22. The nurse plans to conduct a sex education class for 10 year olds. Which one of the following does the nurse recognize as MOST appropriate for this age group?
    A. Present sex information as a normal part of growth and development
    B. Discourage question and answer sessions
    C. Since sexual information supplied by parents usually produces feelings of guilt and anxiety in children, avoid parental assistance in conducting the program
    D. Segregate boys from girls and include information related only to same sex in the discussion

23. List three team membership characteristics that promote child development during the middle years.

    _____

    _____

    _____

24. A factor that MOST influences the amount and manner of discipline and limit-setting imposed on school-age children is:
    A. the age of the parent.
    B. the education of the parent.
    C. response of the child to rewards and punishments.
    D. the ability of the parent to communicate with the school system.

25. To assist school-age children in coping with stress in their lives, the nurse should:
   1. be able to recognize signs that indicate the child is undergoing stress.
   2. teach the child how to recognize signs of stress in herself/himself.
   3. help the child plan a means for dealing with any stress through problem solving.
   4. reassure the child that the stress is only temporary.

   A. 1, 2, 3, and 4
   B. 1, 2, and 3
   C. 1, 2, and 4
   D. 1 and 3

26. Identify which one of the following statements, describing fears in the school-age child, is TRUE.
   A. School-age children are increasingly fearful of body safety.
   B. Most of the new fears that trouble school-age children are related to school and family.
   C. School-age children should be encouraged to hide their fears to prevent ridicule by their peers.
   D. School-age children with numerous fears need continuous protective behavior by parents to eliminate these fears.

27. By the end of middle childhood, children should be able to assume personal responsibility for self-care in the areas of _____, _____, _____, _____, _____, and _____.

28. Sleep problems in the school-age child are often demonstrated by:
   A. delaying tactics because they do not wish to go to bed.
   B. the occurrence of night terrors that awaken the child during the night.
   C. the development of somatic illness that awakens the child during the night.
   D. the increasing need for larger amounts of sleep time as compared to preschool and adolescence.

29. The nurse is planning to advise a school-age child's parents about appropriate physical activity for their child. Which fact does the nurse include?
   A. School-age children have the same stamina and control as 15-year-old teens.
   B. School-age children are prepared for participation in strenuous competitive athletics.
   C. Activities that promote coordination in the school-age child include running and skipping rope.
   D. Most children need continued encouragement to engage in physical activity.

30. List four components included in the content of school health services.

   _____

   _____

   _____

   _____

31. The nurse is planning an educational session for a group of 9-year-olds and their parents which is aimed at decreasing injuries and accidents among this group. The nurse would BEST accomplish this goal by including what topics in the educational session?
    A. Safety rules when dealing with fire to prevent burns
    B. Safety rules when dealing with toxic substances to prevent poisonings
    C. Pedestrian safety rules and skills training programs to prevent motor vehicle accidents
    D. Reviewing the rules for the use of all-terrain vehicles and encouraging their use only with supervision

Critical Thinking • Case Study

Allen Thomas, age 9, is taken to the clinic by his mother for a school physical examination. Allen's mother is concerned because Allen wants to join the school soccer team this year. On physical examination, the nurse discovers that Allen has had an increase of 2 inches in height since last year and has gained 12 pounds since last year. Health history is unchanged from the previous year. Allen tells the nurse that he rides his bike more now than last year because he has a new best friend to go riding with.

32. Based on the above information, the nurse should expand assessment with Allen in which of the following areas at this visit?
    1. his diet
    2. his knowledge and use of safety precautions when riding his bike
    3. his hygiene habits
    4. his reasons for wanting to play soccer

    A. 1, 2, and 3
    B. 2 and 4
    C. 1 and 2
    D. 1 and 4

33. Which of the following would be the nurse's BEST response to the mother's concern about Allen playing soccer?
    A. "Allen is healthy, and playing soccer will allow him to increase strength and develop motor skill performance."
    B. "Allen is overweight for his age and should be encouraged to ride his bike less. Soccer is a better activity for him since it will help decrease his weight."
    C. "Allen is still too young to participate in strenuous sports like soccer. He should be able to participate in another year."
    D. "Let Allen play what he wants to. You worry too much about his activities."

34. Based on the above information, the nurse plans an educational session for Allen and his mother. The knowledge deficit the nurse is most likely to have identified with this family is:
    A. altered nutrition related to improper dietary habits.
    B. altered nutrition related to less than body needs.
    C. lack of proper physical activity related to bike riding.
    D. improper parenting skills related to overprotective mother.

35. Mrs. Thomas asks the nurse how she can foster Allen's development. What should be the response by the nurse?
    A. "Don't interfere with Allen as long as he is doing well in school."
    B. "Give Allen recognition and positive feedback for his accomplishments."
    C. "Always point out to Allen how he incorrectly performs tasks so he can improve his accomplishments."
    D. "Try not to set rules for Allen. He needs to set his own limits during this period of development."

CHAPTER 18
Health Problems of Middle Childhood

1. Functions performed by the skin do NOT include:
   A. protection.
   B. heat regulation.
   C. sensation.
   D. nutrition.

2. The three layers of the skin are the _____epidermis_____, _____dermis_____ and
   _____subcutaneous_____.

3. Match the term related to assessment of the skin with its description.

   A. pruritis
   B. anesthesia
   C. hyperesthesia
   D. paresthesia
   E. erythema
   F. ecchymoses
   G. petechiae
   H. primary lesions
   I. secondary lesions
   J. distribution
   K. configuration

   __E__ reddened area caused by increased amounts of blood
   __F__ localized purple discolorations
   __G__ pinpoint, tiny circumscribed hemorrhagic spots
   __H__ skin changes caused by some causative factor to produce macules, papules, or vesicles
   __I__ changes related to rubbing, scratching, or medication
   __J__ whether the pattern is localized or generalized
   __K__ the size and shape of the lesions or the group of lesions
   __A__ itching
   __C__ excessive sensitiveness
   __B__ absence of sensation
   __D__ abnormal sensation

4. Match the term related to wounds with its description.

   A. acute
   B. chronic
   C. pressure ulcer
   D. abrasion
   E. evulsion
   F. laceration
   G. incision
   H. penetrating
   I. puncture

   __F__ accidental cut, either torn or jagged edges
   __H__ disruption of the skin that extends into the underlying tissue or into a body cavity
   __A__ heals uneventfully within the usual time frame
   __B__ does not heal in the expected time frame and can be associated with complications
   __D__ removal of the superficial layers of skin by scraping
   __C__ often becomes chronic skin injury and is a localized area of cellular necrosis
   __E__ forcible pulling out or extraction of tissue
   __I__ wound with opening that is small compared with the depth
   __G__ division of the skin made with a sharp object

5. Cindy, age 8, is brought to the clinic because of a rash. On examination, the rash is found to consist of irregularly shaped areas of cutaneous edema. The rash has a pale pink appearance and a lighter center. Cindy tells the nurse the rash itches. Which one of the following lesions would the nurse suspect?
   A. Macule
   B. Patch
   C. Plaque
   D. Wheal

6. Match the following skin lesions with its description.

   A.   papule
   B.   vesicle
   C.   bulla
   D.   nodule
   E.   pustule
   F.   cyst
   G.   patch
   H.   macule
   I.   lichenification
   J.   scale
   K.   crust
   L.   keloid

   __F__ elevated, palpable, encapsulated
   __G__ flat, nonpalpable, irregular; greater than 1 cm. in diameter
   __I__ caused by rubbing or irritation; rough, thickened epidermis
   __K__ dried serum, blood or purulent exudate; scab
   __A__ elevated, palpable; firm less than 1 cm. in diameter
   __C__ vesicle greater than 1 cm. in diameter
   __B__ elevated, circumscribed; filled with serous fluid; less than 1 cm. in diameter
   __L__ progressively enlarging scar caused by excess collagen formation
   __J__ heaped-up keratinized cells
   __H__ flat, nonpalpable, circumscribed; less than 1 cm. in diameter
   __E__ elevated, superficial; filled with purulent fluid
   __D__ elevated, firm, palpable; 1 to 2 cm. in diameter

7. During wound healing, immature connective tissue cells migrate to the healing site and begin to secrete collagen into the meshwork spaces. What is this phase called?
   A. Scar contracture
   B. Inflammation
   C. Fibroplasia
   D. Scar maturation

8. Mary, age 7, fell and sustained a deep laceration to her chin. She was taken to the emergency center where the laceration was sutured with the edges well approximated. The nurse expects the repair healing to take place by:
   A. primary intention.
   B. secondary intention.
   C. tertiary intention.

9. The nurse recognizes that a factor that is NOT indicated for use in promoting wound healing is:
   A. nutrition with sufficient protein, calories, vitamin C and zinc.
   B. irrigation of wounds with normal saline.
   C. application of povidone-iodine daily.
   D. application of an occlusive dressing.

10. Jimmy, age 9, has fallen and scraped his knee at school. He is brought to the school nurse for treatment. After cleaning the area and applying an over-the-counter first aide ointment, the nurse applies a gauze dressing. What type of dressing is this considered?
    A. Occlusive
    B. Semiocclusive
    C. Nonocclusive
    D. Impermeable

11. Which one of the following does the nurse include in the educational plan when instructing parents about the use of topical corticosteroids?
    A. Do not use this cream on fungus infection.
    B. Apply a thick layer of the cream and rub into the skin well.
    C. Do not use for longer than three days in chronic conditions.
    D. All of the above

12. Skin disorder assessment includes the objective data collected by inspection and palpation. Which one of the following is NOT objective data?
    A. The lesion has an increased erythema margin edge.
    B. The rash appears as macules and papules.
    C. The lesion is painful and itches.
    D. The lesion is moist.

13. List the objective signs of wound infection.

    _____

    _____

    _____

    _____

14. The nurse is applying wet compresses of Burow's solution to Johnny's wound. Which one of the following does the nurse recognize as CORRECT information about this type of topical therapy?
    A. After application of the compresses the wound is washed with soap and water and rubbed dry.
    B. Compresses will loosen and remove crusts and debris.
    C. Burow's solution is applied directly onto the wound and then covered with a dry soft gauze.
    D. All of the above

15. Care of bacterial skin infections in children may include all of the following EXCEPT:
    A. good handwashing.
    B. keeping the fingernails short.
    C. puncturing the surface of the pustule.
    D. application of topical antibiotics.

16. Lisa, age 7, has been diagnosed with impetigo. Which one of the following does the nurse recognize as being a manifestation of this bacterial infection?
    A. Inflammation of skin and subcutaneous tissues with intense redness
    B. Exudate is honey colored crusts.
    C. Lymphangitis
    D. All of the above

17. Which one of the following is a fungal infection that lives on the skin?
    A. Tinea corporis
    B. Herpes simplex type 1
    C. Scabies
    D. Warts

18. Steve, age 8, has been diagnosed with tinea capitis. Which one of the following does the nurse include in the teaching plan for educating Steve and his parents?
    A. No animal-to-person transmission is associated with this infection.
    B. Steve can continue to share hair grooming articles with his younger brother.
    C. Griseofulvin should be administered with high-fat foods.
    D. Cleanliness is the best way to prevent this disease.

19. Which one of the following statements about scabies is INCORRECT?
    A. Clinical manifestations include intense pruritus, especially at night, and papules, burrows, or vesicles on interdigital surfaces.
    B. Treatment is the application of 5% Elimite for all family members.
    C. After treatment, all previously worn clothing is washed in very hot water and dried at the high setting in the dryer.
    D. The rash and itching will be eliminated immediately after treatment.

20. What would the nurse look for in assessing if a child has pediculosis? "lice"

_____

21. In assisting parents to cope with pediculosis the nurse should emphasize that:
    A. anyone can get pediculosis.
    B. the louse will fly and jump from one person to another.
    C. cutting the child's hair short will prevent reinfestation.
    D. it can be transmitted by pets.

22. The nurse is instructing Angie's parents about using the prescribed Kwell shampoo for pediculosis. Which one of the following is included in these instructions?
    A. Only one application is needed.
    B. The shampoo is toxic when used on children under 2 years.
    C. The shampoo kills the lice and nits on contact.
    D. The shampoo will kill all the nits.

23. Which one of the following products is the drug of choice for treatment of pediculosis capitis in a 2-year-old child?
    A. 5% permethrin cream (Elimite)
    B. 1% lindane shampoo (Kwell)
    C. selenium sulfide shampoos
    D. permethrin 1% cream rinse (Nix)

24. Children with lyme disease do NOT present with which of the following signs and symptoms?
    A. Small erythematous papule that has a circumferential ring with a raised, edematous doughnutlike border
    B. Multiple, small secondary annular lesions with indurated centers on the palms and soles
    C. Flu-like symptoms of headache, malaise, lymphadenopathy
    D. Abdominal pain, splenomegaly, fatigue, anorexia

25. Match the following term with its description.

A. histoplasmosis

B. coccidiodomycosis

C. Rocky Mountain spotted fever

D. epidemic typhus

E. endemic typhus

F. rickettsialpox

___E___ transmission by flea bite; inhaling or ingesting flea excreta

___D___ mammal source, human; patient should be isolated until deloused

___F___ maculopapular rash following primary lesion and eschar at site of bite; mammal source is house mouse

___A___ organism cultured from soil, especially where contaminated with fowl droppings

___C___ transmission tick; maculopapular or petechial rash characteristically on palms and soles

___B___ primary lung disease; endemic in southwestern United States

26. Children with cat scratch fever usually present with:
   A. headache, diarrhea and fever.
   B. regional lymphadenopathy.
   C. maculopapular rash over the entire body.
   D. painful, pruritic papules at the site of inoculation.

27. Billy has come in contact with poison ivy on a school picnic. The BEST intervention for the nurse to implement at this time is:
   A. washing the area with a strong soap and water solution.
   B. applying Calamine lotion to the area.
   C. preventing spread by instructing Billy not to scratch the lesions.
   D. flushing the area immediately with cold water.

28. When advising parents about the use of sunscreen for their children, the nurse should tell them that:
   A. a waterproof sunscreen with a minimum 15 SPF is recommended for children.
   B. the lower the number of SPF the higher the protection.
   C. sunscreens are not as effective as sun blockers.
   D. the sunscreen should be applied one hour before the child is allowed in the sun.

29. Match the following term with the definition.

A. chilblain

B. frostbite

C. sunscreen

D. sunblocker

E. ultraviolet A (UVA)

F. ultraviolet B (UVB)

G. hypothermia

___D___ blocks out UV rays by reflecting sunlight

___C___ partially absorbs UV light

___F___ shorter waves, responsible for tanning, burning and most of the harmful effects attributed to sunlight

___E___ longest waves, causes only minimum burning but plays significant role in photosensitive and photoallergic reactions

___B___ ice crystals form in tissues

___A___ redness and swelling of the skin from cold exposure

___G___ cooling of the body's core temperature below 95° F

30. In caring for the child with frostbite, the nurse remembers that:
    A. slow thawing is associated with less tissue necrosis.
    B. the frostbitten part appears white or blanched, feels solid, and is without sensation.
    C. rewarming produces a small return of sensation with a small amount of pain.
    D. rewarming is accomplished by rubbing the injured tissue.

31. Skin disorders related to drug sensitivity include:
    A. impetigo.
    B. Stevens-Johnson syndrome.
    C. neurofibromatosis.
    D. all of the above.

32. Neurofibromatosis is:
    A. an autosomal dominant genetic disorder.
    B. suspected when the 5-year-old child presents with 6 or more cafe-au-lait spots larger than 5 mm in diameter.
    C. suspected when the infant develops axillary or inguinal freckling.
    D. all of the above.

33. Johnny's mother is calling the clinic because Johnny has developed a rash over his entire body. Two days ago Johnny was prescribed amoxicillin for an ear infection and now the mother tells the nurse she thinks Johnny may have gotten a small rash with this medication when he took it before. Which one of the following would be the BEST intervention by the nurse at this time?
    A. Question Johnny's mother about other symptoms that Johnny may have developed.
    B. Continue the medication and have Johnny come in tomorrow to see the practitioner.
    C. Stop the medication and inform the practitioner.
    D. Decrease the dose of the medication to one-half until Johnny can return to the clinic to see the practitioner.

34. Cindy is 12 years old and presents to the clinic because of a bald spot developing on her head. Cindy wears her hair tightly braided with beads. Which one of the following would the nurse suspect?
    A. Alopecia from trauma
    B. Tinea capitis
    C. Psoriasis
    D. Urticaria

35. The most effective method for tick removal in child is to:
    A. use a curved forcep and pull straight up with a steady, even pressure.
    B. apply mineral oil to the back of the tick and wait for it to back out.
    C. use the fingers to pull the tick out with a straight, steady, even pressure.
    D. place a hot match on the back of the tick and pick it up with gloved hands when the tick falls off.

36. Dog bites in children:
    A. occur most often in girls over 4 years.
    B. occur most often in children less than 4 years of age.
    C. occur most often from stray dogs.
    D. occur most often in school yards and neighborhood parks.

37. Nora has been brought to the emergency room by her father after getting bitten by the family dog. Exam shows three puncture wounds of the hand. Expected therapeutic management for these wounds includes:
    A. suturing the wounds.
    B. prophylactic antibiotics.
    C. hydrogen peroxide irrigations.
    D. administration of a tetanus toxoid booster since Nora's last booster was administered 13 months ago.

38. On a field trip to a remote area with his boy scout troop, Peter is bitten by a snake. Which one of the following actions would be CONTRAINDICATED?
    A. Remove Peter from the area and have him rest.
    B. Feel for a pulse distal to the bite area.
    C. Place ice from the ice cooler on the bite area.
    D. Apply a loose tourniquet above the bite area.

39. The MOST common cause of malocclusion is:
    A. thumb-sucking.
    B. tongue thrusting.
    C. hereditary.
    D. abnormal growth patterns.

40. Emergency care for tooth evulsion includes:
    A. replanting the tooth after bleeding has stopped.
    B. storing the tooth in tap water until it and the child can be transported to the dentist.
    C. holding the tooth by the root.
    D. rinsing the dirty tooth gently under running water before replanting.

41. The major nursing consideration in assisting the family of a child with nocturnal enuresis is to prevent the child from developing alterations in:
    A. body image.
    B. self-esteem.
    C. autonomy.
    D. peer acceptance.

42. The nurse is assisting the family of a child with a history of encopresis. Which one of the following should be included in the nurse's discussion with this family?
    A. Instructing the parents to sit the child on the toilet at twice daily routine intervals
    B. Instructing the parents that the child will probably need to have daily enemas for the next year
    C. Suggesting the use of stimulant cathartics weekly
    D. Reassuring the family that most problems resolve successfully with some relapses during periods of stress

43. Barbara has been diagnosed with attention deficit-hyperactivity disorder and placed on methylphenidate (Ritalin) by her physician. Which one of the following statements, if made by the nurse to Barbara's parents, is CORRECT?
    A. "This drug will ultimately lead to stimulation of the inhibitory system of the central nervous system by increasing dopamine and norepinephrine levels in the body."
    B. "Dosage is usually unchanged until adolescence."
    C. "This medication takes 2 to 3 weeks to achieve an effect."
    D. "Barbara's appetite will be increased with this drug."

44. Therapeutic management for tics in children primarily consists of:
    A. behavioral modification to teach the child to suppress the tic disorder.
    B. administration of haloperidol to suppress the tic disorder.
    C. education and support for the child and family with reassurance about the prognosis.
    D. genetic counseling for the parents.

45. Identify the following statements as TRUE or FALSE.

    __F__ School-phobia is more common in boys than in girls.

    __F__ School-phobia children are correctly viewed as delinquent children.

    __T__ A frequent source of fear in school phobia is separation anxiety based on a strong dependent relationship between the mother and the child.

    __T__ The primary goal for the child with school phobia is to return the child to school.

    __T__ Prevention of dependency problems in childhood is based on encouraging independence at appropriate times during infancy and early childhood.

    __T__ Recurrent abdominal pain of childhood is defined as three or more separate episodes of abdominal pain during a 3-month period.

    __T__ Children at risk for recurrent abdominal pain tend to be high achievers with great personal goals or whose parents have unusually high expectations.

    __T__ Depressed children usually exhibit low-esteem, think of themselves as hopeless, and explain negative events in terms of their personal shortcomings.

    __T__ Three risk factors identified for childhood schizophrenia are genetic characteristics, gestational and birth complications, and winter birth.

Critical Thinking • Case Study

Carol, age 9, went on a picnic yesterday with her family. Today she returns to school and is showing her classmates several leaves that she collected yesterday on her picnic. The teacher notes that three of the leaves are poison ivy. The teacher takes Carol to the school nurse because of a rash that has developed on Carol's arms and legs. Carol tells the nurse that the rash is "very itchy."

46. The nurse completes a diagnostic assessment of the skin rash to include a complete history and physical examination. The nurse knows that this history should include:
    A. inspection of the rash including size and shape of lesions.
    B. symptoms, past and recent exposure to causative agents, medications taken, and history of previous similar rashes.
    C. palpation of the rash for increased heat, edema, and tenderness.
    D. skin scrapings from the site for microscopic examination.

47. The primary action the school nurse should take at this time is:
    A. call Carol's parents to pick her up at school. Isolate Carol from other classmates until her parents arrive.
    B. give the poison ivy leaves to the school janitor so they can be destroyed in the school incinerator.
    C. instruct the teacher to make sure all classmates who had contact with the poison ivy plant wash these areas with mild soap and water.
    D. reassure Carol that everything is going to be fine, apply Calamine lotion to Carol's rash, and instruct Carol not to scratch the rash.

48. The BEST nursing diagnosis for Carol at this time would be:
    A. impaired skin integrity related to environmental factors.
    B. high risk for infection related to presence of infectious organisms.
    C. pain related to skin lesions.
    D. body image disturbance related to presence of rash.

49. Goals for Carol will include which of the following?
    A. Carol will not experience secondary damage, as infection, from scratching.
    B. Child will demonstrate acceptable levels of comfort from itching.
    C. Carol will be able to recognize and avoid precipitating agent in the future.
    D. All of the above

50. In educating Carol and her parents about caring for the rash, the nurse includes which of the following?
    1. bath in tepid or cool water
    2. bath in hot water
    3. apply hydrogen peroxide to the rash daily
    4. apply calamine lotion to the rash
    5. administer over-the-counter diphenhydramine orally to decrease itching
    6. keep fingernails short
    7. wear heavy clothing to prevent contamination
    8. rash will weep and is contagious

    A. 1, 3, 4, 6, and 7
    B. 1, 4, 5, and 6
    C. 2, 5, 6, and 7
    D. 3, 4, 5, and 8

CHAPTER 19

Health Promotion of the Adolescent and Family

1. In the female adolescent who has reached puberty, the lutenizing hormone (LH) initiates which of the following actions?
   A. Production of estrogen
   B. Growth of ovarian follicles
   C. Production of gonadotropin-releasing hormone
   D. Ovulation

2. The hormone in the female that causes growth and development of the vagina, uterus, and fallopian tubes and breast enlargement is:
   A. estrogen.
   B. progesterone.
   C. follicle stimulating hormone.
   D. lutenizing hormone.

3. Identify the following statements regarding adolescence as either TRUE or FALSE.

   ___T___ The adolescent is considered potentially fertile from the first menstrual period or first ejaculation.

   ___T___ Development of secondary sexual characteristics occurs in a predictable sequence.

   ___T___ The Tanner developmental stages is a classification system based on maturity of secondary sex characteristics that can be utilized when assessing adolescent growth.

   ___f___ Hypothalmic-pituitary-gonadal system is maintained in an active state throughout childhood because of the low secretion of gonadotropin-releasing hormone.

   ___T___ The development of small bud of breast tissue is the earliest, most easily visible change of puberty.

   ___f___ The average age for beginning menstruation is 13.

4. Match the term with its description.

A.	thelarche	__D__	menstrual periods begin
B.	adrenarche	__A__	development of breast tissue
C.	physiologic leukorrhea	__E__	male breast enlargement and tenderness
D.	menarche	__B__	development of pubic hair
E.	gynecomastia	__C__	normal vaginal discharge

5. Julie, 12 years old, is brought to the nurse practitioner's office by her mother. Julie has started to develop breast tissue and some pubic hair. Both the mother and Julie are concerned because Julie has been having increased vaginal discharge. Julie tells the nurse, "I wash my private area every day but I still have fluid that comes out." What is the nurse's BEST response?
   A. "It sounds like you have an infection. We'll have the nurse practitioner check you to see what is causing this discharge."
   B. "Have you been using soap when you wash?"
   C. "This sounds like a normal discharge that happens to all girls as they start to mature. It is a sign your body is preparing for your periods to begin."
   D. "This is probably not related to hygiene. Are you concerned that this discharge might be causing an odor?"

6. Girls may be considered to have __pubertal__ __delay__ if breast development has not occurred by age 13 or if menarche has not occurred within 4 years of the onset of breast development.

7. The first pubescent changes in boys is:
   A. appearance of pubic hair.
   B. testicular enlargement with thinning, reddening and increased looseness of the scrotum.
   C. penile enlargement.
   D. temporary breast enlargement and tenderness.

8. Tommy is brought in by his father for his yearly physical. On examination, the nurse notes that since last year Tommy has developed pubic hair, testicular enlargement and related scrotal changes. In planning anticipatory guidance, the nurse recognizes that which one of the following subjects would BEST be discussed with Tommy as soon as possible?
   A. Nocturnal emission
   B. Sexually transmitted disease prevention
   C. Pregnancy prevention
   D. Hygiene needs

9. The __growth spurt__ refers to the increased growth of muscles, skeleton and internal organs that peaks during puberty.

10. During assessment, the nurse observes that Gail has sparse growth of downy hair extending along the labia. Which of the following Tanner stages would be suspected?
    A. Stage 1
    B. Stage 2
    C. Stage 4
    D. Stage 5

11. Which one of the following statements about pattern of growth during adolescence is TRUE?
    A. Knowing the correct sequence of the growth pattern is only useful when assessing abnormal growth patterns versus normal growth patterns.
    B. Girls usually begin puberty and reach maturity about 2 years earlier than boys.
    C. Girls and boys start an increase of muscle mass during early puberty that lasts throughout adolescence.
    D. Girls and boys have an increase in linear growth that begins for both during midpuberty.

12. On the average, girls gain __2__ to __8__ inches in height and __15__ to __55__ pounds during adolescence, while boys gain __4__ to __12__ inches and __15__ to __65__ pounds.

13. Which one of the following BEST describes the formal operational thinking that occurs between the ages of 11 and 14 years?
    A. Thought process includes thinking in concrete terms.
    B. Thought process includes information obtained from the environment and peers.
    C. Thought process includes thinking in abstract terms, possibilities and hypotheses.
    D. Thought process is limited to what is observed.

14. Jimmy, a 13-year-old, is sent to the school nurse because he and some of his peers were caught chewing tobacco while playing baseball. The nurse knows that the BEST way to influence Jimmy's behavior for health promotion would be which of the following?
    A. Tell Jimmy that he will be suspended from school if he continues to chew the tobacco.
    B. Show Jimmy pictures of oral cancers from chewing tobacco.
    C. Tell Jimmy about the dangers of chewing tobacco and stress the fact that girls do not like boys who chew tobacco.
    D. Arrange for a local baseball hero to talk with Jimmy and his friends stressing that he does not use chewing tobacco, his friends do not chew tobacco, and that chewing tobacco causes ugly teeth.

15. Adolescent egocentrism may lead to a pattern of personal fable. An example of a personal fable is:
    A. "Everyone is coming to the play just to see me."
    B. "Mary Sue got pregnant but it won't happen to me."
    C. "I hate taking my clothes off for gym class because everyone stares at me."
    D. "Mary is very envious of how I dress."

16. Adolescents develop the social cognition change of mutual role taking. Which one of the following is the BEST description of this ability?
    A. Heightened sense of self-consciousness
    B. Understands the perspectives of others and that actions can influence others
    C. Beliefs are more abstract and rooted in ideologic principles
    D. Realization that others have thoughts and feelings

17. Elements of principled moral reasonings emerge during adolescence. Which one is the BEST description of this moral development?
    A. Moral guidelines are seen to emanate from authority figures.
    B. Moral standards are seen as objective and not to be questioned.
    C. Absolutes and rules are questioned and subject to disagreement.
    D. Development of a personal value system.

18. According to Erikson, a key to identity achievement in adolescence is BEST described as:
    A. related to the adolescent's interactions with others that serves as a mirror reflecting information back to the adolescent.
    B. linked to the role he/she plays within the family.
    C. related to the adolescent's acceptance of parental guidelines.
    D. related to the adolescent's ability to complete his/her plans for future accomplishments.

19. Expected characteristics of emotional autonomy during early adolescence include:
    A. increased independence from friends.
    B. increased need for parental approval.
    C. views parents as all-knowing and all-powerful.
    D. less emotional dependence on parents.

20. The formation of sexual identity development during adolescence usually involves which of the following?
    A. Forming close friendships with same-sex peers during early adolescence
    B. Developing intimate relationships with members of the opposite sex during the later part of adolescence
    C. Developing emotional and social identities separate from those of families
    D. All of the above

21. Nationally what percentage of boys and girls have had sexual intercourse by the twelfth grade?
    A. 67% of boys and 76% of girls
    B. 84% of boys and 58% of girls
    C. 67% of girls and 76% of boys
    D. 84% of girls and 58% of boys

22. Intimate relationships are NOT necessarily characterized by which one of the following?
    A. Concern for each other's well-being
    B. Sharing of sexual intimacy
    C. A willingness to disclose private, sensitive topics
    D. Sharing of common interests and activities

23. A cognitive coping strategy that is used to deal with feelings of attraction for the same sex and which involves vigorous attempts to find a "cure" is termed:
    A. denial.
    B. repair.
    C. avoidance.
    D. redefinition.

24. Changes in family structure and parent employment have resulted in certain changes for adolescents including:
    A. adolescents having more time unsupervised by adults.
    B. adolescents having more time for communication and intimacy with parents.
    C. adolescents having less time to spend with peers.
    D. adolescents requiring more supervision by outside family members.

25. Adolescents who feel close to their parents show:
    1. more positive psychosocial development.
    2. greater behavioral competence.
    3. less susceptibility to negative peer pressure.
    4. lower tendencies to be involved in risk-taking behaviors.

    A. 1, 3, and 4
    B. 1 and 2
    C. 3 and 4
    D. 1, 2, 3, and 4

26. Describe authoritative parenting and related results from this type of parenting.

_____

_____

_____

27. During adolescence, advances in cognitive development bring which one of the following changes?
    A. Their beliefs become more concrete and less rooted in general ideologic principles.
    B. They show an increasing emotional understanding and acceptance of parents' beliefs as their own.
    C. They encounter few new situations or opportunities for decisions because of their past experiences.
    D. They develop a personal value system distinct from that of significant adults in their lives.

28. As compared to children, adolescent peer groups are:
    A. more likely to include peers from the opposite sex.
    B. less autonomous.
    C. less likely to influence members' socialization roles.
    D. more likely to require parental supervision.

29. The timing of the transition from elementary school to junior high can be advantageous to the adolescent if it:
    A. occurs at the same time as the rapid physical changes of puberty.
    B. precedes the changes of puberty.

30. While Jenny, age 16, is in for her well check-up, her mother asks about Jenny getting a job at the local fast food restaurant. Jenny wants to work there 30 hours a week to earn extra money for clothes. Which one of the following is the nurse's best response?
    A. "Jenny is healthy and there is no reason she could not take the job."
    B. "All adolescents are preoccupied with clothes so let her go ahead."
    C. "Jenny, that is a dead end job, why would you want to work there?"
    D. "Involvement in work may take time away from studies, extracurricular activities and increase fatigue. Looking together at Jenny's future career goals may help identify alternatives."

31. List three primary causes of mortality accounting for 75% of all adolescent deaths.

    _____ injuries _____

    _____ homicide _____

    _____ suicide _____

32. To BEST effect adolescent health promotion activity, the nurse should incorporate which one of the following in the plan?
    A. The adolescent's definition of health
    B. The adolescent's past health promotion activities
    C. A complete assessment of the adolescent's past medical treatment
    D. A complete physical examination

33. Health concerns consistent with middle adolescents include:
    A. school performance.
    B. emotional health issues.
    C. physical appearance.
    D. future career or employment.

34. Adolescents are more likely to participate in health care services when:
    A. they feel confidentiality about sexual activity and substance abuse will be maintained.
    B. they see the health care provider as caring and respectful.
    C. the family has adequate financial resources including health insurance.
    D. all the above.

35. Identify the following statements as TRUE or FALSE.

    __T.__ Protective factors that characterize adolescents who cope successfully with adverse life situations include the ability to adapt to new persons and situations.

    __T__ The nurse involved with adolescent health promotion should plan interventions that decrease exposures to stressful life events and increase sources of emotional support.

    __F__ The most successful adolescent health promotion programs are aimed at single issues presented with a focused educational approach.

    __T__ When interviewing adolescents, the nurse begins with questions of a less sensitive nature and ends with those of a more sensitive area.

    __T__ For black teens the most likely cause of death is homicide.

    __F__ School-based clinics have not proven to increase adolescents' access to preventive services.

    __F__ All adolescents who participate in homosexual activity will become homosexual adults.

36. Three critical elements in establishing trusting relationships with adolescents during the health interview are: __listening__ ; __emotions__ ; __privacy__ .

37. During the adolescent health screening interview, the nurse will focus on which of the following to BEST address injury prevention?
    A. Drownings
    B. Burns
    C. Motor vehicle crashes
    D. Drug use

38. The most appropriate way to prevent firearm injury among adolescents is:
    A. teaching the adolescent proper use of the firearm.
    B. counseling the adolescent on nonviolent ways to resolve conflict.
    C. passing laws to prevent parents from having guns.
    D. telling parents to keep the gun and the ammunition in separate locations within the house.

39. Adolescent girls of low socioeconomic status are particularly at risk for dietary deficiencies of:
    1. calories
    2. sodium
    3. calcium
    4. folic acid
    5. iron

    A. 1, 2, and 3
    B. 2, 3, 4, and 5
    C. 3, 4, and 5
    D. 1, 3, and 5

40. List four risk factors that should be targeted in the adolescent to prevent the development of adult cardiovascular disease.

    _____

    _____

    _____

    _____

41. Susan, age 15 years, comes to the school-based clinic and complains to the nurse practitioner about a vaginal discharge. After establishing a trusting and confidential relationship with Susan, Susan confides in the nurse that she has been active with 3 different partners within the past 6 months. Susan thinks they used condoms every time but she is not sure. Her last menses was three weeks ago and she had a pap test a little over 2 months ago. What tests would the nurse assisting the nurse practitioner expect to prepare for?
    1. Pap test
    2. gonorrhea infection
    3. chlamydial infection
    4. HIV
    5. pregnancy test
    6. syphilis test

    A. 1, 2, 3, and 4
    B. 2, 3, 4, and 6
    C. 2, 3, and 5
    D. 1, 2, 3, and 6

Carol, a 16 year old, visits the nurse practitioner for a routine checkup. She is an A and B student in school and a member of the girls' drill team. Carol matured early and started to menstruate at the age of 10. Her menses are now regular. Carol has a boyfriend and has been dating since the age of 13. She tells the nurse she has no specific concern.

42. Based on risk factors associated with teens Carol's age, the nurse recognizes which one of the following as the MOST important to discuss with Carol at this visit?
    A. Carol's perception and concerns about health
    B. Carol's nutritional habits
    C. Carol's sexual activity
    D. Carol's relationship with her family

43. The nurse establishes a trusting relationship with Carol, and Carol admits to having been sexually active with five boys since she started dating. Besides educating Carol on the risks of sexually transmitted diseases and pregnancy, which one of the following is MOST important for the nurse to include in her plan of care for Carol at this time?
    A. Discuss with Carol how she can tell her parents about her sexual activity.
    B. Explore possible reasons for Carol's behavior with her.
    C. Assess Carol's immunization status for Hepatitis B.
    D. Assess how Carol feels about the possibility of getting pregnant.

44. Mrs. Smith complains to you that her 15-year-old son, Ben, has begun to drift away from the family and find fault with everything she and her husband do. She is worried about the relationship between them and Ben and doesn't understand what she and her husband have done wrong. "Why does Ben seem to suddenly dislike us so much?" Based on your knowledge of the adolescent, which one of the following would be the BEST explanation?
    A. "Ben's behavioral standards are set by his peer group and he is acting this way because of fear of rejection by this group."
    B. "Ben is defining his moral values and parents will need to have the same moral values as Ben if they want to continue to be close to him."
    C. "Ben is developing the capacity for abstract thinking and increasing his concern about social issues. He will return to share parental views shortly."
    D. "Ben is defining independence-dependence boundaries and beginning to disengage from parents."

45. Christy, age 14, comes to the clinic for a physical exam. It has been longer than two years since her last exam. Upon review of Christy's immunization record, the nurse notes that Christy had a diphtheria-tetanus (DT) booster at age 4 years and a measles-mumps-rubella (MMR) vaccine at age 15 months. Christy has been healthy in the past with normal childhood diseases including varicella. Which of the following immunizations would you expect Christy to receive today?
    A. Influenza, pneumococcal, and chickenpox
    B. MMR, hepatitis B, and hepatitis A
    C. MMR, DT, and hepatitis B
    D. Mantoux tuberculin, hepatitis B, and hepatitis A

CHAPTER 20
Physical Health Problems of Adolescence

1. Which one of the following current beliefs about acne formation is TRUE?
   A. Cosmetics containing lanolin and lauryl alcohol are not known to contribute to acne formation.
   B. There is scientific research to support the theory that stress will cause an acne outbreak.
   C. Exposure to oils in cooking grease can be a precursor to acne in adolescents working over fast-food restaurant oils.
   D. Acne usually worsens with dietary intake of chocolates and other foods high in sugars.

2. Nancy, age 16 years, presents to the nurse because of acne on her face, shoulders and neck areas. After talking with Nancy, the nurse makes a nursing diagnosis of knowledge deficit, related to proper skin care. Which one of the following would the nurse include in the instruction plan for Nancy?
   A. Wash the areas vigorously with antibacterial soaps.
   B. Brush the hair down on the forehead to conceal the acne areas.
   C. Avoid the use of all cosmetics.
   D. Gently wash the areas with a mild soap once or twice daily.

3. The practitioner has prescribed Retin-A for Nancy's acne, and Nancy returns for a follow-up visit after one month of treatment. During the nursing assessment, Nancy tells the nurse that she has "done everything" that she was told to do and asks, "Why is my acne no better?" The nurse's BEST reply is:
   A. "Since the medication prevents the formation of new comedones, it will take at least six weeks for improvement to be obvious."
   B. "You must not be using the medication right. Show me how you apply it to your face."
   C. "Acne is caused by dirt or oil on the surface of the skin. You will need to increase the number of times you wash these areas each day."
   D. "You will probably need to ask the practitioner about changing your medicine as soon as possible."

4. The nurse is conducting an educational session with Cindy and her parents on medications used for acne. Which one of the following is CORRECT information?
   A. Tretinoin gel has a bleaching effect on bed coverings and towels.
   B. Topical clindamycin is applied only to the individual lesions.
   C. Oral contraceptive medications contain estrogen which will increase acne formation and should be avoided.
   D. Tretinoin requires that Cindy protect herself from sun exposure.

5. In which of the following adolescents, diagnosed with acne, is the use of Accutane CONTRAINDICATED?
    A. Joseph, age 18, with cystic acne unresponsive to other treatments; past medical history reflects no serious illness; currently on no medications
    B. Janice, age 18, with nodular acne lesions; past medical history reflects no serious illness; history of irregular menses; currently on no medications
    C. Sylvia, age 17, with cystic and nodular acne lesions; past medical history reflects no serious illness; menses regular; current medications includes birth control pills for the past 2 years
    D. All of the above

6. The most common solid tumor in males 15 to 34 years of age is:
    A. varicocele.
    B. testicular torsion.
    C. priapism.
    D. testicular cancer.

7. The adolescent with testicular cancer is MOST likely to present with which one of the following signs and symptoms?
    A. Tender, painful swelling of the testes
    B. A mass in the posterior aspect of the scrotum that transilluminates
    C. Heavy, hard, painless, mass palpable on the anterior or lateral surface of the testicle
    D. Asymptomatic scrotal mass that aches especially after exercise or penile erection

8. In teaching the adolescent male how to perform testicular self-examination, the nurse includes which of the following in the instructions?
    A. Perform the procedure once a month after a warm shower.
    B. A raised swelling palpated on the superior aspect of the testicle indicates an abnormality.
    C. Use the 2nd and 3rd fingers on each hand, holding each testicle between the fingers while it is palpated with the other fingers.
    D. All of the above

9. The nurse knows that which of the following adolescent females should be scheduled for her first pelvic examination?
    1. the 16-year-old who has not become sexually active
    2. the adolescent who has been menstruating for 2 years
    3. the adolescent who wants to start birth control pills
    4. the 18-year-old who has not become sexually acitive
    5. the sexually active adolescent

    A. 1, 3, and 5
    B. 2, 3, and 5
    C. 3 and 5
    D. 3, 4, and 5

10. Match the term with its definition. (Terms may be used more than once.)

A. varicocele

B. epididymitis

C. testicular torsion

D. gynecomastia

___D___ breast enlargement that occurs during puberty

___A___ is palpated as a wormlike mass above the testicle that becomes smaller in size when the adolescent lies down

___D___ treatment includes assurance to the adolescent that the disease is benign and temporary and occurs in about 50% of his peers

___B___ inflammation that is a result of either infection or local trauma

___C___ the testis hangs free from its vascular structure; results in partial or complete venous occlusion

___B___ presents with unilateral scrotal pain, redness, and swelling; may have urethral discharge, dysuria, fever and pyuria; treatment is with antibiotics

___C___ presents with scrotum that is swollen, painful, red, and warm; adolescent will have pain radiating to groin, with nausea, vomiting and abdominal pain; fever and urinary symptoms are usually not present; treatment is immediate surgery

11. ___primary___ ___amenorrhea___ is defined as an absence of menses by age 17.

___secondary___ ___amenorrhea___ is defined as an absence of menses for six months in a previously menstruating female when pregnancy has been excluded.

12. Linda, age 16, started her menses at age 13 years. She now presents at the school-based clinic with a history of secondary amenorrhea. Linda is an honors student and a long distance runner averaging 50 miles per week. The physical exam is normal and Linda has been requested to decrease her running distance and improve nutrition. She is given a follow-up visit and told if her menses are not more regulated, oral birth control pills will be prescribed. Linda wants to know why she would have to take the pills since she is not sexually active. How would you respond?

_____

_____

13. The treatment of choice for adolescents with dysmenorrhea is:

A. acetaminophen.

B. oral contraceptives.

C. nonsteroidal antiinflammatory drugs.

D. estrogen suppression drugs.

14. Adverse effects of exercise on an adolescent's reproductive cycle can include:

A. delayed menarche.

B. anovulation associated with dysfunctional uterine bleeding.

C. amenorrhea.

D. all of the above.

15. Match the term with its description.

A. dysmenorrhea
B. premenstrual syndrome
C. endometriosis
D. dysfunctional uterine bleeding
E. vaginitis candidiasis
F. pelvic inflammatory disease
G. trichomonas vaginalis
H. oligomenorrhea
I. leukorrhea

___B___ It has more than 100 associated physical, psychologic, and behavioral symptoms.

___C___ It may be caused by the presence of endometrial tissue outside the uterine cavity.

___D___ abnormal vaginal bleeding usually associated with anovulation

___A___ painful menses

___H___ abnormally light or infrequent menstruation

___F___ infection of the upper genital tract commonly caused by gonorrhea or chlamydia

___E___ It may present with vaginal pruritus and dysuria and is not an STD.

___G___ anaerobic parasitic protozoan; is an STD

___I___ glutinous, gray-white vaginal discharge caused by physical, chemical or infectious agents

16. Gail has been diagnosed with vaginitis. The nurse is preparing to instruct Gail on prevention. Describe what information the nurse would include in her instructions.

_____

_____

17. Indicate whether the following statements are TRUE or FALSE.

___T___ More than two thirds of high school students report having had sexual intercourse by their senior year in high school.

___T___ The resulting social outcomes of adolescent sexual risk taking are teenage pregnancy and STDs.

___F___ The pregnancies of adolescents less than 15 years old are less frequently complicated by obstetric problems.

___F___ Adolescent mothers are just as likely to complete high school as other adolescents.

___F___ Obstetric risk and risk to the infant during a second pregnancy for the teenager is lower.

___T___ Teens age 12 to 16 years are at high risk for prolonged labor related to fetopelvic incompatibility.

___T___ Pregnant adolescents have diets often deficient in iron, calcium and folic acid.

18. The nurse knows that which of the following adolescents would be at high-risk for pregnancy?
A. Those who have early initiation of sexual activity
B. The adolescent who does not use a reliable method of contraception regularly
C. The adolescent female who has poor school performance
D. All of the above

19. Infants of adolescents are at risk because:
    A. teenage mothers often neglect their infants, leaving them for long periods with grandparents.
    B. teenage mothers supply excessive amounts of cognitive stimulation to their infants.
    C. adolescents lack knowledge of normal infant growth and development.
    D. adolescents are less likely to treat their infant as love objects or playthings.

20. The first goal in nursing care of the pregnant teenager is:
    A. to arrange for the pregnant teen to register for food supplement programs to assure proper nutrition.
    B. to assist the pregnant teen in obtaining prenatal care.
    C. to involve the boyfriend and parents in the pregnancy so the pregnant teen will have support during her pregnancy.
    D. to educate the pregnant teen regarding child care.

21. Postpartum care of adolescents should be directed toward:
    A. preventing subsequent pregnancies.
    B. reestablishment with high school counselors for completion of education.
    C. arranging for childcare classes.
    D. increasing father interactions with the new mother and the newborn.

22. Emily is an unmarried 17-year-old who is six weeks pregnant and who has decided to have an abortion. One nursing action used to assist Emily would be:
    A. explaining to Emily that it is wrong for her to have an abortion and arranging for Emily to visit an adoption center.
    B. referral of Emily to an appropriate abortion agency when Emily is four months pregnant.
    C. providing Emily with relaxation strategies to be used during the procedure.
    D. calling Emily's parents so they can be present for the abortion.

23. In discussing prevention of sexually transmitted diseases, the nurse tells the adolescent that which one of the following is MOST effective?
    A. Birth control pills
    B. Norplant
    C. Spermicides
    D. Condoms

24. Nancy, age 17, is brought to the family planning clinic by her mother for birth control. Which one of the following does the nurse recognize as being MOST important to include in her plan with Nancy at this time?
    A. Discussion of the effectiveness rates for various methods and importance of compliance
    B. Including Nancy's partner in the discussions
    C. Discussion of Nancy's perception of likelihood of getting pregnant and her desire to prevent pregnancy versus her desire for pregnancy
    D. Cost of the various methods of contraception

25. Which of the following is NOT recommended as a method of birth control in Nancy, age 17 years?
    A. Intrauterine device
    B. Sponge
    C. Depo-Provera
    D. Diaphragm

26. The nurse is conducting a sexual education program. What technique has been found helpful when dealing with the subject of sexual abstinence?

_____

27. Rape victims display a variety of manifestations. Which of the following might the nurse see in 16-year-old Sally as she arrives at the emergency center for treatment?
    A. Hysterical crying or giggling
    B. Calm and controlled behavior
    C. Anger and rage alternating with helplessness and agitation
    D. All of the above

28. The primary goal of nursing care for the adolescent rape victim is:
    A. not to inflict further stress on the victim.
    B. obtaining a complete history of the incident.
    C. assisting in the physical examination.
    D. notifying the police and the parents of the victim before proceeding with assessment.

29. Identify the following statements about sexually transmitted diseases in adolescence as TRUE or FALSE.

    ___F___ Adolescent females are at a lower risk for chlamydia and human papilloma virus because of the immature adolescent endocervix.

    ___F___ In the adolescent, the immune system provides excellent localized antibody response to infectious agents at the cervical level.

    ___T___ Research has demonstrated that as the use of hormonal contraception increases, the use of condoms declines among adolescents.

    ___T___ Adolescents age 15 to 19 have the highest overall incidence of gonococcal infection.

    ___T___ Symptoms of gonorrhea can occur 1 day to 16 days after sexual contact, or there may be no symptoms.

    ___T___ Use of ciprofloxacin for treating gonorrhea is contraindicated in the adolescent with incomplete sexual development.

    ___F___ Collection of a specimen from the cervix for gonorrhea must be delayed until the adolescent is not on her menses.

    ___F___ Treatment for gonorrhea includes both the partner and the client and provides life-long immunity.

    ___T___ A major effect of sexually transmitted diseases among adolescent females is impairment of fertility as a result of scarring of the fallopian tubes.

30. Therapeutic management for chlamydia includes:
    A. doxycycline, 100 mg bid for 7 days in the pregnant adolescent and her partner.
    B. intramuscular injection of ceftriaxone (rocephrin) 125 mg for the client and partner.
    C. intramuscular injection of penicillin 2.4 million units for the client and partner.
    D. azithromycin 1 gram po in a single dose for the client and her partner.

31. Shirley, age 17, has been diagnosed with pelvic inflammatory disease caused by gonorrhea. The nurse can expect treatment to include which one of the following?
    A. Immediate inpatient hospitalization
    B. Shirley to be given ceftriaxone (rocephrin) intramuscularly with oral antibiotics as outpatient treatment for 14 days
    C. No treatment of Shirley's partner will be necessary
    D. Shirley to be placed on oral contraceptives

32. The most common STD in the United States is _____. These individuals are at risk for development of _____ and _____.

33. One STD for which there is an immunization recommended for all adolescents is:
    A. human immunodeficiency virus.
    B. hepatitis B virus.
    C. syphilis.
    D. herpes simplex type 2 virus.

34. Connie, age 15 has requested information about prevention of sexually transmitted diseases. As the nurse begins to discuss HIV and AIDS, Connie tells the nurse to skip information on this topic. Based on knowledge about adolescents, which one of the following is the MOST likely reason for Connie's response?
    A. Connie does not think she has at risk behavior for AIDS.
    B. Connie already knows as much about AIDS as is necessary.
    C. Connie is not sexually active.
    D. Connie wants information about birth control but is afraid to ask.

Critical Thinking • Case Study

Bryan, age 14, has come to the clinic because he has started breaking out on his face, chest, and shoulders with acne. He says he is embarrassed to go out because his friends stare at him and that girls avoid him. The physician has started medical treatment and sent him to you for further guidance.

35. Based on the above information, a priority nursing diagnosis for Bryan at this time would be:
    A. altered family process related to the adolescent with a skin problem.
    B. body image disturbance related to perception of acne lesions.
    C. bathing/hygiene self-care deficient related to skin care.
    D. altered role performance related to perceived peer separation.

36. The BEST goal for Bryan would be which of the following?
    A. Will have a positive body image
    B. Will receive appropriate education for hygiene
    C. Will have a reduction in dietary fat and calories
    D. Will receive appropriate referral to skin specialist

37. Subjective data collection should include which of the following?
    A. Family history of acne
    B. Location and size description of visible lesions
    C. Culture and sensitivity for identifying organism
    D. All of the above

38. The nurse has established a plan of care with Bryan. Which one of the following would be an expected component of the plan to improve Bryan's body image?
    A. Help adolescent find mechanisms to reduce emotional stress.
    B. Explain the disorder and therapy prescribed to increase family understanding.
    C. Emphasize the positive aspects, as well as limited nature of the disorder, and assist with grooming to enhance appearance.
    D. Discourage peer relationship until the adolescent has improved facial appearance from medication.

Sixteen-year-old Jenny is pregnant and coming to the school-based clinic for prenatal care. Jenny and the baby's father, Doug, are still seeing each other but their relationship has "cooled" since Jenny found out she was pregnant.

39. As the nurse assists Jenny to prepare for the physical exam, the nurse notes that Jenny does not mention her infant but only talks about herself. Based on knowledge about pregnant adolescents the nurse would:
   A. bring Jenny's behavior to the immediate attention of the practitioner.
   B. call Jenny's parents and boyfriend to see how she has been behaving at home.
   C. realize that adolescents have egocentrism behaviors that focus mainly on themselves.
   D. discuss with Jenny why she does not care about her baby.

40. The nurse is planning for prenatal and child rearing classes that could include both Jenny and Doug attending. Based on knowledge of adolescent fathers the nurse would:
   A. realize that adolescent fathers have little association with their infants.
   B. understand that adolescent fathers want to start breaking the contact with the adolescent mother and Doug will refuse to go.
   C. realize that Doug is still most influenced by his male peer friends and is embarrassed by getting Jenny pregnant and will not go.
   D. realize that active participation in the pregnancy by the adolescent father may enhance his ability to define his role in the life of the child.

41. Which one of the following statements if made by Jenny would reflect the concept of personal fable and could lead to risk taking behaviors?
   A. "I don't want to get a STD, so it won't happen to me."
   B. "Only girls that are permissive get STDs."
   C. " Abstinence is the only way to prevent an STD."
   D. "All my friends have sex."

CHAPTER 21
Behavioral Health Problems of Adolescence

1. Identify the following statements as either TRUE or FALSE.

   A. _____ The number of fat cells may be established at an early age, and overfeeding during this time may have a significant influence on the development of obesity at a later age.

   B. _____ Obesity is the most common nutritional disturbance of children.

   C. _____ During the adolescent growth spurt, the distribution of fat in girls decreases sharply.

   D. _____ Obesity refers to the state of weighing more than average for height and body build and may or may not include an increased amount of fat.

   E. _____ Birth weight is an indicator of childhood obesity.

   F. _____ In Prader-Willi syndrome, children manifest slow intellectual development, short stature, obesity, and will go to great lengths to obtain food.

   G. _____ Obesity in adolescents can be caused by overeating or low activity levels.

   H. _____ Obese persons eat more at a given sitting and tend to eat more rapidly than those who are not obese.

   I. _____ Obese adolescents are characteristically night eaters and skip meals, especially breakfast.

   J. _____ Obese children are often from families in which large meals are emphasized or children are scolded for leaving food on their plates.

   K. _____ Being obese in childhood and adolescence is a significant risk factor for adult obesity.

2. Gail, age 14, comes to the school nurse's office because she is obese and wants to lose weight. The nurse's assessment will include:
   A. Gail's physical activity.
   B. dietary intake and meal patterns for Gail.
   C. eating patterns of Gail's family.
   D. all of the above.

3. Adolescents with obesity have common emotional problems of:
   A. poor body image.
   B. low self-esteem.
   C. social isolation and feelings of rejection.
   D. all of the above.

4. List three factors that can contribute to the development of a disturbed body image in the obese adolescent.

   _____

   _____

   _____

5. Using standard growth charts, ideal body weight is estimated as _____ percentile weight for the child's age, gender and height.

Obesity is often defined as the child's actual body weight greater than _____ percent of the ideal body weight for height and age.

Percent of _____ _____ _____ is calculated by dividing the child's actual weight in kilograms by the growth chart's 50th percentile weight or the child's age.

6. Weight reduction management in adolescent should include:
   A. significant caloric restriction.
   B. elimination of physical hunger cues.
   C. regular physical activity.
   D. appetite-suppressant drugs.

7. Janie, age 14 years, wants to discuss with the nurse how to modify her eating habits to reduce her weight. Which one of the following methods does the nurse recognize as LEAST helpful in assisting Janie to meet her goals?
   A. Have Janie keep a list of everything she eats.
   B. Request that Janie's parents remind Janie not to eat junk foods.
   C. Establish a system of rewards for changes in eating habits.
   D. Discuss with Janie methods other than eating than can be used to deal with emotional stress.

8. The age range for anorexia nervosa is _____ to _____ years. This disorder is characterized by _____ .

9. Individuals with bulimia are classified into two categories: those that _____ and those that _____.

10. Cindy, age 16, has been sent to the school nurse because her gym teacher has noticed a marked decrease in Cindy's weight since vacation. Which one of the following does the nurse recognize as a common finding among adolescent girls with anorexia nervosa?
    A. Wears form-fitting clothes like tank tops and jeans
    B. Has strong peer relationships with classmates and several best friends
    C. Has poor schoolwork performance because of little interest in school
    D. Is present at meals, selects foods, and appears to family and friends to be eating appropriately

11. Cindy has been diagnosed with anorexia nervosa. Her therapeutic management plan includes hospitalization. Which one of the following would the nurse recognize as a possible reaction of Cindy to the treatment plan?
    A. High energy level activity participation, especially with marked preoccupation with food preparation
    B. Becoming dependent on her parents, especially her mother
    C. Attempts to control the situation and views the treatment plan as an attempt to remove her autatomy
    D. Regards her appearance as abnormal or ugly

12. Cindy is about to be discharged after treatment for anorexia nervosa. The nurse has formulated a nursing diagnosis related to family coping with a goal that the family will be prepared for home care. Which one of the following interventions would best help meet this goal?
   A. Make certain both patient and family understand the therapeutic plan.
   B. Observe family interaction for assessment of family coping patterns.
   C. Explore feelings and attitudes of family members.
   D. Convey an attitude of caring and acceptance to family and patient.

13. Bulimia is observed most frequently in _____ _____.
   _____ bulimics are uncommon.

14. Which one of the following does the nurse recognize as being an adolescent group at high risk for bulimia?
   A. Adolescents in the lower socioeconomic level
   B. Adolescents who want to be tough muscular football players
   C. Adolescents who aspire to careers that require low weight
   D. Adolescents with good self-image

15. Karen is suspected of being bulimic. The nurse recognizes which of the following as clinical manifestations of this disease?
   A. Often starts with decreased dietary intake because of poor relationships with family members
   B. Once started, the binges decrease in frequency to only about 2 to 3 times per day
   C. Insulin production is decreased because of excessive self-induced vomiting
   D. May have a caloric intake of 20,000 to 30,000 calories per day

16. The patient with bulimia must be watched by the nurse for medical complications. Which one of the following does the nurse recognize as needing IMMEDIATE intervention?
   A. Backs of the hands scarred and cut from self-induced vomiting
   B. Potassium depletion from diuretic abuse
   C. Erosion of teeth enamel from self-induced vomiting
   D. Chronic esophagitis from self-induced vomiting

17. In treating the adolescent with bulimia, the integration of medical, psychologic and nutritional approaches are essential. What group of antidepressants has been shown to diminish the obsessive-compulsive urge to binge and vomit in some adolescent patients?

   _____

18. Identify the following statements about substance abuse as either TRUE or FALSE.
   A. _____ A person may be physically dependent on a narcotic without being addicted.
   B. _____ The adolescent abusing drugs has often adopted the use of a substance as a means of coping with feelings of depression, boredom, and emptiness.
   C. _____ Identification of the pattern of drug use in the adolescent is essential but offers little help in developing a successful approach to the problem.
   D. _____ The usual goal for the compulsive drug user is one of peer acceptance.
   E. _____ One of the hazards associated with drug use is the risk of injury while driving under the influence of the drug.

19. Which one of the following adolescents does the nurse recognize as LEAST likely to begin smoking?
    A. Johnny, age 16 years, whose Dad quit smoking 2 years ago
    B. Karen, age 13 years, whose older sister smokes
    C. Ted, age 17 years, who smoked a cigarette at home in front of his parents
    D. Lilly, age 12, who feels uncomfortable with her early maturing body

20. Johnny, age 16, has tried his first cigarette because of peer pressure to "look cool." What stage of becoming a smoker might the nurse label Johnny?
    A. Preparation
    B. Initiation
    C. Experimentation
    D. Regular smoking

21. The school nurse is planning an educational program centered on smoking prevention for junior high school adolescents. Which of the following methods does the nurse recognize as the MOST effective way to present this program?
    A. Ban smoking in the school.
    B. Teach methods of resistance to peer pressure.
    C. Use peer-led programs that emphasize social consequences.
    D. Use media videotapes and films on smoking prevention.

22. Identify one of the following statements as TRUE.
    A. Smokeless tobacco is a safe alternative to cigarette smoking.
    B. Smokeless tobacco is often linked to periodontal disease and lesions in the oral soft tissue.
    C. Smokeless tobacco is not addictive.
    D. Smokeless tobacco users are less likely to become cigarette smokers.

23. Adolescent alcoholics are often described as:
    A. hard to live with and indecisive.
    B. good students with a strong desire to complete school.
    C. rarely denying their problem.
    D. having poor role models but excellent peer relations.

24. Protective factors have been identified as helping adolescents at risk to resist pressures to use drugs and alcohol. List 5 recognized protective factors.

    _____

    _____

    _____

25. The motivation phase of treatment and rehabilitation of young drug users is directed toward:
    A. assessment of the drug habits and amount of drugs used.
    B. exploring the factors that influence drug use.
    C. prevention of relapse into drug use.
    D. all of the above.

26. Complete the following statements about drug abuse.

   A. The form of cocaine known as the purer and more menacing form is _____.

   B. Cocaine taken by _____ is associated with the highest levels of dependence.

   C. Cocaine is a potent _____ and the crash after a cocaine high usually consists of _____ .

   D. Physical signs of narcotic abuse include: _____ _____.

   E. _____ also known as the "date rape drug" is 10 times more powerful than diazepam and produces short-term memory loss.

   F. _____ with the street name of "crank" and "crystal" produces more excitement than cocaine and the user can remain "up" for hours.

   G. Inhalant abuse usually gives the child an inexpensive euphoria but is extremely dangerous and can cause _____.

27. The increase in suicide and depression during adolescence may be due to:
   A. expected low self-esteem among this population.
   B. the importance of peer pressures among this group.
   C. cognitive development and the ability to observe one's self.
   D. higher substance abuse among this group.

28. Jim, who has no history of previous suicide attempt, is talking with the school nurse about his feelings of despair and hopelessness about the future. He tells the nurse he would be better off dead. The nurse's BEST response is which one of the following?
   A. Recognize that Jim is going through a common phase of adolescence.
   B. Recognize that Jim is at low risk for suicide since he has not previously attempted suicide.
   C. Explain to Jim that suicide never solved anything and that he will feel better tomorrow.
   D. Take Jim seriously, allow time for Jim to verbalize his feelings, and stay with Jim until referral.

29. The nurse has been asked to present an educational program on prevention of adolescent stress and suicide. In planning the program the nurse should include:
   A. the importance of being supportive and establishing positive communication patterns between family and teens.
   B. the precipitating factors for suicide.
   C. effective coping mechanisms and problem-solving skills.
   D. all of the above.

30. Mark, age 14 years, has been rushed to the emergency department because of illegal drug ingestion at a party. Which of the following data is MOST important for the nurse to collect to assist in the emergency treatment plan?
    1. the type and amount of drug taken
    2. the time the drug was taken and mode of administration
    3. number of times Mark has previously overdosed
    4. why the drug was taken

    A. 1 and 2
    B. 1, 2, and 3
    C. 1 only
    D. 1, 2, 3, and 4

31. Match the term with its description.

    A. suicidal ideation
    B. suicide attempt
    C. parasuicide
    D. suicide
    E. contagion suicide
    F. obesity
    G. overweight
    H. anorexia nervosa
    I. bulimia

    _____ behaviors ranging from gestures to serious attempts to kill oneself
    _____ increase in body weight from excess fat
    _____ deliberate act of self-injury with death as result
    _____ deliberate act of self-injury but is unsuccessful
    _____ weighing more than average for height and body build
    _____ thoughts about killing oneself
    _____ results because of excessive media coverage after an adolescent suicide
    _____ deny the existence of hunger
    _____ binge eating followed by purging

Critical Thinking • Case Study

Kenny, 16 years of age, visits the clinic for follow-up of a recent infection. While talking with the nurse, he tells her that he has recently broken up with his girlfriend after going steady for 11 months. Kenny has a history of having a difficult home situation. His recent school performance has declined, and this has further upset Kenny's parents and their expectations for Kenny. Physical exam of Kenny reveals an expressionless face with a slight smell of alcohol on his breath and signs consistent with depression.

32. You suspect that Kenny might be suicidal. Which factors in the above data might support this assumption?
    1. alcohol consumption
    2. recent break up with girlfriend
    3. history of difficult home situation
    4. depression
    5. age and gender

    A. 1, 2, 3, and 4
    B. 2, 3, and 4
    C. 2, 4, and 5
    D. 1, 2, 3, 4, and 5

33. Upon questioning by the nurse, Kenny admits to suicidal ideation. What should the nurse first assess to determine risk?
    A. History of suicide attempts within the family
    B. Past methods of coping with stress by the individual
    C. Whether Kenny has a plan for suicide
    D. Whether Kenny has a gun available to him

34. Which one of the following nursing diagnoses would the nurse develop to BEST deal with Kenny's suicide thoughts?
    A. High risk for injury related to feelings of rejection
    B. Sleep pattern disturbance related to inability to sleep
    C. Social isolation related to withdrawal from friends
    D. High risk for self-directed violence related to excessive alcohol use

35. The MOST important goal in the nursing management for Kenny at this time should focus on:
    A. reestablishing Kenny's relationship with his girlfriend.
    B. teaching Kenny how to cope with the stress of being an adolescent.
    C. maintaining physical safety for Kenny.
    D. assisting Kenny to express his emotional pain and regain his ability to perform assigned tasks.

CHAPTER 22
Family-Centered Care of the Child with Chronic Illness or Disability

1. Match the term or definition with the best description of that term. Use each term only once.

   A. chronic illness   D. handicap   G. home care
   B. developmental delay   E. impairment   H. normalization
   C. disability   F. technology dependent   I. mainstreaming

   ___D___ a barrier imposed by society

   ___H___ principle that permits disabled children to remain a part of their community

   ___F___ a child that requires the routine use of a medical device for support of a bodily function

   ___A___ a condition that interferes with daily functioning for more than three months

   ___C___ physical or mental impairment substantially limiting one or more major life activities

   ___G___ a system of care that minimizes the disruptive impact of the child's condition on the family

   ___B___ a maturational lag

   ___I___ process that has largely resulted from the passage Public Law 94-142, the Education for All Handicapped Children Act of 1975

   ___E___ a loss or abnormality of a structure or function

2. Programs for Individuals with Special Needs—Matching

   A. Education for all   C. Individual Education   E. Individual Family
       Handicapped Children   Program (IEP)   Service Plan (IFSP)
       Act of 1975   D. The Education of the   F. Americans with
   B. Individuals with   Handicapped Act   Disabilities Act (ADA)
       Disabilities Education   Amendments of 1986
       Act (IDEA)

   ___B___ the 1990 amendment to the Education of all Handicapped Children Act of 1975 that changed its name

   ___F___ requires daycare providers to make "reasonable modifications" for equal access to program participation

   ___C___ the approach where a multi disciplinary team designs special education and therapeutic strategies and goals for each eligible child

   ___E___ developed jointly by families and professionals; includes information about the infant/toddler's present level of development, family strengths and needs relating to enhancing development, major outcomes expected, services needed, identification of a case manager, and transition steps to preschool services

   ___A___ the Public Law that is largely responsibly for the development of a variety of supplemental programs in the school system to accommodate children with special needs

   ___D___ directs states to develop and implement statewide comprehensive, coordinated, multi disciplinary interagency programs of early intervention services for infants and toddlers with disabilities as well as support services for their families

3. The Impact on the Child and Family—Matching

A. Special Olympics
B. Very Special Arts
C. Coping Health Inventory For Parents (CHIPS)
D. approach behaviors
E. avoidance behaviors
F. trajectory model
G. family management styles
H. guilt
I. anger/bitterness
J. overprotection
K. rejection
L. denial
M. gradual acceptance
N. chronic sorrow
O. functional burden
P. Programs for Children with Special Health Needs

__B__ normalization that offers disabled children an opportunity to celebrate and share their accomplishments in a variety of expressive activities such as art, music, poetry, dance and drama

__N__ an emotional response of parents manifested throughout the life span of the disabled or chronically ill child; acceptance is interspersed with periods of intensified grieving for the loss; typically seen at each period of the child's development, when the parent is again reminded of what could have been

__C__ an 80 item checklist providing self-report information about how parents perceive their overall response to the management of family life with a child with a chronic illness

__A__ a program that offers children with physical disabilities an opportunity to compete with their peers and to achieve athletic skill

__D__ those coping mechanisms that result in movement toward adjustment and resolution of the crisis

__F__ a theory about chronic illness that acknowledges that the condition has a course that varies and changes over time

__H__ self accusation; a feeling that is often greatest when the cause of a disorder is directly traceable to the parent such as in genetic disease

__O__ a concept that considers the issues related to caring for and living with the chronically ill/disabled child in relation to the family's resources and ability to cope

__I__ common and normal reactions of families to a chronic illness diagnosis; parents, the ill child and siblings are all apt to respond in this way; manifestations include: verbal self degrading and arguments, withdrawal, and complaints about nursing care

__L__ Parents act as if the disorder does not exist or attempt to have the child overcompensate for it.

__G__ a theory about chronic illness that emphasizes the family's role in actively responding to a child's illness

__J__ Parents avoid all discipline and cater to the child's desires to prevent frustration.

__E__ result in movement away from adjustment to the crisis

__K__ Parents detach themselves emotionally from the child, but usually provide adequate physical care or constantly nag and scold the child.

__P__ formerly Crippled Children's Services; provides financial assistance for children with many disabling conditions

__M__ Parents place necessary and realistic restrictions on the child, encourage self-care activities, and promote reasonable physical and social abilities.

4. Which one of the following diseases is the most common chronic childhood illness?
A. Asthma
B. Congenital heart disease
C. Cancer
D. Spina bifida

5. Which of the following chronic disorders have had markedly improved survival rates in recent years?
   1. Hodgkin's disease and leukemia
   2. cystic fibrosis and spina bifida
   3. asthma and muscular dystrophy
   4. premature and low birth weight infants

   A. 4 only
   B. 1 and 2
   C. 1, 2 and 4
   D. 2, 3, and 4

6. Emphasizing the child's abilities and strengths rather than viewing the disabilities within a pathological framework BEST describes which one of the following approaches to care of the disabled child?
   A. Chronological
   B. Developmental

7. A goal that would be considered INAPPROPRIATE for family-centered care would be to:
   A. maintain the integrity of the family.
   B. empower the family members.
   C. support the family during stressful times.
   D. maintain a high level of professional control.

8. The Individual Family Service Plan (IFSP) is:
   A. developed jointly by families and professionals.
   B. a comprehensive insurance plan for families with a disabled child.
   C. developed by a team of professionals for the disabled child.
   D. built of strategies for the school-aged disabled child.

9. When working with people of other cultural backgrounds who are caring for a child with a disability, the nurse always:
   A. promotes independent living.
   B. refers the family to a support group.
   C. promotes normalization.
   D. incorporates traditional family beliefs into the treatment plan.

10. Match the developmental stage with the particular challenge/risk that a disability would usually impart at this age.

    A. infant   __E__ self image
    B. toddler   __C__ social development
    C. preschooler   __A__ attachment
    D. school-aged child __B__ mobility
    E. adolescent   __D__ participation

11. According to Sorenson (1990), which one of the following coping mechanisms is more characteristic of a well child rather than a child with a disability?
    A. Develops competence
    B. Submission or endurance
    C. Complies with treatment
    D. Seeks support

12. The child who is disabled tends to develop appropriate independence and achievement when the parents:
    A. protect the child from all dangers.
    B. establish reasonable limits.
    C. emphasize their limits.
    D. isolate the child to avoid peer rejection.

13. Which one of the following strategies would be INAPPROPRIATE for the nurse to use when teaching families with children who are disabled?
    A. Give information that meets the current needs of the child.
    B. Give as much information as possible at the time of diagnosis.
    C. Describe the therapeutic plan thoroughly.
    D. Repeat information as often as needed.

14. When should the adolescent client with a disability or chronic illness be transferred to an adult provider?
    A. When the client reaches the age of 18 years
    B. When the client reaches the age of 16 years
    C. When the client knows about his/her condition and is prepared for the transition
    D. It is better not to change providers

15. The purpose of the initial assessment of the coping mechanisms of a child who is disabled is for the nurse to:
    A. determine help that the family may want or need.
    B. establish a rapport with the child and family.
    C. provide care from stage to stage of development.
    D. provide care from phase to phase of the disorder.

16. Which one of the following statements is FALSE about family members' perceptions of a child's illness or disability?
    A. Children may interpret the reason for the illness/disability as a punishment.
    B. Family members are usually shocked to learn that their child has a serious illness/disability.
    C. Parents may interpret illness/disability as a punishment.
    D. Family members usually have no knowledge about the disorder when they learn their child has it.

17. Which of the following statements about the time of diagnosis is FALSE?
    A. Parents may not remember all that is said.
    B. Parents remember the tone of the communication.
    C. Parents cannot sense the tone of communication.
    D. Parents may not hear all that is said.

18. The primary purpose of including both parents in the initial informing interview is to:
   A. observe the interaction between the parents.
   B. provide mutual support.
   C. avoid marital conflict.
   D. permit expression of their emotions.

19. Describe at least 3 guidelines for the nurse to use when providing ongoing information to the family with a disabled or chronically ill child.

   _____

   _____

   _____

20. Parents in thriving families:
   A. stress normalcy and feel confident.
   B. have an enduring management style.
   C. feel competent but burdened.
   D. feel dominated by the illness.

21. The two most important environments of the child who is disabled or chronically ill are:
   _____home_____ and _____school_____.

22. Which one of the following factors is more characteristic of a father's than a mother's pattern of adjusting to a child's chronic illness? The father is more likely to:
   A. feel a threat to his self esteem.
   B. report a periodic crisis pattern.
   C. forfeit personal goals.
   D. seek immediate professional counseling.

23. Which one of the following situations is most often true of the father of a disabled child?
   A. Is directly involved in the provision of care
   B. Is socialized to express his concerns
   C. Is without adequate emotional support
   D. Is directly involved in the medical decision making

24. Define "courtesy stigma".

   _____

   _____

25. Which one of the following characteristics would indicate that a sibling of a child with a disability is having difficulty?
   A. Sharing
   B. Withdrawal
   C. Competing
   D. Compromising

26. Describe an example of how an extended family member may be a source of stress to the parents of the disabled or chronically ill child.

_____

_____

27. Identify each one of the following coping behaviors as either an *approach* behavior or an *avoidance* behavior.

___Ap___ A. A father stops at a friend's house and talks about his child's poor prognosis.

___Av___ B. A father's alcohol use increases to the point of being excessive.

___Ap___ C. A mother tells the nurse that she is afraid to tell her child about his/her poor prognosis.

___Av___ D. A mother never carries a glucose source for her toddler who takes insulin for Type 1 diabetes mellitus.

___Ap___ E. A mother begins to cry in the nurse's office at school saying that she always gets depressed at the beginning of the new year.

___Ap___ F. A father asks the nurse to explain the diagnosis again.

___Ap___ G. A mother asks her neighbor to watch her older child for a few hours while she is at the clinic.

28. Corbin and Strauss's "chronic illness trajectory" model is based on the idea that the:
    A. family understands the meaning of the illness situation.
    B. course of the illness changes over time.
    C. family member roles do not change with illness.
    D. coping patterns for the illness can be learned.

29. The adaptive coping process includes:
    A. cognitive tasks.
    B. behavioral tasks.
    C. emotional tasks.
    D. all of the above.

30. If the reaction of a family member to the diagnosis of a chronic illness is denial, the nurse would recognize that denial is:
    A. an abnormal response to grieving this type of loss.
    B. preventing treatment and rehabilitation.
    C. necessary to prevent a crisis.
    D. necessary for the child's optimum development.

31. Health professionals work with people in denial frequently, but many health professionals typically do NOT:
    A. actively attempt to remove the denial behaviors.
    B. repeatedly give blunt explanations.
    C. label denial as maladaptive.
    D. understand the concept of denial.

32. Hope in the terminally ill child's family would be considered:
    A. a way to absorb stress in a manageable way.
    B. negative coping with a serious diagnosis.
    C. a maladaptive mechanism for dealing with the inevitable death.
    D. to have the same meaning for the nurse and the family.

33. Describe at least two effective methods of support that would help families manage their emotional response to the diagnosis of a disability or chronic illness in their child.

    _____

    _____

34. The BEST sign that a young child has adjusted to his/her terminal illness is that he/she:
    A. believes that procedures are inflicted as a punishment.
    B. talks about the disease and its effect on his/her life.
    C. passively accepts painful procedures.
    D. expresses anger about the restrictions imposed by the disease.

35. Which of the following types of parental reactions to the child with a chronic illness is characterized by the parents who detach themselves emotionally but provide adequate physical care?
    A. Overprotection
    B. Denial
    C. Gradual acceptance
    D. Rejection

36. The nurse should respond to anger in parents of the disabled child with:
    A. reciprocal anger.
    B. disapproval.
    C. acceptance.
    D. avoidance.

37. List at least five characteristics of parental overprotection.

    _____

    _____

    _____

38. When the parents of a child with special needs experience chronic sorrow, the process:
    A. of grief is pronounced and self limiting.
    B. involves social reintegration after grieving.
    C. is characterized by realistic expectations.
    D. is interspersed with periods of intensified grief.

39. Which one of the following stressors can usually be estimated in a child with special needs?
    A. The approximate cost of the yearly medical bills
    B. The future needs for residential care
    C. The types of schooling and vocational training that will be needed
    D. The developmental milestones and the start of school will cause stress of some kind.

40. The adjustment process for families with a disabled child is MOST significantly influenced by the:
    A. functional burden.
    B. severity of the condition.
    C. family's perception of the condition.
    D. available resources.

41. The effectiveness of the family's support system depends upon the:
    A. sources of the support and their availability.
    B. sources of the support and their communication.
    C. extended family and their availability.
    D. extended family and their resources.

42. Which one of the following characteristics is NOT necessary to consider when identifying parents to offer support to other parents of children with disabilities?
    A. Advocacy and problem-solving skills
    B. A child with the same diagnosis
    C. Nonjudgmental approach to problem solving
    D. A good listener

43. Fill in the blanks in the following statements.

    A. ___recipients___ ___of___ ___care___ parents usually have a high level of trust in the nurse with a low level of need for information.

    B. Parents who fit in the ___silent___ ___in___ ___care___ category do not initiate relationships with nurses; are difficult to engage in decision making.

    C. If the parent is in control of health-related decisions and uses the nurse for consultation and direct care, he/she can be said to follow the pattern of ___managers___ ___of___ ___care___.

    D. Parents who keep track of the staff and seek detailed information would be referred to as ___monitors___ ___of___ ___care___.

    E. Nurses who use a ___facilitative___ approach try to remove barriers to parents' participation.

    F. A nurse who seeks a high degree of control over his/her work may take the role of ___rule___ ___enforcer___ with parents.

44. Nurses who provide support to parents of a child with a disability should develop an attitude that has all of the following characteristics EXCEPT the belief that:
    A. every person has burdens to bear.
    B. trust is a foundation for good communication.
    C. parents are experts about their own child.
    D. parents and professionals are colleagues.

45. Out of home placement of a child with a disability:
    A. occurs if the integrity of the family unit is in jeopardy.
    B. occurs if coping strategies are not employed within the home.
    C. is becoming increasingly more difficult to accomplish.
    D. demonstrates that the family is maladjusted.

46. The Crippled Children's Services, which provides financial assistance for children with many disabling conditions is now known as:
    A. Programs for Children with Special Health Needs.
    B. National Information Center for Children and Youth With Disabilities.
    C. Association for the Care of Children's Health.
    D. Alliance for Health, Physical Education, Recreation and Dance.

Critical Thinking • Case Study

Jerome Thomas is a 15-month-old infant who was born prematurely and was discharged from the hospital at age 3 months after multiple invasive procedures, including intubation, ventilation and surgery. He is delayed in his motor development, but other areas of development are progressing as would be expected for a prematurely born infant of his age. Jerome has recently been diagnosed with cerebral palsy. He is at the physician's office for a routine health check. His mother is with him.

47. In order to assess the family's adjustment to the diagnosis the nurse would gather more information. One area that could be deferred to a later date would be the assessment of his:
    A. developmental level.
    B. available support system.
    C. family's coping mechanisms.
    D. family's goals for the future.

Jerome's mother has returned to work part time as a partner in a computer consulting firm. Jerome's father is a marketing consultant in the food industry and travels frequently. The couple has hired a woman whom they trust with Jerome's many needs to come into the home. Jerome goes out of the home several times a week for therapy. Jerome is an only child. His parents are in their late thirties.

48. Based on the information given above, select the BEST nursing diagnosis for Jerome?
    A. High risk for injury
    B. Altered family processes
    C. Altered growth and development
    D. Impaired social interaction

49. With the selected diagnosis in mind, what is the expected outcome with the highest priority for Jerome?
    A. Jerome will achieve physical development of a 15-month-old.
    B. Jerome will achieve psychosocial and cognitive development of a 15-month-old.
    C. Jerome's parents express both positive and negative reactions to Jerome's progress.
    D. Jerome's parents will set realistic goals for themselves and Jerome.

50. Which one of the following interventions would be appropriate for Jerome's parents to begin at this time?
    A. Expose infant to pleasurable experience through all of his senses.
    B. Encourage mastery of self help skills
    C. Help Jerome deal with criticism.
    D. Help Jerome realize that his disability is not a punishment

51. Between now and Jerome's next visit at 24 months, the nurse should provide anticipatory guidance to the parents about Jerome's growth toward developing:
    A. a sense of trust and attachment to his parents.
    B. mastery of self care skills.
    C. a sense of body image.
    D. through sensorimotor experiences.

CHAPTER 23
Family-Centered Care of the Child with Life-Threatening Illness/Unexpected Death

1. Terms—Matching

   A. small deaths
   B. grief
   C. mourning
   D. Leukemia Society of America/American Cancer Society

   E. Candlelighters Childhood Cancer Foundation
   F. palliation
   G. comfort care
   H. Mothers Against Drunk Driving

   I. hospice
   J. DNR
   K. The Compassionate Friends
   L. burnout
   M. detached concern

   __B__ the internal thoughts and feelings about the deceased

   __G__ occurs when treatment is only prolonging death, continuing (and perhaps increasing) suffering, and is no longer providing benefit to the child (Martinson, 1995)

   __D__ support organizations; the nurse may consider referring families who need financial help

   __F__ the use of procedures and medications to support life in a child for whom cure is not possible but for whom the quality of life remains good and dying is not immediate

   __A__ Those events such as the seasons in nature, the death of a pet, flowers or a television character may each help children become familiar and more comfortable with loss and present an opportunity for discussion about death.

   __E__ support organization; the nurse may consider referring families for information and psychological support

   __C__ the outward expression of thoughts or feelings about the deceased

   __H__ resource group for some families who experience a child's sudden death; other groups that may also be resources are: Sudden Infant Death Syndrome Alliance, National Sudden Infant Death Syndrome Resource Center, American Sudden Infant Death Syndrome Institute and National Organization of Parents of Murdered Children, Inc.

   __M__ the level of involvement which allows sensitive, understanding care as a result of being sufficiently neutral to make objective rational decisions

   __I__ holistic care for the patient and family that is intended to maximize the present quality of life whenever there is not reasonable expectation of cure

   __L__ a state of physical, emotional and mental exhaustion that occurs as a result of prolonged involvement with individuals in situations that are emotionally demanding; an occupational hazard that nurses are susceptible to

   __J__ no code; withholding cardiopulmonary resuscitation in response to cardiac arrest

   __K__ an international organization for bereaved parents and siblings

2. Which one of the following causes of death has increased in incidence in all age groups of children in the years from 1985 to 1990?
   A. Acquired Immunodeficiency Syndrome (AIDS)
   B. Sudden Infant Death Syndrome
   C. Injuries
   D. Malignant neoplasms

3. Describe 3 ways in which nurses can provide anticipatory guidance to families of children about death.

_____

_____

_____

4. Match the cognitive stage with the child's concept of death at that stage.

A. sensorimotor
B. preoperational
C. concrete operations
D. early formal operations
E. later formal operations

_E___ mature understanding of death; may deny mortality through risk taking; may be unable to cope or accept support

_D___ death is irreversible, interested in details of death and funerals

_B___ Death is temporary and reversible, like sleep.

_C___ death is irreversible; sees death as naturalistic; comprehend their own mortality

_A___ There is no concept of death, but child reacts to loss.

5. Fear of the unknown is one of the greatest threats to seriously ill children of which age group?
   A. Toddlers
   B. Preschoolers
   C. School-age children
   D. Adolescents

6. Immobilization is one of the greatest threats to seriously ill children of which age group?
   A. Toddlers
   B. Preschoolers
   C. School-age children
   D. Adolescents

7. Fear of punishment is one of the greatest threats to seriously ill children of which age group?
   A. Toddlers
   B. Preschoolers
   C. School-age children
   D. Adolescents

8. Inability to use their parents for emotional support is one of the greatest threats to seriously ill children of which age group?
   A. Toddlers
   B. Preschoolers
   C. School-age children
   D. Adolescents

9. Which one of the following age groups will be most likely to suffer negative reactions to an altered body image as a result of a life threatening illness?
   A. Young children
   B. School aged children
   C. Adolescents
   D. All age groups are affected equally.

10. Which of the following strategies would enhance compliance in adolescents?
    A. Include the adolescent in the treatment discussions.
    B. Help the family set clear expectations.
    C. Clarify roles and provide written instructions.
    D. All of the above.

11. When assisting parents in supporting their dying child, the nurse should stress the importance of honesty, because if parents are honest and openly discuss their fears the child is more likely to:
    A. discuss his/her fears.
    B. ask fewer distressing questions.
    C. lose his/her sense of hope.
    D. all of the above

12. The sibling of a dying child may feel:
    A. left out and unimportant.
    B. concern for his/her own health.
    C. physical symptoms similar to his/her sibling's.
    D. all of the above.

13. The nurse should recommend to the parents of a child who is dying that the sibling may benefit from being:
    A. protected from the reasons for the death.
    B. involved in funeral arrangements.
    C. observed for the abnormal signs of anger or jealousy.
    D. excused from any of the care or chores related to the sick child.

14. List at least three of the tasks that Baker's research (1992) suggests children must accomplish in their process of grief.

    _____

    _____

    _____

15. List at least three reasons that a nurse becomes an important part of the therapeutic team when the child has a life threatening disease.

    _____

    _____

    _____

16. Parents of a child who is in remission from cancer and going home should be advised to:
    A. schedule return appointments to give the child a break in the routine.
    B. resume rules and limits in effect before the illness.
    C. increase vigilance and liberalize the discipline.
    D. indulge in the child now while they can.

17. Because many children with cancer are treated in tertiary centers, they will:
    A. have one primary nurse to act as liaison.
    B. be assured continuity of care.
    C. often lack preventive interventions.
    D. be only a short distance from their home.

18. During Phase III, the cessation of cancer therapy and possible cure, many parents:
    A. express ambivalence.
    B. readily give up the medical regimen.
    C. have a psychologic need for the child's sick role.
    D. need less support than at the time of diagnosis.

19. The families' reactions during the terminal stage of a life-threatening illness involve a period of intense anticipatory grieving characterized by the reaction of:
    A. depression.
    B. loss of hope.
    C. pessimism.
    D. all of the above.

20. Which one of the following interventions is MOST important for the dying child?
    A. Emotional support
    B. Preparing parents to deal with fears
    C. Relief from pain
    D. Control of pain

21. When the parent of a child who is dying tells the nurse the child is in pain, even when the child appears comfortable, the nurse should be sure that:
    A. p.r.n. pain control measures are instituted.
    B. pain control is administered on a preventive schedule.
    C. parents understand that pain is a physical process.
    D. parents understand that the child is probably in less pain than the parents think.

22. Which one of the following strategies would be BEST for the nurse to use to support the family's spiritual needs when their child's death is imminent and a clergy member is unavailable?
    A. Pray appropriately with the family.
    B. Implement relaxation techniques.
    C. Make an appointment for the family to speak with an expert.
    D. Review the physical signs of death with the family.

23. List at least five physical signs of approaching death.

_____

_____

_____

24. The extended phase of mourning:
    A. usually takes about a year.
    B. is accompanied by support of the family at the funeral.
    C. may extend over years.
    D. can be eliminated if the family is well prepared.

25. When a child dies suddenly, which one of the following interventions would be LEAST beneficial?
    A. Avoid having the family view the body of a disfigured child.
    B. Inform the family of what to expect when they see the disfigured body of their child.
    C. Offer the parents the opportunity to see the child's body even after resuscitation was performed.
    D. Arrange to have a health care worker with bereavement training meet with the family.

26. List the 3 basic ways of providing hospice care.

    _____

    _____

    _____

27. Describe at least 3 benefits of implementing the hospice concept in the child's home environment.

    _____

    _____

    _____

28. Answer TRUE or FALSE.
    _____ Children with cancer, chronic disease, or infection or who have suffered prolonged cardiac arrest are excellent candidates for organ donation.
    _____ The nurse should never inquire if organ donation was discussed with the child, but allow the family to come forward with this information on their own.
    _____ If organs are donated the family will most likely need to choose a closed casket funeral service.
    _____ Most families choose not to donate organs because of the high cost.
    _____ Many body tissues and organs can be donated, but their removal may cause mutilation of the body.

29. In regard to whether a child should attend the funeral of a loved one, the nurse should consider:
    A. the age of the child.
    B. that it will be a frightening experience.
    C. their responsibility to protect the child from distressing events.
    D. that attending the funeral may be useful to the child.

30. Which one of the following techniques would be considered an example of the MOST therapeutic communication to use with the bereaved family?
   A. Cheerfulness
   B. Interpretation
   C. Validating loss
   D. Reassurance

31. Which one of the following helping statements would be LEAST therapeutic for the nurse to use with the bereaved family?
   A. "You can stay with him and hold him if you wish."
   B. "It must be painful for you to return to the doctors office without her."
   C. "Fortunately his suffering is over now."
   D. "Will your husband return to be with you soon?"

32. Which one of the following symptoms would be considered normal grief behavior?
   A. Depression
   B. Obsessive compulsive behavior
   C. Hearing the dead person's voice
   D. All of the above

33. The resolution of grief usually:
   A. occurs in sequential phases.
   B. is completed in about two years.
   C. is completed in about three years.
   D. may take years with periods of intensification of grief.

34. Reorganization after the death of a child means that the:
   A. loved one is forgotten.
   B. pain is gone.
   C. survivors have "let go".
   D. survivors have recovered from their loss.

35. List at least 3 of the reactions that nurses have when caring for children with fatal illnesses.

   _____   _____

   _____   _____

36. Intervening therapeutically with terminally ill children and their families requires:
   A. self awareness.
   B. nursing practice that is based on a theoretical foundation.
   C. years of experience.
   D. all of the above

Critical Thinking • Case Study

Julie Casswell is a 6-year-old child with leukemia. She has undergone a bone marrow transplant with associated complications and has had several remissions. After the last remission she deteriorated rapidly. Her parents tell the nurse that they believe that Julie is now in the final stages of her illness. Her parents also express their feelings of discouragement and depression.

37. How should the nurse approach the parents in regard to their feelings about Julie's impending death?
    A. The nurse should begin by assessing the reason for the depression.
    B. The nurse should be sure that Julie's parents know that repeated relapses with remissions are associated with a better prognosis.
    C. The nurse should begin to help the parents work through their depression.
    D. The nurse should use heavy sedation to help Julie and her parents cope with this phase.

38. As Julie's parents express their concerns, it becomes very clear that pain control is a fear for Julie and her parents. What strategy should the nurse use to help them deal with this fear?
    A. The nurse should assure the parents that all of Julie's pain will be eliminated.
    B. The nurse should use heavy sedation to help Julie and her parents cope with this phase.
    C. A preventive medication schedule should be adopted as pain develops.
    D. The pain medications should be given only intravenously when Julie is near death.

39. After Julie's death at Christmas time, which one of the following evaluation strategies is MOST likely to help support and guide the family through the resolution of their loss?
    A. A written questionnaire
    B. A telephone call placed in early January
    C. A meeting with the family at the time of death
    D. A telephone call placed in early February

40. Which one of the following choices would be the BEST expected outcome for the nursing diagnosis of fear/anxiety when planning care for Julie in this terminal stage?
    A. Julie will discuss her fears without evidence of stress.
    B. Julie will exhibit no evidence of loneliness.
    C. Julie's parents are actively involved in Julie's care.
    D. Julie's parents demonstrate ability to provide care for her.

CHAPTER 24
The Child with Cognitive, Sensory, or Communication Impairment

1. Matching—Cognitive Impairment Terms

A. cognitive impairment
B. educable mentally retarded
C. trainable mentally retarded
D. Bayley Mental and Motor Scales

E. Wechsler Preschool and Primary Scales of Intelligence (WPPSI-R)
F. Vineland Social Maturity Scale
G. primary prevention strategies
H. secondary prevention activities

I. tertiary prevention strategies
J. negative reinforcement
K. trisomy 21
L. translocation of chromosome 21
M. mosaicism
N. atlantoaxial instability
O. fragile site

_H_ identification and early treatment of conditions; in regard to mental retardation this would include prenatal diagnosis or carrier detection of disorders, such as Down syndrome, and newborn screening for treatable inborn errors of metabolism such as congenital hypothyroidism, phenylketonuria and galactosema

_A_ a general term that encompasses any type of mental deficiency; mental retardation

_C_ comprises about 10% of the mentally retarded population; moderately mentally retarded

_B_ comprises about 85% of all people with mental retardation; mildly retarded

_E_ used during the preschool years to make the diagnosis of mental retardation

_D_ along with the Cattell Infant Intelligence Scale is one of the most commonly used tests used to make the diagnosis of mental retardation in infants

_F_ along with the AAMR Adaptive Behavior Scale is used to assess adaptive behaviors

_I_ treatment to minimize long-term consequences; in regard to mental retardation this would include early identification of conditions and appropriate therapies and rehabilitation services; such as medical treatment of coexisting problems such as hearing and visual impairment in Down syndrome and programs for infant stimulation, parent treating, preschool education, and counseling services to preserve the integration of the family unit

_G_ interventions designed to preclude the occurrence of the condition; in regard to mental retardation this would include rubella immunization, genetic counseling, especially in terms of Down or fragile X syndrome, preventing neural tube defects by the use of folic acid supplements during pregnancy

_M_ refers to cells with both normal and abnormal chromosomes; associated with 1-3% of persons with Down syndrome; the degree of impairment is related to the percentage of cells with the abnormal chromosome makeup

_J_ the process of consistently ignoring undesirable behavior

_L_ a genetic aberration that is usually hereditary and associated with 3-6% of Down syndrome cases

_K_ an extra chromosome 21 (Group G), 92-95% Down syndrome cases have this genetic pattern

_N_ occurs in 15-20% of children with Down syndrome; symptoms include neck pain, weakness and torticollis; most affected children are asymptomatic

_O_ a region on the chromosome that fails to condense during mitosis; characterized by a nonstaining gap or narrowing

2. Matching—Hearing Impairment Terms

A. deaf
B. hard of hearing
C. conductive hearing loss
D. sensorineural hearing loss
E. mixed conductive-sensorineural hearing loss
F. central auditory imperception

G. organic type of central auditory imperception
H. aphasia
I. agnosia
J. dysacusis
K. functional type of hearing loss
L. decibel (dB)
M. hearing-threshold level

N. cochlear implants
O. tactile devices
P. acoustic feedback
Q. ASL/SEE/BSL
R. telecommunications devices for the deaf (TDD)
S. closed captioning

_____ refers to a person whose hearing disability precludes successful processing of linguistic information through audition, with or without a hearing aid

_____ middle-ear hearing loss; results from the interference of transmission of sound to the middle ear; most common of all types of hearing loss; frequently a result of recurrent serious otitiis media; mainly involves interference with loudness of sound

_____ refers to a person who, generally with the use of a hearing aid, has residual hearing sufficient to enable successful processing of linguistic information through audition

_____ includes all hearing losses that do not demonstrate defects in the conductive or sensorineural structures; divided into organic or functional

_____ perceptive deafness; nerve deafness; involves damage to the inner ear structures and/or the auditory nerve; commonly caused by congenital defects or a consequence of an acquired condition such as kernicterus; results in distortion of sound and problems in discrimination

_____ results from interference with transmission of sound in the middle ear and along neural pathways; frequently caused by recurrent otitis media and its complications

_____ defect involves the reception of auditory stimuli along the central pathways and the expression of the message into meaningful communication; examples are aphasia, agnosia, and dysacusis

_____ hearing loss with no organic lesion; examples are conversion hysteria, infantile autism and childhood schizophrenia

_____ inability to express ideas in any form either written or verbally

_____ the measurement of an individual's hearing threshold by means of an audiometer

_____ inability to interpret sound correctly

_____ provides a vibrotactile or electrotactile signal to transmit impulses to a point of stimulation, usually the fingers or hands and then to the language processing center in the brain

_____ difficulty in processing details or in discrimination among sounds

_____ a unit of loudness measured in frequencies; cycles per second

_____ a surgically implanted prosthetic device that converts sound to electrical impulses and feeds them directly to the auditory nerve

_____ visual-gestural languages that use hand signals and concepts in the English language that roughly correspond to specific word; signing

_____ a special decoding device that translates the audio portion of a television program into subtitles that appear written on the television screen

_____ an annoying whistling sound usually caused by improper fit of the ear mold of the hearing aid

_____ special teletypewriters that help deaf people communicate over the telephone

3. Matching—Visual Impairment Terms

A.	legal blindness	G.	penetrating wounds of the eye	L.	braille
B.	partially sighted	H.	nonpenetrating wound of the eye	M.	braille writer
C.	visual impairment			N.	braille slate/stylus
D.	refraction	I.	tapping method	O.	Library of Congress
E.	myopia –	J.	guides	P.	finger spelling
F.	hyperopia –	K.	blindisms	Q.	Tadoma method
				R.	John Tracy Clinic

_____ trauma to the eye that is most often a result of sharp instruments such as sticks, knives or scissors

_____ portable system for written communication used by the blind person

_____ a human or dog used to help a person who is visually impaired move around in the environment and avoid obstacles

_____ a general term that includes both school vision and legal blindness

__E___ the light rays enter the lens and rather than falling directly on the retina, they fall in front it   *eyeball is too long – farsighted   nearsighted – too short*

_____ a system that uses six raised dots to represent each letter and number

_____ the light rays enter the lens and rather than falling directly on the retina they fall beyond it

_____ may be a result of foreign objects in the eye, lacerations, a blow from a blunt object such as a baseball or fist, or thermal or chemical burns

_____ communication technique where the letters are spelled into the deaf-blind child's hand and the child spells out ideas to the other person

_____ school vision; defined as visual acuity above 20/200 but worse than 20/70 in the better eye with correction   *too long – farsighted*

__F___ use of a cane to survey the environment for direction and avoid obstacles   *eyeball is too short   nearsighted*

_____ refers to the bending of light rays as they pass through the lens of the eye

_____ self stimulatory activities such as body rocking, finger flicking, or arm twirling; as a habit they retard the child's social acceptance and are discouraged

_____ a small typewriter like device that enables the blind child to write a message

_____ offers a home correspondence course for parents of the deaf blind child

_____ has talking books, braille books and a special record program available for no cost to the blind person

_____ defined as visual acuity of 20/200 or less and/or a visual field of 20 degrees or less in the better eye

_____ a type of tactile communication that involves the child placing the hand over the speaker's face and neck to monitor facial movements associated with speech production

NTD – largest group of congenital anomalies that is consistent
c̄ multifactorial inheritance
girls > boys
nutritional &
Prevention – folic acid

Hydro – ↓ eyes, irritable, swallowing difficulties

VP shunt – ventricular tap
Nembutal & chloral hydrate
Keep flat on unoperated side   observe for abd. distention
observe for signs of ↑ ICP   I & O   NPO 24-48 hrs. p̄ surgery

4. Matching—Communication Impairment Terms

A. language
B. receptive language
C. expressive language
D. speech
E. developmental language disorder
F. articulation errors

G. dysfluencies
H. stuttering/stammering
I. block
J. voice disorders
K. blissymbols
L. direct observation
M. indirect assessment

N. Denver Articulation Screening Examination
O. Early Language Milestone Scale (ELM)
P. Denver II
Q. Peabody Picture Vocabulary Test-Revised

___O___ a standardized screening instrument for assessing language development in children less than 3 years of age

___L___ a method of assessing speech and language development that uses spontaneous language interaction between the child and nurse for children less than 3 years of age

___C___ speaking verbal symbols

___E___ a communication impairment that occurs without impairment in other developmental realms

_____ understanding the spoken word

_____ rhythm disorders; usually consist of repetitions of sounds, words, or phrases

_____ primarily refers to the symbol system used to convey thoughts or feelings to others

_____ the oral production of language including articulation of sounds, rhythm, and tone

___H___ one of the most common and potentially serious dysfluencies characterized by tense repetition of sounds or complete blockages of sound or words; a normal characteristic of language development during the preschool years

_____ sounds that a child makes incorrectly or inappropriately

_____ a highly stylized communication system consisting of graphic symbols that represent words, ideas, and concepts

_____ a useful screening instrument for word comprehension used for children ages 2 1/2 to 18 years

___N___ a reliable effective screening test to measure speech development that takes about 10 minutes to administer

_____ a stutter that is characterized by no sound coming out when the person tries to speak

___P___ a revision of the Denver Developmental Screening Test that includes an expanded section with language items

_____ characterized by differences in pitch, loudness and/or quality

_____ a method of evaluating speech and language development that relies on parental information obtained through a history

5. Match the level of retardation/IQ range to the appropriate example of maturation and/or development.

A. mild (50-55 to about 70)
B. moderate (35-40 to 50-55)
C. severe (20-25 to 35-40)
D. profound (below 20-25)

_____ a preschool-age child with noticeable delays in motor development and in speech

_____ an adolescent who may walk, but needs complete custodial care

_____ a school-age child who is able to walk and who can profit from systematic habit training

_____ a preschool-age child who may not be noticed as retarded but is slow to walk, feed self, and talk

6. The American Association on Mental Retardation's definition of *mental retardation* includes:
   A. an intelligence quotient that is lower than 50.
   B. adaptive limitation in the criteria.
   C. only intelligence and no other criteria.
   D. an age limit of 12.

7. List at least 4 early behavioral signs that are suggestive of cognitive impairment.

   _____ _____

   _____ _____

8. When teaching a child with a cognitive impairment, the BEST strategy for the nurse to use to present symbols in an exaggerated concrete form is:
   A. singing.
   B. memorizing.
   C. verbal explanation.
   D. ignoring the child.

9. Define the term *fading*.

   _____

   _____

10. Define the term *shaping*.

    _____

    _____

11. Acquiring social skills for the child who is mentally retarded includes:
    A. learning acceptable sexual behavior.
    B. being exposed to strangers.
    C. greeting visitors without being overly friendly.
    D. all of the above.

12. Describe the pro's and con's involved in the advisability of a marriage between two individuals with significant cognitive impairment.

    _____

    _____

    _____

13. The reasons that parents often give for seeking sterilization for their child who is mentally retarded include:
    A. contraception.
    B. eliminating menses.
    C. avoiding hygiene problems.
    D. all of the above.

14. The BEST contraceptive choice for the child who is cognitively impaired that would require little compliance, produce amenorrhea, and provide long term protection from pregnancy is:
    A. the intrauterine device.
    B. levonorgestrel implant (Norplant).
    C. the diaphragm.
    D. oral contraception.

15. Define *task analysis* and describe its use when teaching a child who is mentally retarded.

    _____

    _____

16. The primary purpose of recordkeeping for seven days prior to toilet training a mentally retarded child is to:
    A. determine patterns of behavior and parents' response.
    B. determine the amount of urinary output.
    C. determine parental responses to the child's toileting behaviors.
    D. all of the above are equally important.

17. Describe the conditions necessary for a child with cognitive impairment to begin learning how to dress.

    _____

    _____

    _____

18. The mutual participation model of care for the child who is cognitively impaired who needs hospitalization would include:
    A. isolating the child from others to avoid conflicts.
    B. encouraging the parents to room in.
    C. having the parents perform all activities of daily living.
    D. having the nurse perform all activities of daily living.

19. Another name for trisomy 21 is:
    A. phenylketonuria.
    B. Turner syndrome.
    C. Down syndrome.
    D. galactosemia.

20. Testing of the parents is necessary to identify the carrier and offer genetic counseling when Down syndrome is caused by:
    A. mosaicism.
    B. translocation.
    C. maternal age over 40.
    D. paternal age over 40.

21. List 5 physical features that are found in the infant with Down syndrome.

    _____   _____

    _____   _____

    _____

22. Some research has shown that families who keep the Down syndrome child at home report having:
    A. negative feelings for the child.
    B. a more accepting attitude toward others.
    C. higher divorce rates.
    D. more sibling problems.

23. Decreased muscle tone in the infant with Down syndrome:
    A. indicates inadequate parenting.
    B. is a sign of infant detachment.
    C. compromises respiratory expansion.
    D. predisposes the infant to diarrhea.

24. Fragile X syndrome is:
    A. the most common inherited cause of mental retardation.
    B. the most common inherited cause of mental retardation next to Down syndrome.
    C. caused by an abnormal gene on chromosome 21.
    D. caused by a missing gene on the X chromosome.

25. Genetic counseling for parents of a child with fragile X syndrome is recommended whenever there is:
    A. permutation.
    B. translocation.
    C. It is always necessary.
    D. It is never necessary.

26. The correct term to use for a person whose hearing disability precludes successful processing of linguistic information through audition is:
    A. deaf-mute.
    B. mute.
    C. deaf.
    D. deaf and dumb.

27. Conductive hearing loss in children is most often a result of:
    A. the use of tobramycin and gentamicin.
    B. the high noise levels from ventilators.
    C. congenital defects.
    D. recurrent serous otitis media.

28. At what decibel (dB) level would a hearing loss be considered profound?
    A. Less than 30 dB
    B. 55-70 dB
    C. 70-90 dB
    D. Greater than 90 dB

29. One behavior associated with hearing impairment in the child is:
    A. a monotone voice.
    B. consistent lack of the startle reflex.
    C. a louder than usual cry.
    D. inability to form the word "da-da" by 6 months.

30. In the assessment of the child to identify whether a hearing impairment has developed the nurse would look for:
    A. a loud monotone voice.
    B. consistent lack of the startle reflex.
    C. a high level of social activity.
    D. attentiveness especially when someone is talking.

31. All of the following strategies will enhance communication with a child who is hearing impaired EXCEPT:
    A. touching the child lightly to signal presence of a speaker.
    B. speaking at eye level or a 45-degree angle.
    C. using facial expressions to convey message better.
    D. moving and using animated body language to communicate better.

32. In order to BEST promote socialization for the child with a hearing impairment, teachers should:
    A. discourage hearing impaired children from playing together.
    B. use frequent group projects to promote communication.
    C. use audio visual assisted instruction as much as possible.
    D. minimize background noise.

33. Care for the hearing impaired child who is hospitalized should include:
    A. supplementing verbal explanations with tactile and visual aids.
    B. communicating only with parents to assure accuracy.
    C. discouraging parents from rooming in.
    D. sending non-vocal communication devices home to avoid loss.

34. Which of the following situations would be considered abnormal?
    A. A newborn who lacks binocularity
    B. A toddler whose mother says he looks cross eyed
    C. A five-year-old who has hyperopia
    D. Presence of a red reflex in a 7 year old

35. If a child has a penetrating injury to the eye, the nurse should:
    A. apply an eye patch.
    B. attempt to remove the object.
    C. irrigate the eye.
    D. use strict aseptic technique to examine the eye.

36. Match the type of visual impairment with its description.

A. astigmatism   _F_ increased intraocular pressure
B. anisometropia   _D_ squint or cross eye; malalignment of eyes
C. mblyopia   _B_ different refractive strength in each eye
D. strabismus   _A_ unequal curvatures in refractive apparatus
E. cataract   _E_ opacity of crystalline lens
F. glaucoma   _C_ lazy eye; reduced visual acuity in one eye

37. List at least eight of the strategies that the nurse can use during hospitalization with a child who has lost his sight.

_____   _____

_____   _____

_____   _____

_____   _____

38. Which of the following statements is CORRECT about eye care and sports?
A. Glasses may interfere with the child's ability in sports.
B. Face mask and helmet should be required gear for softball.
C. Contact lenses provide less visual acuity than glasses for sports.
D. It is usually very difficult to convince children to wear their glasses to play sports.

39. The method of communication used with the deaf-blind child that involves spelling into the child's hand is called:
A. finger spelling.
B. the Tadoma method.
C. blindism.
D. the tapping method.

40. In order to help the deaf-blind child establish communication, parents should:
A. always place the child in the same place in the room to help identify surroundings.
B. select a cue that is always used to help the child discriminate one person from another.
C. limit the cues that are sent and received.
D. limit stimulation to allow the child to feel safe.

41. Which one of the following examples would be MOST indicative of a language disorder?
A. A 22-month-old child who has not uttered his first word
B. A 38-month-old who has not uttered his first sentence
C. An 18-month-old who uses short "telegraphic" phrases
D. A 4-year-old who stutters

42. Which of the following statements about stuttering is CORRECT?
A. Stuttering is normal in the school-age child.
B. Stuttering occurs because children do not know what they want to say.
C. Undue emphasis on a stutter may cause an abnormal speech pattern.
D. Chances for reversal of stuttering are good until about age 3 years.

43. The parents of a child who is stuttering should be encouraged to:
    A. have the child start again more slowly.
    B. give the child plenty of time.
    C. show concern for the hesitancy.
    D. reward the child for proper speech.

44. Define the term *situated approach*.

    _____

    _____

45. Detecting communication disorders during early childhood:
    A. adversely affects the child's social relationships.
    B. increases the child's difficulty with academic skills.
    C. increases the child's ability to correct deficit skills.
    D. adversely affects the child's emotional interactions.

46. Following assessment and detection of a language problem, the nurse should advise the family to:
    A. wait and see what happens.
    B. wait, because the child will grow out of it.
    C. obtain a specialized evaluation.
    D. repeat words so that the child will learn more language.

47. Which one of the following findings would indicate a need for referral regarding a communication impairment?
    A. A 5-year-old who stutters
    B. A 3-year-old who omits word endings
    C. A 2-year-old with unintelligible speech
    D. A 3-year-old who substitutes easier sounds for hard ones

Critical Thinking • Case Study

Paula Larson is a 9-month-old infant with Down syndrome (DS) who is also blind and deaf and is admitted to the hospital with pneumonia. She holds her head steady, but cannot sit without support or pull up on the furniture. Paula squeals and laughs, but does not imitate speech sounds or have any words, not even "da-da" or "ma-ma". She can shake a rattle but cannot pass a block from one hand to the other. She smiles spontaneously and holds her own bottle, but she does not play "pattycake" or wave "bye-bye".

Along with the developmental deficits, she has congenital heart anomalies and has been hospitalized many times for pneumonia and bronchiolitis.

Paula's parents knew that she would be born with DS. They have chosen to care for Paula at home. Paula's care has become increasingly more time consuming. During the admission assessment interview, Mr. and Mrs. Larson state they are both exhausted.

48. The nurse determines that Paula's developmental lag is LEAST pronounced in the area of:
    A. gross motor skills.
    B. language skills.
    C. fine motor skills.
    D. personal-social skills.

49. Paula's parents have cared for her at home since her birth. Mrs. Larson expresses concern that she is not doing a good enough job and that perhaps it is time to consider placement out of the home for Paula. The nurse responds based on the knowledge that:
   A. the potential for development varies greatly in DS.
   B. every available source of assistance to help Mr. and Mrs. Lawson with the care of Paula should be explored.
   C. the nurse's responses may influence Mr. and Mrs. Larson's decisions.
   D. all of the above.

50. Which one of the common nursing diagnoses used in planning care for mentally retarded children should take priority in Paula's current situation?
   A. Altered growth and development
   B. Altered family processes
   C. Anxiety related to the hospitalization
   D. Impaired social interaction

51. Mr. and Mrs. Larson make the decision to explore residential care for Paula. The BEST expected outcome during this time for Paula Larson would be for the parents to:
   A. demonstrate acceptance of Paula.
   B. express feelings and concerns regarding the implications of Paula's birth.
   C. make a realistic decision based on Paula's needs and capabilities as well as their own.
   D. identify realistic goals for Paula's future home care.

CHAPTER 25
Family-Centered Home Care

1. Matching—Terms

   A. home care
   B. hospice
   C. impetus for home care
   D. cost of care
   E. Individualized Home Care Plan (IHCP)
   F. care coordination
   G. nurse case manager
   H. American Nurses' Credentialing Center
   I. The Hospice Nurses' Association

   ___I___ offers certification in hospice nursing

   ___G___ a single person who works with the family to accomplish the many tasks and responsibilities involved; should have a minimum of a baccalaureate degree in nursing and 3 years experience; needs to be knowledgeable about community resources

   ___A___ care provided for a child with complex healthcare needs and their families in the place of residence for the purpose of promoting, maintaining, or restoring health or for maximizing the level of independence while minimizing the effects of disability and illness, including terminal illness

   ___C___ parents' desire and the efforts to improve the quality of life for both children and their families

   ___H___ a subsidiary of the American Nurses Association; offers generalist and clinical specialist certification in both home health and community health

   ___B___ a program of palliative and supportive care services that provides physical, psychologic, social, and spiritual care for dying persons, their families, and their loved ones

   ___D___ a critical factor that influences the numbers of technology dependent children that are returned home more quickly than ever

   ___F___ the coordination of care across hospital, home, educational, therapeutic and other settings to ensure continuity for the child and family; general focus is cost control, attainment of desired clinical outcomes and the monitoring and evaluation of care provided

   ___E___ a general plan developed before discharge that ideally is developed with multi disciplinary input; should address the range of needs identified as part of the comprehensive predischarge assessment

2. Name at least two major reasons why care for complex medical conditions has moved from the hospital to the home setting.

   _____

   _____

3. The increase in the number of children who are cared for at home has probably been most influenced by:
   A. increased survival rates for children with leukemia.
   B. open heart surgery advances for congenital heart defects.
   C. advances in neonatal intensive care.
   D. consumer efforts to increase the quality of life.

4. The cost of home care for children dependent on medical technology is usually more than hospital care for:
   A. third party payers.
   B. the government.
   C. the family.
   D. all of the above.

5. Some of the nursing care of children at home is provided by:
   A. registered nurses.
   B. home health aides.
   C. the family.
   D. all of the above.

6. Which one of the following situations would be of MOST concern to the nurse who was evaluating a family for the possibility of a discharge with home care?
   A. The preterm infant who will be managed with home care is stable after surgery for his congenital heart anomaly.
   B. The family of a child who will be on a ventilator at home has no telephone.
   C. The parents are asking about the availability of respite care.
   D. The mother plans to stop working outside the home to be with the infant.

7. List 4 major areas of predischarge assessment for the child who is dependent on medical technology.

   _____

   _____

   _____

   _____

8. List all of the minimum contents of any written home care instructions for the child with complex home care requirements.

   _____

   _____

   _____

   _____

9. The BEST strategy to use when planning for transition from hospital to home for the child with complex home care requirements would be to:
   A. give the parents a trial period at home during which the parents provide some of the care.
   B. teach a family member all aspects of the child's care.
   C. allow the parents to provide total care in the hospital with support from the staff as needed.
   D. arrange a predischarge visit during the hospitalization by the home care nurse.

10. Ideally home care of the child who is technology dependent should be based on the concept of:
    A. traditional case management.
    B. independent care.
    C. primary care management.
    D. case management with care coordination.

11. According the American Nurses Association, the qualifications of the nurse case manager should include:
    A. a baccalaureate degree in nursing.
    B. three years of experience.
    C. knowledge about community resources.
    D. all of the above.

12. List at least five aspects of care coordination in pediatric home care.

    _____

    _____

    _____

13. The pediatric home care nurse's practice includes all of the following EXCEPT:
    A. consultation with peers to make most daily decisions.
    B. a high level of technical clinical expertise.
    C. knowledge of child development.
    D. the ability to support family autonomy.

14. The pediatric nurse in home care practice would be expected to adhere to standards of practice developed by:
    A. the World Health Organization.
    B. the American Nurses Association.
    C. the Society for Pediatric Nurses.
    D. the National League for Nursing.

15. Strategies that promote the central goal of family-centered home care would include all of the following EXCEPT:
    A. emphasizing family strengths.
    B. identifying family coping mechanisms.
    C. developing unidirectional communication.
    D. promoting family empowerment.

16. The LEARN framework for communication (Berlin and Fowles, 1983) with families involves:

    L _isten_____

    E _xplain_____

    A _cknowledge_____

    R _ecommend_____

    N _egotiate_____

17. Basic principles used to communicate with the family include all of the following EXCEPT:
    A. informing families who will have access to the information.
    B. assuring families that they have the right to confidentiality.
    C. collecting all information firsthand.
    D. restricting communications with other professionals to clinically relevant information.

18. The nurse should use all of the following guidelines for communication with family members EXCEPT:
    A. give information slowly and repeat it as necessary.
    B. answer questions honestly.
    C. use medical terminology.
    D. encourage family members to ask questions.

19. When conflict occurs between the family and the treatment nurse about the child's treatment, the nurse should first:
    A. call the physician and negotiate a change.
    B. contact the home care supervisor.
    C. respect parental preferences if no danger is posed.
    D. explain the correct way and have the family return a demonstration.

20. The nursing process in home care nursing practice integrates:
    A. normalization.
    B. various disciplines.
    C. family priorities.
    D. all of the above.

21. In home nursing practice the nurse allows the family to maintain control over their:
    A. home.
    B. child's care.
    C. personal lives.
    D. all of the above.

22. When a family chooses NOT to pursue developmental intervention, the nurse should:
    A. develop an Individual Family Service Plan.
    B. assure that developmental needs have been explained in a meaningful way.
    C. notify child protective services.
    D. all of the above

23. Describe at least three of the general guidelines a nurse should use when a disagreement between the nurse and the family arises in regard to the care of the child at home.

    _____

    _____

    _____

24. The school-age child who is physically able may be expected to participate in his/her own care by:
    A. doing no more than holding equipment and discarding used supplies.
    B. administering his/her own medicines with supervision.
    C. assuming responsibility for scheduling home visits.
    D. The school aged child is too young to participate in his/her own care.

25. Laws that ensure that children who are dependent on medical technology are mainstreamed into the school system always result in:
   A. a free, appropriate public education.
   B. payment for health care services in the school setting.
   C. the need for educational planning and coordination.
   D. all of the above.

26. One safety issue, specific to the home care child who is dependent on electrical equipment, is the need to:
   A. have a telephone on site.
   B. be cared for by trained individuals.
   C. notify the telephone and electric companies that the family needs to be placed on a priority service list.
   D. have someone in the house at all times who knows how to perform cardiopulmonary resuscitation.

27. At night the care of the child dependent on medical technology poses the safety concern that:
   A. the child may become frightened from the strange noises.
   B. accidental strangulation on equipment wires can occur during sleep.
   C. the lights must be kept brightly lit all night so that procedures can be performed correctly.
   D. all of the above

28. Family-to-family support:
   A. promotes family strength through shared experiences.
   B. often relieves the health professional from their role in the primary support system.
   C. meets the specific emotional needs of all families.
   D. all of the above.

Critical Thinking • Case Study

William Patterson who is now 18 months old was born with Werdnig-Hoffman Disease, a congenital neuromuscular disorder. His disease has developed to the point that he is unable to breath for more than a few hours without ventilator assistance.

William's older brother George died two years ago from complications of the same disease. His parents took care of him at home until his death. William's parents are preparing for a similar progression of the disease, which means that William will probably be maintained at home on a ventilator for many months until his death.

The case manager assigned to William is the same nurse who was assigned to his brother two years ago. This nurse, Ruth, was instrumental in helping the family cope with the technical issues of home ventilator management and total parenteral nutrition as well as the stressors of caring for their dying child.

29. Ruth is concerned about the boundary between collaborating with the Patterson family and becoming enmeshed in the family system as she did when George was dying. She knows that the family is able to technically care for William, but she is feeling as if she also needs to be involved again in some way. Ruth has consulted her supervisor for advice. Based on the above information the supervisor is MOST likely to suggest:
    A. reassignment.
    B. psychological counseling for Ruth.
    C. assessment of the therapeutic relationship.
    D. psychological counseling for the Pattersons.

30. At William's stage of development, the home care plan should include ways to promote:
    A. oral-motor development.
    B. mobility and exploration.
    C. self-care.
    D. independence in home management.

31. The quality of William's home care would BEST be evaluated by asking:
    A. Ruth to review the goals.
    B. the Pattersons to review the goals.
    C. Ruth and the Pattersons to jointly review the goals.
    D. the Pattersons to complete an evaluation questionnaire.

CHAPTER 26
Family-Centered Care of the Child During Illness and Hospitalization

1. Matching—Stressors Related to Hospitalization

A. stressors	D. despair	G. anger, guilt
B. anaclitic depression	E. detachment	H. fear, anxiety, frustration
C. protest	F. disbelief	I. depression
		J. presence

___J___ defined as spending time being physically close to the child while using a quiet tone of voice, appropriate choice of words, eye contact, and touch in ways that establish rapport and communicate empathy

___I___ usually occurs when the acute crisis is over, may be related to concerns for the child's future well-being, including negative effects produced by hospitalization and financial burden incurred

___H___ common feelings expressed by parents as they respond to their child's illness; often related to the type of trauma and pain inflicted on the child and lack of information provided to the parents

___G___ reactions that parents have following the realization of their child's illness; characterized by questioning their adequacy as caregivers

___F___ the characteristic initial reaction parents have to their child's illness, especially if the illness is sudden and severe

___E___ also called denial, this is the uncommon third phase of separation anxiety where superficially the child appears to have finally adjusted to the loss. The behavior is a result of resignation and is not a sign of contentment.

___D___ the phase of separation anxiety in which the crying stops; the child is much less active and withdraws from others.

___C___ a phase of separation anxiety in which children cry loudly, scream for the parent, refuse the attention of anyone else, and are inconsolable in their grief

___B___ separation anxiety; the major stress from middle infancy throughout the preschool years

___A___ events that produce stress

2. Matching—Pain Management

A. pain	J. nonopioids	S. EMLA
B. narcotic addiction	K. opioids	T. iontopheresis
C. drug tolerance	L. coanalgesics	U. intradermal route
D. physical dependence	M. placebos	V. buffered lidocaine
E. QUESST	N. first pass effect	W. around the clock (ATC)
F. CHEOPS	O. equianalgesia	X. respiratory depression
G. pain assessment record	P. patient-controlled analgesia	Y. constipation
H. behavioral cognitive pain control strategies	Q. epidural route	Z. pruritus
I. physical methods of pain control	R. oral transmucosal/ trandermal routes	AA. nausea/vomiting and sedation

___D___ physiologic, involuntary effect manifested by withdrawal symptoms when chronic use of opioid is abruptly discontinued or opioid antagonist, such as naloxone is administered

___O___ equal analgesic effect; conversion factors have been developed for selected opioids when a change is made from intravenous to oral to account for the first pass effect

___A___ defined as "whatever the experiencing person says it is, existing whenever the person says it does"; implying the attitude toward patients that they are believed

___I___ a type of nonpharmacologic pain intervention; an example is transcutaneous electrical nerve stimulation (TENS)

___F___ a pain rating scale that monitors six behaviors—cry, vocalization, facial expressions, torso and leg movements, verbal report of pain and touching of incision or location of discomfort—that are perceived to be associated with feelings of pain

___B___ behavioral, voluntary pattern characterized by compulsive drug-seeking behavior leading to overwhelming involvement with use and procurement of drug for purposes other than such medical reasons, such as pain relief

___J___ suitable for mild to moderate pain; includes acetaminophen, nonsteroidal anti-inflammatory drugs

___G___ used to monitor the effectiveness of pain interventions and evaluate regimens to provide maximum pain relief with minimum side effects

___E___ an approach to pain assessment that provides qualitative and quantitative information

___C___ physiologic involuntary need for larger dose of opioid to maintain original analgesic effect

___H___ a type of nonpharmacologic pain intervention; mind-body techniques

___K___ needed for moderate to severe pain; act primarily at site of the central nervous system

___S___ anesthetic cream; a eutectic mixture of local anesthetics (lidocaine 2.5% and prilocaine 2.5%); penetrates intact skin

___Q___ epidural; a catheter is placed in the epidural or caudal space of the spinal column; may be used to administer analgesia

___M___ an unethical and unjustified approach to pain management

___Y___ a common, sometimes serious side effect of opioids which decreases peristaltic activity and increase anal sphincter tone, central nervous system

___T___ *Numby Stuff*; uses low voltage current to enhance penetration of lidocaine and epinephrine through intact skin

___R___ provide non traumatic preoperative and preprocedural analgesia and sedation

___P___ administration of parenteral analgesics in which the patient controls the amount and frequency of the analgesic

___V___ reduces the stinging sensation that initially occurs with injection

___L___ adjuvant analgesics; may be used alone or with opioids to control pain symptoms, although they may or may not have analgesic properties; Valium, Versed

___N___ the rapid absorption from the gastrointestinal tract and partial metabolism in the liver before the drug reaches the central circulation thus causing the loss of some of the drug's potency

___W___ a preventive schedule of medication that is more effective than sporadic administration for continuous pain control

___AA___ side effects of opioid administration that subside after about 2 days

___X___ the most serious complication of pain medication administration; is most likely to occur in sedated patients

___Z___ a common side effect from epidural or IV infusions for pain; treated with low doses of naloxone infused slowly, with IV nalbuphine, or oral antihistamines

___U___ often used to inject a local anesthetic, typically lidocaine into the skin to reduce pain from a procedure such as lumbar puncture, bone marrow aspiration or venous arterial access

3. Matching—Terms—Hospitalization

A. play therapy   C. Childlife specialists   E. Interdisciplinary team
B. therapeutic play   D. postvention   approach

_____B_____ an effective non-directive modality for helping children deal with their concerns and fears; often helps the nurse to gain insights into the child's needs and feelings

_____E_____ a shift from the multi-disciplinary team approach; team members typically share leadership and decisions are made by consensus

_____A_____ technique used as an interpretive method with emotionally disturbed children by trained and qualified therapists

_____D_____ counseling subsequent to the event

_____C_____ health care professionals with intensive knowledge of child growth and developmental and the special psychosocial needs of children who are hospitalized and their families; help prepare children for hospitalization, surgery and procedures

4. Separation anxiety would be MOST expected in the hospitalized child at age:
A. 3 to 6 months.
B. 15 to 30 months.
C. 30 months to 2 years.
D. 2 to 4 years.

5. Match the phase of separation anxiety with the behaviors that are typical of that phase.

A. protest   B. despair   C. detachment

_____B_____ inactive; withdraws from others; depressed; sad; uninterested in environment; uncommunicative; regression behaviors

_____C_____ increased interest in surroundings; interacts with care givers; appears happy; forms new but superficial relationships; rarely seen in hospitalized children

_____A_____ cries; screams; attacks stranger physically and verbally; attempts to escape; continuous crying

6. One difference between the toddler and the school-age child in their reactions to hospitalization is that the school-age child:
A. does not experience separation anxiety.
B. has coping mechanisms in place.
C. relies on his/her family more than the toddler.
D. experiences separation anxiety to a greater degree.

7. A toddler is most likely to react to short term hospitalization with feelings of loss of control which are manifested by:
A. regression.
B. withdrawal.
C. formation new superficial relationships.
D. self assertion and anger.

8. The technique to prepare a child for a painful procedure that is most appropriate for the preschool age is to:
   A. encourage the child to act grown up.
   B. demonstrate the procedure.
   C. verbally instruct the child.
   D. allow structured choices.

9. Which one of the following statements about getting a cold is MOST characteristic of the toddler? "I got this cold:
   A. because I did not wear my hat."
   B. by breathing in bacteria."
   C. because I feel sick."
   D. from harmful germs."

10. The MOST consistent indicator of distress in infants is:
    A. initial cry.
    B. heart rate.
    C. facial expression.
    D. uncooperativeness.

11. School-age children with chronic illness are MOST likely to be concerned about which one of the following stressors?
    A. Pain
    B. Their physical symptoms
    C. Strange surroundings
    D. Intrusive procedures

12. Which one of the following risk factors makes a child more vulnerable to the stresses of the hospitalization?
    A. Urban dweller
    B. Strong willed
    C. Female gender
    D. Passive temperament

13. The pediatric population in the hospital today is different from the pediatric population of ten years ago in that the usual length of stay has:
    A. decreased and the acuity has increased.
    B. increased and the acuity has decreased.
    C. increased and the acuity has increased.
    D. decreased and the acuity has decreased.

14. Describe at least one of the possible psychological benefits a child might gain from hospitalization.

    _____

    _____

15. Which one of the following factors, according to Craft's 1993 framework, would be considered MOST likely to negatively influence the reactions of siblings to the hospitalized child?
    A. The sibling is an adolescent.
    B. Care providers are not relatives.
    C. The sibling has received information about the ill child.
    D. The ill child is cared for in the hospital.

16. Which one of the following statements is TRUE in regard to parent participation in the hospitalized child's care?
    A. The parents need 24-hour responsibility to help maintain their feeling of importance to the child.
    B. Fathers and mothers need the same kind of support during the hospitalization of their child.
    C. Nurses may express support of parent participation but may not foster an environment that encourages parental involvement.
    D. Mothers feel comfortable assuming responsibility for their child's care.

17. List 3 strategies nurses can use to help minimize stresses for the parents of the hospitalized child.

    _____

    _____

    _____

18. To help the parent deal with issues related to separation while their child is hospitalized the nurse should NOT suggest:
    A. using associations to help the child understand time frames.
    B. ways to explain departure and return.
    C. quietly leaving while the child is distracted or asleep.
    D. short frequent visits over an extended stay if rooming in is impossible.

19. Which one of the following strategies should the nurse use to help the hospitalized child adjust to the strange environment?
    A. Discontinue school lessons.
    B. Evaluate stimuli from the adult point of view.
    C. Send personal items home to prevent loss.
    D. Combine familiar sights with the unfamiliar.

20. Which one of the following age groups is MOST affected by the hospitalization in regard to their feelings of loss of control?
    A. Infant
    B. Toddler
    C. Preschooler
    D. School-aged

21. The Joint Commission on Accreditation of Healthcare Organizations recommends that children's rights and responsibilities during the hospitalization be:
    A. the same as those of adults.
    B. the same throughout the agency.
    C. different from those of adults.
    D. prominently displayed as a "Bill of Rights" for parents.

22. Whenever performing a painful procedure on a child, the nurse should attempt to:
    A. perform the procedure in the playroom.
    B. standardize techniques from one age to the next.
    C. perform the procedure quickly and safely.
    D. have the parents leave during the procedure.

23. After administering an intramuscular injection the nurse would BEST reassure the young child with poorly defined body boundaries by:
    A. telling the child that the bleeding will stop after the needle is removed.
    B. using a large bandage to cover the injection site.
    C. using a small bandage to cover the injection site.
    D. using a bandage but removing it a few hours after the injection.

24. One way to evaluate whether a child fears mutilation of body parts is to:
    A. explain the procedure.
    B. ask the child to draw a picture of what will happen.
    C. stress the reason for the procedure.
    D. investigate the child's individual concerns.

25. Which of the following reactions to surgery is MOST typical of an adolescent's reaction of fear of bodily injury?
    A. Concern about the pain
    B. Concern about procedure itself
    C. Concern about the scar
    D. Understanding explanations literally

26. List the six strategies used in the QUESTT approach to pain assessment.

    Q uestion
    U se pain scale
    E valuate
    S ecure parents' involvement
    T ake cause of pain into account
    T ake action + evaluate results

27. In regard to pain management, nurses tend to:
    A. over treat children's pain more often than adults'.
    B. under treat children's pain more often than adults'.
    C. overestimate the existence of pain in children, but not in adults.
    D. overestimate the existence of pain in both children and adults.

28. Identify the following statements about pain in children as TRUE or FALSE.
   A. _____ Children may not realize how much they are hurting when they are in constant pain.
   B. _____ Children always tell the truth about pain.
   C. _____ Narcotics are no more dangerous for children than they are for adults.
   D. _____ Neonates have the mechanisms to transmit noxious stimuli by 20 weeks gestation.
   E. _____ Children cannot tell you where they hurt.
   F. _____ Younger children tend to rate procedure-related pain higher than older children.
   G. _____ A three-year-old child can use a pain scale.
   H. _____ Meperidine (Demerol, pethidine) is less dangerous for children than morphine.
   I. _____ Children tolerate pain better than adults.
   J. _____ Children may not admit having pain in order to avoid an injection.
   K. _____ Infants do not feel pain if they are asleep.
   L. _____ Children may believe that the nurse knows if they are hurting.
   M. _____ Children become accustomed to pain or painful procedures.
   N. _____ Children's signs of discomfort often increase with repeated painful procedures.
   O. _____ The active resistant child may rate pain lower than the passive accepting child.
   P. _____ Addiction from opioids used to treat pain is rare in children.
   Q. _____ Respiratory depression from opioids is uncommon in children.
   R. _____ The child's behavior indicates the intensity of the pain.
   S. _____ Infants 6 months of age or older metabolize opioids similarly to older children.
   T. _____ An effective and safe combination of drugs for conscious sedation is Demerol, Phenergen, and Thorazine.
   U. _____ A benefit of the sublingual route is direct absorption of the drug into the blood stream.

29. The Wong-Baker FACES pain rating scale:
   A. is easy to use but less reliable than other methods.
   B. is a rating of how children are feeling.
   C. has a coding system from .04 to .97
   D. consists of six cartoon faces.

30. The Oucher rating scale:
   A. consists of six cartoon faces.
   B. consists of six photographs of faces.
   C. uses descriptive words.
   D. uses a straight line.

31. The Poker Chip Tool:
   A. is recommended for children who understand the value of numbers.
   B. does not offer an option for "no pain".
   C. uses a picture of four different colored poker chips.
   D. is recommended for children under 3 years of age.

32. In regard to behavioral and physiologic responses to pain, children:
    A. remain consistent from age to age.
    B. vary widely in their responses.
    C. exhibit typical behaviors at each developmental stage.
    D. are unaffected by temperament.

33. Which one of the following characteristics is MOST likely to be exhibited by an adolescent who is in pain?
    A. Decreased verbal expression and withdrawal
    B. Requests to terminate the procedure
    C. Verbal expression such as "You're hurting me!"
    D. Facial expression of pain and anger

34. Which one of the following persons can provide the BEST indicator of the child's pain experience?
    A. Father
    B. Mother
    C. Nurse
    D. Child

35. Which one of the following pain assessment scales uses blood pressure as a variable?
    A. Behavior Pain Score (BPS)
    B. Children's Hospital of Eastern Ontario Pain Scale (CHEOPS)
    C. Nurses Assessment of Pain Inventory (NAPI)
    D. Objective Pain Score (OPS)

36. Which one of the following statements is TRUE in regard to nonpharmacologic pain management?
    A. When used properly, nonpharmacologic measures are a good substitute for analgesics.
    B. Whenever possible nonpharmacologic and pharmacologic measures should be combined to manage pain.
    C. Nurses and physicians are well educated about nonpharmacologic approaches to pain management.
    D. Nonpharmacologic approaches to pain management are not effective with children.

37. Identify 3 specific nonpharmacologic strategies that can be used to manage pain.

    _____

    _____

    _____

38. Which one of the following statements is TRUE in regard to mind body methods of pain management?
    A. Behavioral cognitive techniques can produce a cooperative child who continues to suffer.
    B. Most mind body techniques are effective in children.
    C. Distraction techniques work well with most children.
    D. Sensory focusing is a technique that works well in most children.

39. Which one of the following opioids is the BEST choice for pain management?
    A. Hydromorphone
    B. Fentanyl
    C. Oxycodone
    D. Morphine

40. If oral hydromorphone is NOT controlling the child's pain, which action should occur FIRST?
    A. Change to morphine.
    B. Increase the dose.
    C. Change to fentanyl.
    D. Change to intravenous hydromorphone.

41. Describe the 3 typical methods of drug administration used with PCA devices.

    _____

    _____

    _____

42. When using Patient Controlled Analgesia (PCA) with children, the:
    A. drug of choice is meperidine.
    B. parent should control the dosing.
    C. nurse should control the dosing.
    D. drug of choice is morphine.

43. Which one of the following methods of analgesic drug administration is a liquid gel that provides anesthesia to non-intact skin in about 15 minutes?
    A. Midazolam
    B. EMLA
    C. LAT
    D. Numby Stuff

44. The anesthetic cream EMLA is applied:
    A. before invasive procedures.
    B. as preoperative oral sedation.
    C. for chronic cancer pain.
    D. postoperatively.

45. Which one of the following guidelines should be followed when using EMLA?
    A. Explain that it is like "magic cream that takes hurt away".
    B. Apply a thin layer over intact skin.
    C. Leave the cream in place for about 20 to 30 minutes.
    D. Leave the cream in place for about 60 to 90 seconds.

46. For postoperative or cancer pain control, analgesics should be administered:
    A. whenever needed.
    B. around the clock.
    C. before the pain escalates.
    D. after the pain peaks.

47. The MOST common side effect from opioid therapy is:
    A. respiratory depression.
    B. pruritus.
    C. nausea and vomiting.
    D. constipation.

48. Treatment of tolerance to opioid therapy includes:
    A. discontinuing the drug.
    B. decreasing the dose.
    C. increasing the dose.
    D. increasing the duration between doses.

49. List 3 functions of play in the hospitalized child.

    _____

    _____

    _____

50. When helping parents to select activities for their hospitalized child, the nurse should recommend:
    A. simpler activities than would normally be chosen.
    B. new toys and games to help distract the child.
    C. small colorful toys that can be played with in bed.
    D. games that can be played with adults.

51. List at least 2 ways drawing or painting may be used by the nurse in caring for the hospitalized child.

    _____

    _____

    _____

52. The nurse can facilitate the hospitalized child's feelings of self mastery by:
    A. acknowledging uncooperative behavior.
    B. acknowledging negative behavior.
    C. emphasizing aspects of the child's competence.
    D. providing emotional support to the family.

53. Preparation for hospitalization reduces stress in which of the following age groups?
    A. Infancy
    B. Toddlerhood
    C. Preschool
    D. All of the above

54. Define the role of a child-life specialist.

    _____

    _____

    _____

55. Questions related to activities of daily living at the time of admission are:
    A. inappropriate and should be saved for later.
    B. directed toward evaluation of the child's preparation for hospitalization.
    C. asked directly and in the order provided on the assessment form.
    D. designed to help the nurse develop appropriate routines for the hospitalized child.

56. Describe at least 3 strategies that can be used in the intensive care unit to support the child and family.

    _____

    _____

    _____

57. The question "How does your child act when annoyed or upset?" would be asked on admission to assess the child's:
    A. health perception-health management pattern.
    B. cognitive-perceptual pattern.
    C. activity-exercise pattern.
    D. self perception-self concept pattern.

58. The question "How does your child usually handle problems or disappointments?" would be asked on admission to assess the child's:
    A. role-relationship pattern.
    B. sexuality-reproductive pattern.
    C. coping-stress tolerance pattern.
    D. value-belief pattern.

59. The advantages of a hospital unit specifically for adolescents include:
    A. exclusive group membership.
    B. fewer preparation requirements.
    C. increased socialization with peers.
    D. all of the above.

60. The benefit of the ambulatory/outpatient setting is reduction of:
    A. stressors.
    B. infection risk.
    C. cost.
    D. all of the above.

61. Discharge instructions from the ambulatory setting should always include all of the following EXCEPT:
    A. guidelines for when to call.
    B. dietary restrictions.
    C. activity restrictions.
    D. referral to a home health agency.

62. When caring for the child in isolation, the nurse should:
    A. spend as little time as possible in the room.
    B. teach the parents to care for the child to decrease the risk of spreading infection.
    C. let the child see the nurse's face before donning the mask.
    D. all of the above.

63. Define postvention and describe a situation in which it would be therapeutic.

_____

_____

64. The MOST ideal way to support parents when they first visit the child in the intensive care unit is:
   A. for the nurse to accompany them to the bedside.
   B. to use picture books of the unit in the waiting area.
   C. to limit the visiting hours so that parents are encouraged to rest.
   D. expect parents to stay with their child continuously.

65. Transfer from the intensive care unit to the regular pediatric unit can be BEST facilitated by:
   A. discussing the details of the transfer at the bedside where the child can listen.
   B. establishing a schedule that mimics the child's home schedule.
   C. assigning a primary nurse from the regular unit who visits the child before the transfer.
   D. explaining to the family that there are fewer nurses on the regular unit.

66. Transitional care which is a trial period for the family to assume the child's care with minimum supervision may take place:
   A. on the nursing unit.
   B. during a home pass.
   C. in a motel near the hospital.
   D. any of the above.

Peter Chen is an 8-year-old child who is admitted to the pediatric unit for an appendectomy. He is in the third grade and is very active in after-school activities. Recently he began to take karate lessons and he also plays baseball. Peter loves school, particularly when he is able to read. He awakens every morning at 6 am to read, and reading is the last thing he does before he falls asleep.

Peter's parents are with him during the admission interview. His mother works, but she has made arrangements to take some time off after surgery and during his hospital stay to be available to him.

67. Based on the above information, the nurse should expect:
    A. a normal response to hospitalization.
    B. more anxiety than would normally be seen.
    C. difficulty with the parents.
    D. cultural factors to take precedence.

68. The nurse identifies which of the following nursing diagnoses after surgery for Peter?
    A. Diversional activity deficit and powerlessness
    B. Activity intolerance and high risk for injury
    C. Anxiety/fear and self care deficit
    D. Any of the above are possible

69. One reasonable expected outcome for Peter's diagnosis of powerlessness would be which one of the following?
    A. Peter will tolerate increasingly more activity.
    B. Peter will remain injury-free.
    C. Peter will play and rest quietly.
    D. Peter will help plan care and schedule.

70. Which one of the following interventions would be BEST for the nurse to incorporate into Peter's plan related to the diagnosis of diversional activity deficit?
    A. Organize activities for maximum sleep time.
    B. Keep side rails up.
    C. Choose an appropriate roommate.
    D. Assist with dressing and bathing.

CHAPTER 27
Pediatric Variations of Nursing Interventions

1. Matching—General Concepts Related to Pediatric Procedures

A.	mature minors doctrine	E.	nitrous oxide	I.	educational strategies
B.	emancipated minor	F.	malignant hyperthermia (MH)	J.	treatment strategies
C.	fentanyl oralet			K.	behavioral strategies
D.	conscious sedation	G.	compliance	L.	contracting
		H.	organizational strategies		

_____ those interventions used to improve compliance that are designed to modify behavior directly, such as positive reinforcement and contracting

_____ an oral transmucosal preparation that provides an effective and atraumatic form of prepoperative sedation; consists of a lozenge on a plastic holder that is sucked by the child to produce sedation

_____ one who is legally under the age of majority but is recognized as having the legal capacity of an adult under circumstances prescribed by state law

_____ adherence; refers to the extent to which the patient's behavior in terms of taking medication, following diets, or executing other lifestyle changes

_____ permits some minors to give consent even though they are not technically adults as long as they understand the consequences of their decisions

_____ those interventions used to improve compliance that are related to the child's refusal or inability to take the prescribed medication or prescribed treatment regimen

_____ used for conscious sedation; used in a concentration of 50% or less with the balance of the mixture oxygen

_____ a medically controlled state of depressed consciousness that allows protective reflexes to be maintained, retains the patient's ability to maintain a patent airway independently and continuously, and permits appropriate response by the patient to physical stimulation or verbal comment

_____ those interventions used to improve compliance that are concerned with instructing the child and family about the treatment plan

_____ a potentially fatal genetic myopathy that occurs in the perioperative period and demands immediate attention; characterized by hypermetabolism, muscle rigidity and an elevated temperature

_____ a process in which the exact elements of desired behavior are explicitly outlined in the form of a written agreement; a very effective method of shaping behavior especially with older children who are involved in the process of defining the rules of the agreement; coincides with the prescribed regimen

_____ those interventions used to improve compliance that are concerned with the care setting and the therapeutic plan

2. Matching—General Hygiene and Care

A. pressure ulcers
B. pressure reduction device
C. pressure relief device
D. friction

E. shear
F. epidermal stripping
G. set point
H. fever

I. hyperthermia
J. chill phase
K. plateau
L. defervescence

_____ hyperpyrexia; an elevation in set point such that the body temperature is regulated at a higher level; may be arbitrarily defined as temperature above 38° C (100° F)

_____ the point in the febrile state where shivering and vasoconstriction generate and conserve heat and raise the central temperatures to a level of the new set point

_____ the point during the febrile state when the temperature stabilizes at the higher range

_____ can develop when the pressure on the skin and underlying tissues is greater than the capillary closing pressure causing capillary occlusion results in tissue anoxia and cellular death; most commonly occurs over a bony prominence

_____ the result of the force of gravity pulling down on the body and friction of the body against a surface; for example when a patient is in the semi fowler position and begins to slide to the foot of the bed

_____ product that reduces pressure more than what would usually occur with a regular hospital bed or chair; usually an overlay that is placed on top of the regular mattress

_____ occurs when the surface of the skin rubs against another surface, such as the sheets on the bed

_____ maintains pressure below that which would cause capillary closing; usually a high-technology bed that is used for patients who have multiple problems and cannot be turned effectively

_____ a situation in which body temperature exceeds the set point, which usually results from the body or external conditions creating more heat than the body can eliminate, such as in heat stroke, aspirin toxicity, or hyperthyroidism

_____ the point when the temperature is greater than the set point or when the pyrogen is no longer present

_____ results when the epidermis is unintentionally removed with tape removal

_____ the temperature around which body temperature is regulated by a thermostat-like mechanism in the hypothalamus

3. Matching Terms—Safety and Collection of Specimens

A.	nosocomial	E. droplet precautions	I. bladder catheterization
B.	Standard precautions	F. contact precautions	J. suprapubic aspiration
C.	Transmission-based precautions	G. Direct contact transmission	K. Allen test
D.	airborne precautions	H. Indirect contact transmission	L. gastric washings
			M. nasal washings

_____ lavage; used to collect a sputum specimen from infants and small children who are unable to follow directions to cough and may swallow sputum produced when they do

_____ designed to reduce the risk of transmission of infection agents that involve contact of the conjunctiva or the mucous membrane of the nose or mouth of a susceptible person with large particles generated during coughing, sneezing, talking; suctioning or bronchoscopy

_____ designed to reduce the risk of transmission of microorganisms transmitted by direct or indirect contact

_____ synthesize the major features of universal (blood and body fluid) precautions and body substance isolation (BSI); involve the use of barrier protection; designed for the care of all patients to reduce the risk of transmission of microorganism from both recognized and unrecognized sources of infection

_____ used to obtain a urine specimen when the child is unable to void or otherwise provide an adequate specimen; used to obtain a sterile urine specimen; a sterile procedure where a feeding tube or a Foley catheter is inserted into the urethra to obtain urine

_____ hospital-acquired

_____ involves skin-to-skin contact and physical transfer of microorganisms to a susceptible host from an infected or colonized person

_____ designed for patients documented or suspected to be infected or colonized with highly transmissible or epidemiologically important pathogens for which additional precautions beyond standard precautions are needed to interrupt transmission in hospitals

_____ involves contact of a susceptible host with a contaminated intermediate object, usually inanimate in the patient's environment

_____ used to obtain a urine specimen when the child is unable to void or otherwise provide an adequate specimen; useful in clarifying the diagnosis of suspected urinary tract infection in acutely ill infants; mainly used when the bladder cannot be accessed through the urethra or to reduce the risk of contamination that may be present when passing a catheter; involves aspirating bladder contents by inserting a needle in the midline above the symphysis pubis and vertically downward into the bladder

_____ usually obtained to diagnose an infection of respiratory syncytial (RSV); 1-3 ml of sterile normal saline is instilled into one nostril; then aspirated

_____ a procedure that assesses the circulation of the radial ulnar or brachial arteries

_____ designed to reduce the risk of those infectious agents that are transmitted by dissemination of droplets that may remain suspended in air or dust particles containing the infectious agent

4. Terms—Matching—Administration of Medication and Feeding Techniques

A. body surface area (BSA)
B. West nomogram
C. needleless injection system

D. subcutaneous injections
E. intradermal injection
F. orogastric/nasogastric gavage
G. enteral gavage

H. gastrostomy
I. jejunostomy
J. skin level device
K. Familial adenomatous polyposis (FAP)

_____ MIC-KEY, Bard Button, Gastroport; a long term gastrostomy feeding device; a small flexible silicone device protruding slightly from the abdomen affords increased comfort and mobility to the child, is easy to care for, and is fully immersible water; has a one-way valve to minimize reflux and eliminates the need for clamping; requires a well-established gastrostomy site; expensive

_____ The lateral side of the volar surface of the forearm is used.

_____ used as the basis for calculating children's drug dosages from a standard adult dose in the most reliable way

_____ feeding by a tube inserted directly into the stomach

_____ feeding by way of a tube inserted orally or nasally into the duodenum/jejunum

_____ usually used to determine body service area

_____ These children may require a colectomy with ileoanal reservoir to prevent or treat carcinoma of the colon.

_____ Biojector; delivers intramuscular or subcutaneous injections without the use of a needle; eliminates the risk of accidental needle puncture

_____ feeding by way of a tube inserted orally or nasally into the stomach

_____ common injection sites include the center third of the lateral aspect of the upper arm, the abdomen, and the center third of the anterior thigh

_____ feeding by a tube inserted directly into the jejunum

5. An informed consent is required for:
   A. an emergency appendectomy.
   B. a cutdown for intravenous medications.
   C. release of medical information.
   D. all of the above.

6. When the parents are divorced, who is eligible to consent to medical treatment of the child?
   A. Only the custodial parent may consent.
   B. Only the noncustodial parent may consent.
   C. Both parents must consent.
   D. Either parent may consent.

7. The mature minors doctrine permits minors to give consent for treatment in relation to:
   A. psychiatric care.
   B. health care of any kind.
   C. sexually transmitted diseases.
   D. routine physical exams only.

8. Emancipated minors are usually recognized as having the legal capacity of an adult in all matters after they:
   A. have acquired a sexually transmitted disease.
   B. use contraceptives.
   C. use drugs or alcohol.
   D. become pregnant.

9. When preparing a child for a procedure, the nurse should:
   A. use abstract terms.
   B. teach based on the child's developmental level.
   C. use phrases with dual meanings.
   D. introduce anxiety laden information first.

10. If a child needs support during an invasive procedure, the nurse should:
    A. inform the parents about how the child did after the procedure.
    B. ask the parents to stay in the room where they can have eye contact with the child.
    C. respect the parents' wishes and give appropriate explanations.
    D. encourage the parents to stay close by to console the child immediately following the procedure.

11. Which one of the following guidelines would be MOST appropriate to use to prepare a toddler for a procedure?
    A. Give one direction at a time.
    B. Always restrain the child.
    C. Use only verbal directions.
    D. Ask for the child's thoughts about why the procedure is being performed.

12. Which one of the following words or phrases would be considered nonthreatening?
    A. "A little stick"
    B. "Boo-boo"
    C. Dye
    D. Deaden

13. According to Zain and colleagues (1996), who is likely to believe that parents' presence during a procedure is LEAST helpful?
    A. The child
    B. The mother
    C. The father
    D. The physician

14. List at least five strategies the nurse can use to support the child during and after a procedure.

    _____

    _____

    _____

15. Describe at least one play activity for each of the following procedures.

A. Ambulation _____

B. Range of motion _____

C. Injections _____

D. Deep breathing _____

E. Extending the environment _____

F. Soaks _____

G. Fluid intake _____

16. The MOST effective method of preoperative preparation is:
A. consistent supportive care.
B. systematic preparation at specific stress points.
C. offering parents the option of attending the induction of anesthesia.
D. a single session of preparation.

17. Which one of the following statements about the school-age child's perception of the surgical experience is TRUE?
A. Fear is a major concern.
B. Most fearful events are remembered.
C. Children often remember waking up in pain.
D. Parental presence often increases the child's anxiety.

18. To prepare a breast-fed infant physically for surgery, the nurse would expect to:
A. permit breast-feeding up to three hours before surgery.
B. withhold breast-feeding from midnight the night before surgery.
C. withhold breast-feeding from four to eight hours before surgery.
D. replace breast milk with formula and permit feeding up to two hours before surgery.

19. Preoperative sedation in children is BEST accomplished by:
A. intravenous conscious sedation.
B. oral transmucosal conscious sedation.
C. intravenous opioids.
D. oral analgesics.

20. According to the Acute Pain Management Guidelines (1992), meperidine should be used when the patient:
A. needs chronic dosing.
B. has impaired renal function.
C. needs preprocedural sedation.
D. is allergic to other opioids.

21. Fear of induction of anesthesia by mask can be minimized by applying:
A. the mask quickly and with assurance.
B. an opaque mask.
C. the mask while the child is sitting.
D. the mask while the child is supine.

22. A change in vital signs of the young child in the postanesthesia recovery room that demands immediate attention is:
    A. increased temperature.
    B. tachycardia.
    C. muscle rigidity.
    D. all of the above.

23. Which one of the following statements about non-compliant families is TRUE?
    A. Non-compliant families share typical characteristics.
    B. Non-compliant families have less education than compliant families.
    C. Non-compliant families often have complex medical regimens.
    D. Non-compliant families often have an increased loss of control.

24. Which one of the following interventions to improve compliance would be considered an organizational strategy?
    A. Incorporate teaching principles that are known to enhance understanding.
    B. Encourage the family to adapt hospital medication schedules to their home routine.
    C. Evaluate and reduce the time the family waits for their appointment.
    D. All of the above are organizational strategies.

25. In planning strategies to improve the child's compliance with the prescribed treatment, the nurse knows that:
    A. an every-8-hour schedule should be implemented.
    B. an every-6-hour schedule should be implemented.
    C. the child may not be able to drink liquid medication.
    D. the family usually does not remember or understand the instructions given.

26. General guidelines for care of a child's skin would include:
    A. covering the fingers of the extremity used for an intravenous line.
    B. lifting the child under the arms to transfer the child from the bed to a stretcher.
    C. placing a pectin-based skin barrier directly over excoriated skin.
    D. keeping the skin moist at all times.

27. Stage III pressure ulcers usually present as:
    A. a deep crater.
    B. an abrasion.
    C. non-blanchable erythema.
    D. reactive hyperemia.

28. To prevent injuries from shearing, the nurse should avoid:
    A. using sheepskin over the elbows.
    B. pulling the patient up in bed without a lift sheet.
    C. pulling the patient up in bed with a lift sheet.
    D. using Montgomery straps.

29. Which one of the following disadvantages is associated with the gel/water filled pressure reduction devices?
    A. Cost of electricity
    B. Difficult to transfer the patient
    C. Difficult to keep clean
    D. Cold to touch

30. When bathing an uncircumcised male child under the age of 3, the nurse should:
    A. gently remind the child to clean his genital area.
    B. not retract the foreskin.
    C. retract the foreskin.
    D. avoid cleansing between the skinfolds of the genital area.

31. Care for a black child's hair includes braiding the hair:
    A. when it is damp.
    B. tightly.
    C. when it is dry.
    D. after petroleum jelly is applied.

32. To avoid dehydration from diarrhea the nurse should offer:
    A. gelatin.
    B. plain water.
    C. flavored fluids.
    D. carbonated beverages.

33. Which one of the following examples of a child's food intake would be the BEST sample of adequate documentation?
    A. Child ate one bowl of cereal with milk.
    B. Child ate an adequate breakfast.
    C. Child ate 80% of the breakfast served.
    D. Parent states that child ate an adequate breakfast.

34. During the chill phase of the febrile state:
    A. heat is generated and conserved.
    B. the temperature stabilizes at a higher range.
    C. a crisis of the temperature is occurring.
    D. the temperature is greater than the set point.

35. The MOST effective intervention for the treatment of fever in a 4-year-old child is to:
    A. administer a tepid sponge bath.
    B. administer ibuprofen.
    C. reduce the room temperature.
    D. administer acetaminophen.

36. Of the following strategies the BEST intervention for the treatment of hyperthermia in a 4-year-old child is to administer:
    A. a tepid sponge bath.
    B. acetaminophen.
    C. an alcohol sponge bath.
    D. aspirin.

37. The strength of the liquid form of infant acetominophen contains:
    A. 160 mg/5 ml
    B. 160 mg/ml
    C. 100 mg/ml
    D. 80 mg/ml

38. The revised "CDC Guidelines for Isolation Precautions in Hospitals" now contain:
    A. two levels: standard precautions and transmission based precautions.
    B. two levels: direct contact transmission and indirect contact transmission.
    C. three levels: airborne, droplet, and contact precautions.
    D. three levels: universal precautions, body substance isolation, and blood and body fluid precautions.

39. Which one of the following recommendations about contamination of the hands during procedures is MOST important for the nurse to adhere to?
    A. Follow disease specific infection control guidelines.
    B. Wear vinyl gloves.
    C. Avoid wearing nail polish.
    D. Wash the hands routinely after each patient contact.

40. List three acceptable methods to transport infants and children.

    _____

    _____

    _____

41. List 5 nursing interventions for the child who is restrained.

    _____

    _____

    _____

42. After mouth or lip surgery, the nurse would choose to restrain the child using:
    A. arm and leg restraints.
    B. elbow restraints.
    C. a jacket restraint.
    D. a mummy restraint.

43. Which one of the following restraint techniques for performing venipuncture on a toddler is CORRECT?
    A. A simple explanation is usually sufficient to have the child hold still.
    B. Extend the neck and maintain head alignment to expose the jugular vein.
    C. Place the child prone with legs in a frog position to expose groin the area.
    D. Lean across the child's upper body to prevent movement.

44. The BEST positioning technique for a lumbar puncture in a neonate is a:
    A. side-lying position with neck flexion.
    B. sitting position.
    C. side-lying position with modified neck extension.
    D. side-lying position with knees to chest.

45. The MOST frequently used site for bone marrow aspiration in children is the:
    A. femur.
    B. sternum.
    C. tibia.
    D. iliac crest.

46. To facilitate urination in a 4-year-old child who is toilet trained, the nurse could:
    A. wipe the abdomen with alcohol and fan it dry.
    B. elicit the Perez reflex.
    C. apply a urine collection device.
    D. wash and dry the genitalia thoroughly.

47. When applying a urine specimen bag to an infant, it is sometimes necessary to:
    A. oil the surface of the skin.
    B. place the scrotum inside the bag.
    C. remove and replace the bag often.
    D. restrain all four extremities tightly.

48. To obtain a sterile catheterized urine specimen from a female infant, the nurse will MOST likely choose to use:
    A. size 8 French sterile feeding tube.
    B. size 14 French Foley catheter.
    C. size 8 French coude' tipped catheter.
    D. 20 gauge needle.

49. Suprapubic aspiration has a HIGHER/LOWER success rate than catheterization of the bladder through the urethra.

50. Which one of the following techniques is CORRECT in regard to obtaining blood culture specimens from an intermittent infusion device?
    A. Use the first sample of blood.
    B. Discard the first sample of blood.
    C. Irrigate the device with D5W first.
    D. Use a heparinized collection tube.

51. In order to avoid the complication of necrotizing osteochondritis, the nurse should:
    A. warm the site with moist compresses.
    B. cleanse the site with alcohol.
    C. use an automatic lancet device.
    D. use the inner aspect of the heel.

52. After a venipuncture is performed in the young child, the nurse should:
    A. use "spot" bandage for the day.
    B. extend the arm while pressure is applied.
    C. avoid the use of any bandage.
    D. flex the arm while pressure is applied.

53. To obtain a sputum specimen for tuberculosis or respiratory syncytial virus (RSV) in an infant the nurse may need to:
    A. have the infant cough.
    B. obtain mucous from the throat.
    C. insert a suction catheter into the back of the throat.
    D. perform gastric lavage.

54. The MOST accurate method for determining the safe dose of a medication for a child is to use:
   A. a Body Surface Area formula.
   B. Clark's rule.
   C. Wright's rule.
   D. milligrams per kilogram.

55. To ensure that medication administration is LEAST traumatic for the child the nurse should:
   A. administer the drug quickly.
   B. leave the drug with the parent at the bedside.
   C. supervise the parent administering the drug.
   D. ask the parent to assist by restraining the child.

56. To administer 1 teaspoon of medication at home, the BEST device for the parent to use would be the:
   A. household soup spoon.
   B. household measuring spoon.
   C. hospital's molded plastic cup.
   D. household teaspoon.

57. All of the following techniques for medication administration in the infant are acceptable EXCEPT:
   A. adding the medication to the infant's formula.
   B. allowing the infant to sit in the parent's lap during administration.
   C. allowing the infant to suck the medication from an empty nipple.
   D. inserting a needleless syringe into the side of the mouth while the infant nurses.

58. When determining the needle length for intramuscular injection into a child, the nurse should:
   A. grasp the muscle and use a length that is half the distance.
   B. use a needle length that is too short rather than one that is too long.
   C. choose a half inch needle for a 4-month-old infant.
   D. grasp the muscle and use a length that is less than half the distance.

59. Which of the following intramuscular injection sites is generally reserved for children who have been walking for more than a year?
   A. Deltoid muscle
   B. Vastus lateralis
   C. Dorsogluteal
   D. Ventrogluteal

60. Which one of the following guidelines should the nurse use when administering intramuscular medications to infants and small children?
   A. The maximum volume to administer in a single syringe is 1 ml.
   B. The dorsogluteal muscle is the most commonly used site.
   C. Instruct the small child to stand; leaning against his/her parent for support.
   D. Inject the medication slowly.

61. Which one of the following intravenous medication administration guidelines is CORRECT?
    A. Check site for patency before each dose.
    B. Administer medication through the large bore blood line.
    C. Combine antibiotics to avoid fluid overload.
    D. Use the maximum dilution of the drug permitted by the manufacturer.

62. When administering medications to a child through a gastric tube, the nurse should:
    A. use oily medications to ease passage through the tube.
    B. mix the medication with the enteral formula.
    C. use a syringe with the plunger in place to administer the drug.
    D. flush the tube well between each medication administration.

63. The rectal route of medication administration is used in children when the child:
    A. is not responding to oral antiemetic preparations.
    B. needs a reliable route of administration.
    C. is constipated.
    D. all of the above.

64. To instill eyedrops in an infant whose eyelids are clenched shut, the nurse should:
    A. apply finger pressure to the lacrimal punctum.
    B. place the drops in the nasal corner where the lids meet and wait until the infant opens the lid.
    C. administer the eye drops before nap time.
    D. use any of the above mentioned techniques.

65. During continuous enteral feedings, the nurse should:
    A. use the same pole as the intravenous line.
    B. use a burette to calibrate the feeding times.
    C. give the infant a pacifier for sucking.
    D. all of the above.

66. In the small infant, a feeding tube is usually inserted through the:
    A. nose.
    B. mouth.

67. One of the MAJOR advantages of the recently developed skin level devices for feeding children is that the button device:
    A. does not clog as easily as other devices.
    B. eliminates the need for frequent bubbling.
    C. is less expensive than the traditional devices.
    D. eliminates the need for clamping.

68. When administering an enema to a small child, it is advisable to use:
    A. a pediatric Fleet enema.
    B. a commercially prepared solution.
    C. an isotonic solution.
    D. plain water.

69. A young child with an ostomy pouch may need to:
    A. wear one-piece outfits.
    B. begin toilet training at a later than usual age.
    C. use an alcohol based skin sealant.
    D. use a rubber band to help the appliance fit.

Critical Thinking • Case Study

Janis Smith is a 6-year-old child admitted to the hospital for an emergency appendectomy. She is accompanied by her mother. Her parents have been divorced for four years. Janis has a sister who is 7 years old.

70. The nurse's plan for preparing Janis for surgery based on her developmental characteristics should include:
    A. an emphasis on privacy.
    B. the correct scientific medical terminology.
    C. ways to help Janis accept new authority figures.
    D. teaching sessions no longer than 5 minutes.

71. One of the nursing diagnoses identified by the nurse for Janis is high risk for injury related to the surgical procedure and anesthesia. During the assessment interview, which of the following sets of facts would be MOST pertinent to this diagnosis?
    A. The nurse auscultated vesicular breath sounds.
    B. Janis' mother tells the nurse that the child's father who is 27 years old and in good health had some heart problems with anesthesia after a minor surgical procedure last year.
    C. Janis' mother tells the nurse not to expect the child's father to participate in the preoperative preparation, because he lives in another state.
    D. The nurse assesses that the child has moist mucous membranes and no tenting of the skin.

72. The nursing diagnosis of anxiety related to the surgery and hospitalization is identified by the nurse. Which one of the following strategies would be BEST for the nurse to incorporate into the surgical care plan to address this diagnosis?
    A. Discuss events that the child remembers.
    B. Administer analgesics around the clock.
    C. Teach the child to use the incentive spirometer.
    D. Ambulate the child as early as possible.

73. To evaluate the care plan in regard to the nursing diagnosis of high risk for fluid volume deficit, the MOST appropriate measurable data that demonstrates that the nurse's goal was met would include the point that:
    A. the child has vesicular breath sounds.
    B. the child's father who is 27 years old and in good health had some heart problems with anesthesia after a minor surgical procedure last year.
    C. the child's father lives in another state.
    D. the child has moist mucous membranes and no tenting of the skin.

CHAPTER 28
Balance and Imbalance of Body Fluids

1. Match the term with its definition.

A. total body water
B. intracellular fluid
C. extracellular fluid
D. osmotic pressure
E. diffusion
F. aldosterone

G. antidiuretic hormone
H. intravascular
I. interstitial
J. transcellular
K. insensible water loss

L. third-spacing
M. peripheral edema
N. ascites
O. pulmonary edema
P. oral rehydration
    solution

_____ fluid compartment, constitutes about half of the total body water at birth

_____ fluid within the cells

_____ 45% to 75% of body weight

_____ enhances sodium reabsorption in renal tubules

_____ released from the posterior pituitary gland in response to increased osmolality and decreased volume of intravascular fluid

_____ the physical pull created by a solution of higher concentration across a semipermeable membrane

_____ random movement of molecules from a region of greater concentration to regions of lesser concentration

_____ fluid loss through the skin and respiratory tract

_____ pooling of body fluids in a body space

_____ localized or generalized swelling of the interstitial space

_____ used to successfully treat loss infants with dehydration

_____ surrounding the cell and the location of most extracellular fluid

_____ accumulation of fluid in the abdomen

_____ fluid contained within the body cavities as cerebrospinal

_____ occurs when there is an increase in the interstitial volume

_____ fluid contained within the blood vessels

2. The nurse would expect which one of the following conditions to produce an increased fluid requirement?
   A. Congestive heart failure
   B. High intracranial pressure
   C. Mechanical ventilation
   D. Tachypnea

3. The nurse recognizes which individual as having the LEAST water content in relation to weight?
   A. Obese adolescent female
   B. Thin adolescent female
   C. Obese adolescent male
   D. Thin adolescent male

4. Infants and young children are at high risk for fluid and electrolyte imbalances. Which one of the following factors contributes to this vulnerability?
   A. Decreased body surface area
   B. Lower metabolic rate
   C. Mature kidney function
   D. Increased extracellular fluid volume

5. ___Isotonic___ dehydration occurs when electrolyte and water deficits are present in balanced proportion.

6. ___Hypotonic___ dehydration occurs when the electrolyte deficit exceeds the water deficit. There is a greater proportional loss of extracellular fluid, and plasma sodium concentration is usually __less__ than 130 mEq/L.

7. ___Hypertonic___ dehydration results from water loss in excess of electrolyte loss. This is often caused by a large __loss__ of water and/or a large __intake__ of electrolytes. Plasma sodium concentration is __greater__ than 150 mEq/L.

8. In infants and young children, the MOST accurate means of describing dehydration or fluid loss is:
   A. as a percentage.
   B. milliliters per kilogram of body weight.
   C. by the amount of edema present or absent.
   D. degree of skin elasticity.

9. An infant with moderate dehydration has what clinical signs?
   A. Mottled skin color, decreased pulse and respirations
   B. Decreased urine output, tachycardia and fever
   C. Tachycardia, oliguria, capillary filling 2-3 seconds
   D. Tachycardia, bulging fontanel, decreased blood pressure

10. Johnny, age 13 months, is being admitted for parenteral fluid therapy because of excessive vomiting. The nurse would recognize which one of the following as MOST essential in implementing care for Johnny?
    A. Give Johnny oral fluids until the parenteral fluid therapy can be established.
    B. Question the physician's order for parenteral fluid therapy of glucose 5% in 0.22% sodium chloride.
    C. Withhold the ordered potassium additive until Johnny's renal function has been verified.
    D. Replace half of Johnny's estimated fluid deficit over the first 24 hours of parenteral fluid therapy.

11. Rapid fluid replacement is CONTRAINDICATED in which one of following types of dehydration?
    A. Isotonic
    B. Hypotonic
    C. Hypertonic

12. Water intoxication can occur in children from:
    1. excessive intake of electrolyte-free formula.
    2. administration of inappropriate hypotonic solutions.
    3. dilution of formula with water.
    4. isotonic dehydration.
    5. vigorous hydration with water following a febrile illness.
    6. fluid shifts from intracellular to extracellular spaces.

    A. 1, 2, 3, and 4
    B. 1, 2, 3, and 5
    C. 2, 3, and 4
    D. 2, 3, 5, and 6

13. Severe generalized edema in all body tissues is called _____.

14. Edema formation can be caused by which one of the following?
    A. Decreased venous pressure
    B. Alteration in capillary permeability
    C. Increased plasma proteins
    D. Increased tissue tension

15. Match the following term with its description.

    A. respiratory acidosis   _____ occurs when there is a reduction of hydrogen ion
    B. respiratory alkalosis   concentration or an excess of base bicarbonate
    C. metabolic acidosis   _____ caused by any process that reduces base
    D. metabolic alkalosis   bicarbonate concentration or increases metabolic
                                            acid formation
                                    _____ results from factors that depress the respiratory
                                            center, factors that affect the lung, and factors that
                                            interfere with the bellows action of the chest wall
                                    _____ results primarily from central nervous system
                                            stimulation

16. To obtain relevant information from the mother of a child with fluid and electrolyte
    disturbances, the nurse should question the parent about:
    A. the type and amount of intake and output.
    B. observations of general appearance.
    C. weight of the child.
    D. if the parents have taken the child's temperature within the last 24 hours.

17. In measuring intake and output, the nurse often has to weigh the diaper. As a general rule,
    what is the wet diaper weight equivalent to in ml of urine?

    _____

18. Which symptoms would the nurse expect in a child with hypocalcemia?
    A. Abdominal cramps, oliguria
    B. Muscle cramps, hypertonic
    C. Thirst, low urine specific gravity
    D. Flushed, mottled extremities and weight gain

19. Joan, age 3, is admitted for fluid and electrolyte disturbances. The nurse's assessment should include:
    1. general appearance observation.
    2. vital signs.
    3. intake and output measurements.
    4. daily weights.
    5. review of laboratory results.

    A. 1, 2, 3, and 4
    B. 2, 3, and 4
    C. 3, 4, and 5
    D. 1, 2, 3, 4, and 5

20. Johnny, age 2, presents with moderate dehydration from diarrhea. What would the expected recommendation for replacement of fluid consist of?

    _____ Oral rehydration solution _____

    _____

21. _____ The American Academy of Pediatrics no longer advises withholding food and fluids for 24 hours after the onset of diarrhea, or the administration of the BRAT diet (bananas, rice, applesauce, and tea or toast). TRUE or FALSE?

22. Billy, age 3, has just been ordered NPO. To prevent intake of fluids the nurse should do which of the following?
    A. Place an NPO sign over his bed and remove fluids from the bedside.
    B. Place him in a private room away from other children.
    C. Apply an elbow restraint jacket to keep Billy from being able to drink by himself.
    D. Provide administration of ice chips every 30 minutes.

23. In starting an IV infusion in most children, the nurse recognizes the plan of care should include which of the following?
    A. Interruptions during the procedure are kept to a minimum.
    B. Use of a 20 gauge over-the-needle catheter is preferred.
    C. Allow the child to handle the equipment before procedure.
    D. Preparation of the IV fluid and tubing, that delivers 20 drops/ml, before the procedure begins

24. Identify the following statements about parenteral fluid therapy as TRUE or FALSE.
    __F__ Glucose 10% in water is a hypotonic solution.
    __T__ One molecule of glucose has half the osmolality of one molecule of sodium chloride.
    __T__ IV solutions given to infants and young children should contain at least 0.2% NaCl to prevent brain edema.
    __T__ IV infusion for children must be given with an apparatus that delivers a microdrop factor of 60 drops/ml and contains a calibrated volume control chamber.
    __F__ Pediatric patients receiving IV fluids via continuous infusion pumps need less monitoring.
    __F__ The IV infusion must be monitored every 4 hours for proper infusion rate and for site assessment.

25. Intraosseous infusions are _____.
    They are used when _____.

26. What nursing action should be included in the plan of care for 10-year-old Debbie, who requires intravenous fluid therapy?
    A. Position the extremity in a natural anatomic position with the fingers and thumb immobilized.
    B. Use an ace bandage and completely encircle the extremity with tape to secure the IV line, insertion site and extremity.
    C. Teach Debbie how to safely manipulate the IV when getting out of bed and ambulating.
    D. Use Debbie's dominant hand for the IV placement or the same extremity where her identification bracelet is located.

27. Which one of the following alerts the nurse to a potential problem in a child receiving IV fluids?
    A. Edema, blanching and cool skin at the IV insertion site
    B. The IV tubing is not changed or replaced for 16 hours.
    C. Blood appears in the tubing when the IV bag is held below the IV site level.
    D. Unrestricted flushing of the catheter

28. Match the term with its definition. (A term may be used more than once.)

    A. peripheral intermittent   _____ includes implanted infusion ports; most contact
       infusion device   sports are prohibited

    B. short-term or   _____ peripherally inserted central catheters placed by
       nontunneled catheters   specially trained nurses

    C. peripherally inserted   _____ A chest x-ray film should be taken to verify
       central catheters (PICCs)   placement of the catheter tip before administration
                                              of medication.
    D. long-term, tunneled
       catheters   _____ used for infusion when extended access is necessary
                                              without the need for continuous fluid

                                      _____ If catheter is threaded midline, TPN is not
                                              administered because it irritates the vessel.

29. Discuss ways to prevent catheter-related infections with the use of central line catheters.

    _____

    _____

30. Jamie, age 12, is receiving parenteral hyperalimentation. The nurse knows that which one of the following serum levels must be carefully monitored?
    A. White blood cell
    B. Calcium
    C. Bicarbonate
    D. Glucose

Critical Thinking • Case Study

Jennifer, age 4 months, is admitted to the hospital because of dehydration caused by diarrhea. Her mother has been giving her electrolyte-free solutions for volume replacement. Parenteral fluids have been ordered for Jennifer.

31. What type of dehydration does Jennifer MOST likely have?
   A. Isotonic
   B. Hypertonic
   C. Hypotonic
   D. Water intoxication

32. Diarrhea most commonly causes which one of the following?
   A. Respiratory acidosis
   B. Respiratory alkalosis
   C. Metabolic acidosis
   D. Metabolic alkalosis

33. Which of the following questions should the nurse ask in obtaining the admission history?
   A. Type of food and fluid intake and amount
   B. Urinary output amount or number
   C. Number and consistency of stools passed in the past 24 hours
   D. All of the above

34. Which of the following observations does the nurse recognize as the BEST indicator that Jennifer's dehydration is becoming more severe?
   A. Jennifer's cry is whining and low pitched.
   B. Jennifer's activity level is decreased.
   C. Jennifer's appetite is diminished.
   D. Jennifer is becoming more irritable and lethargic.

35. A priority goal in the management of acute diarrhea is:
   A. determining the cause of the diarrhea.
   B. preventing the spread of the infection.
   C. rehydration of the child.
   D. managing the fever associated with the diarrhea.

36. What is the MOST critical nursing responsibility when administering IV fluids to Jennifer?
   A. Prevent IV infiltration
   B. Assurance of sterility
   C. Prevent cardiac overload
   D. Maintenance of the fluid at body temperature

37. Tim is a one-month-old infant admitted for uncontrolled vomiting. The nurse will observe Tim for signs of which one of the following?
   A. Alkalosis
   B. Acidosis
   C. Hypocalcemia
   D. Hemodilution

38. An infant is to receive 500 ml of IV fluid per 24 hours. The drop factor of the microdropper is 60 gtts/ml. The nurse should regulate the IV to run at how many drops per minute?
   A. 15 gtts/min
   B. 60 gtts/min
   C. 21 gtts/min
   D. 27 gtts/min

CHAPTER 29
Conditions that Produce Fluid and Electrolyte Imbalance

1. Match the term with its description.

   A.   secretory diarrhea   C.   osmotic diarrhea   E.   chronic diarrhea
   B.   cytotoxic diarrhea   D.   dysenteric diarrhea

   ___D___   associated with inflammation of the mucosa and submucosa in the ileum and colon by infectious agents such as Salmonella or Shigella

   ___C___   commonly seen in malabsorption syndromes such as lactose intolerance; the intestine cannot absorb nutrients

   ___A___   usually due to bacterial enterotoxins which stimulate fluid and electrolyte secretion from the small intestine

   ___B___   viral destruction of the mucosal cells within the small intestine resulting in a smaller intestinal surface area and decreased absorption of fluid and electrolytes

   ___E___   may be the result of inadequate management of acute diarrhea; increase in stool frequency and increased water content with a duration of more than 14 days

2. Which one of the following is MOST likely to develop acute diarrhea?
   (A) The 2-month-old infant who attends daycare each day
   B.   The 18-month-old infant who stays at home each day with his mother
   C.   The 6-year-old child who attends public school
   D.   The 24-month-old infant with two older brothers, aged 5 years and 8 years

3. Identify the following statements as TRUE or FALSE.
   ___T___   Rotavirus is the most common pathogen identified in young children hospitalized for diarrhea and dehydration in this country.

   ___T___   Acute diarrhea in children may be associated with respiratory infections, otitis media infections, and urinary tract infections.

   ___T___   Excessive ingestion of apple juice can cause osmotic dietary diarrhea.

   ___F___   Ampicillin, amoxicillin, cephalothin, and cefaclor are seldom associated with diarrhea in children because of their lower specific gravity.

   ___F___   Clostridium difficile produces a protective mechanism against diarrhea because it alters the intestinal flora increasing absorption surfaces.

   ___F___   Because the infant's metabolic rate is lower than the adult's metabolic rate, the infant is more rapidly depleted of nutritional reserves during periods of malabsorption and decreased intake and therefore more prone to the development of dehydration.

4. Johnny, age 2 years, is diagnosed with uncomplicated diarrhea with no signs of dehydration. Diagnostic evaluation should include which one of the following?
   A.   Cultures of the stool
   (B) Presence of associated symptoms
   C.   Complete blood count
   D.   Urine specific gravity

5. Based on the following subjective and objective findings, what would be the suspected cause of diarrhea?

    A. administration of cefaclor for one month for recurrent ear infections _____
    B. neutrophils or red blood cells in the stool _____
    C. watery, explosive stools _____
    D. foul-smelling, greasy, bulky stools _____
    E. high numbers of esinophils in the stools _____

6. The four major goals in the management of acute diarrhea are:

    _____   _____

    _____   _____

7. The MOST appropriate therapeutic management for rehydration of Jenny, age 8 months, who has been diagnosed with acute diarrhea and has evidence of mild dehydration, is:
    A. oral rehydration therapy of 50 ml/kg within 4 hours.
    B. restarting lactose-free formula.
    C. encouraging intake of clear fluids by mouth, such as fruit juices and gelatin.
    D. BRAT diet which consists of bananas, rice, apples and toast or tea.

8. Drug therapy for acute infectious diarrhea in young children should include:
    A. Kaopectate administered until the diarrhea has stopped.
    B. continuation of antibiotics for the presence of C. difficile.
    C. administration of sedatives to decrease bowel motility.
    D. antibiotic therapy based on culture results.

9. Which one of the following nursing interventions is NOT appropriate for 6-month-old Terry, admitted to the pediatric unit with acute diarrhea and vomiting?
    A. Ongoing assessment of Terry's intake and output and physical appearance
    B. Education of the parents about the necessity of oral rehydration solution administration
    C. Rectal temperatures at least every four hours to monitor fever elevations
    D. Gentle cleansing of perianal areas and application of protective topical ointments

10. Diarrhea that occurs in the first few months of life, persists for longer than 2 weeks with no recognized pathogens, and is refractory to treatment is termed _____.

11. The therapeutic management of chronic nonspecific diarrhea in children includes:
    A. increasing dietary intake of foods and liquids with sorbitol and fructose.
    B. increasing dietary fiber.
    C. decreasing dietary fat content.
    D. increasing total fluid intake.

12. The major emphasis of nursing care of the vomiting infant or child is:
    A. determining prior treatments utilized for the vomiting.
    B. preventing the spread of the infection.
    C. managing the fever associated with the vomiting.
    D. observation and reporting of vomiting behavior and associated symptoms.

13. Fill in the blank in the following statements.
   A. __hypovolemic__ shock follows a reduction in circulating blood volume, plasma volume or extracellular fluid loss.
   B. __Cardiogenic__ shock results from impaired cardiac muscle function resulting in reduced cardiac output.
   C. __Vasogenic__ shock results from a vascular abnormality that produces maldistribution of blood supply throughout the body.
   D. __anaphylactic__ shock is characterized by a hypersensitivity reaction causing massive vasodilation and capillary leak.
   E. __septic__ shock is characterized by decreased cardiac output and derangements in the peripheral circulation in response to a severe, overwhelming infection.

14. Match the term with its description.

   A. compensated shock   D. colloids   G. enteral
   B. uncompensated shock   E. acidosis   H. parenteral
   C. irreversible shock   F. alkalosis   I. enteritis

   __G__ by way of the alimentary tract
   __E__ serum pH equal to or less than 7.35
   __F__ serum pH equal to or greater than 7.45
   __B__ cardiovascular efficiency diminished; microcirculatory perfusion marginal despite compensatory adjustments; tissue hypoxia, metabolic acidosis, and impairment of organ systems function
   __D__ protein-containing fluids, often administered to children in shock; albumin
   __H__ not in or through the digestive tract
   __A__ Vital organ function is maintained by intrinsic compensatory mechanism; blood flow is usually normal or increased, but generally uneven or maldistributed in the microcirculation.
   __I__ inflammation of the intestine
   __C__ condition in which actual damage to vital organs occurs and the disruption or death occurs even if measurements return to normal with therapy

15. Clinical manifestations of pronounced tachycardia, narrowed pulse pressure, poor capillary filling, and increased confusion would suggest which of the following?
   A. Compensated shock
   B. Decompensated shock
   C. Irreversible shock

16. The position of choice for the child in shock is:
   A. Trendelenberg.
   B. head-down with feet straight.
   C. flat with the legs elevated.
   D. semi-fowler's.

17. Match the stage of septic shock with its characteristics.

    A. hyperdynamic stage
    B. normodynamic stage
    C. hypodynamic stage

    __C__ lasts for only a few hours with respiratory distress, narrow pulse pressure, severe hypotension, profound hypothermia

    __A__ warm, flushed skin with tachypnea, chills and fever, and normal urinary output

    __B__ cool shock with depressed sensorium, oliguria, slightly elevated systemic blood pressure, cool extremities, and normal pulses

18. The MOST common initial sign of anaphylaxis is:
    (A.) cutaneous signs and the child may complain of feeling warm.
    B. bronchiolar constriction with wheezing.
    C. vasodilation and hypotension.
    D. laryngeal edema and stridor.

19. To prevent toxic shock syndrome, what should be included in the teaching plan for adolescent females about tampon use?

    _____

    _____

    _____

20. Burns are caused by _____, _____, _____ and _____ agents.

21. __Scald__ burns are the most common cause of burn injuries in children under the age of 4. Burn injury from child abuse is seen most often in children under 2 years of age and includes injury most often caused by __immersion in hot H2O - cigs__.

22. Identify the following statements as either TRUE or FALSE.

    __T__ The single most important factor in the decrease in fire related deaths since 1978 is the use of smoke detectors.

    __T__ Since electric current travels through the body on the path of least resistance, the area surrounding the long bones would be expected to experience the most damage.

    __T__ An area of concern for electrical burns in the very young child is chewing on electrical cords.

    __T__ The physiologic responses, therapy, prognosis, and disposition of the injured child with burns is all directly related to the amount of tissue destroyed.

23. The standard adult rule of nines cannot be utilized to determine the total body surface area of a burn in a child because:
    (A.) the child has different body proportions than the adult.
    B. the child has different fluid body weight than the adult.
    C. the child's proportions of trunk and arms are larger than the adult.
    D. as the infant grows, percentage for head increases while percentages for arms decrease.

24. Burns involving the epidermis and part of the dermis, that exhibit blister and edema formation, and that are extremely sensitive to temperature changes, exposure to air, and light touch are termed:
    A. superficial first-degree burns.
    B. partial-thickness second degree burns.
    C. full-thickness third degree burns.
    D. fourth degree burns.

25. The severity of the burn injury is determined by which of the following?
    1. pain associated with the burn measured on a scale of one to ten
    2. percentage of body surface area burned
    3. level of consciousness of the victim
    4. depth of the burn
    5. measuring vital signs

    A. 1, 2, and 3
    B. 1, 2, 3 and 5
    C. 2, 3, 4 and 5
    D. 2 and 4

26. The expected predominant symptom of a superficial burn is:
    A. pain.
    B. significant tissue damage.
    C. absence of protective functions of the skin.
    D. blister formation.

27. The nurse recognizes that which one of the following pediatric clients is at higher risk of complications from burn injury?
    A. The 12-month-old infant who pulled a pan of hot water over on his chest
    B. The 12-month-old infant who is burned on his chest by gasoline
    C. The 9-month-old infant who is burned on the hands and feet with scalding water as a punishment
    D. The 12-year old child who is burned on one side of the face as a result of playing with cigarettes

28. Jordan, age 12 years, has suffered severe burns and now his chest appears constricted. What procedure should the nurse prepare for?
    A. Intubation
    B. Chest tube insertion
    C. Escharotomy
    D. Hydrotherapy

29. Systemic response to thermal injury would include:
    A. hypoglycemia.
    B. increased capillary permeability.
    C. myoglobinuria.
    D. decreased metabolic rate.

30. Following a major burn injury, which of the following is the MOST common gastrointestinal systemic response?
   A. Gastric ileus
   B. Gastric ulcers
   C. Severe diarrhea
   D. Ulcerative colitis

31. Thermally injured children have an immediate threat to life related to _____ and _____. During healing, _____ is the primary complication.

32. What should be included in the plan for emergency care of the burned child?
   A. Apply large amounts of cold water over denuded areas.
   B. Apply ointments to the burned area.
   C. Removal of jewelry and metal
   D. Application of neutralizing agents to the skin of chemical burn areas

33. Bobby, age 2 years, has suffered a minor burn injury. Expected management would include:
   A. redress the wound with a gauze dressing every five days.
   B. soak stuck dressings in hydrogen peroxide before removal.
   C. administration of oral antibiotics.
   D. watching wound margins for redness, edema or purulent drainage.

34. In major burn injuries of children weighing less than 30 kg, adequate fluid replacement during the emergent phase is BEST assessed by which one of the following?
   A. Maintaining an hourly urinary output of 30 ml an hour
   B. Urinary output of 1 to 2 ml/kg per hour
   C. Increasing hematocrit
   D. Normal blood pressure

35. To maintain adequate nutrition and promote healing in the child with a major burn injury, the nurse would recommend which one of the following nutrition plans?
   A. Diet high in proteins and calories
   B. Diet high in calories, low in proteins
   C. Diet high in fats and carbohydrates
   D. Diet high in vitamins A and D

36. Johnny, age 8 years, suffered partial-thickness second degree burns of his chest, abdomen and upper legs while on a recent camping trip. He is scheduled for hydrotherapy each morning for 20 minutes followed by further debridement. The BEST nursing action to assist Johnny at this time would be:
   A. ensure that pain medication is given before treatment.
   B. hold Johnny's breakfast until he returns from treatment.
   C. offer sedation after the procedure to promote rest.
   D. reassure Johnny that hydrotherapy and debridement are not painful.

37. A temporary graft obtained from human cadavers and used in burn treatment is:
   A. Allograft.
   B. Xenograft.
   C. Autograft.
   D. Isograft.

Kenny, age 5 years, is brought to the emergency center after his clothes caught on fire while he was playing in the family garage with matches. He has partial-thickness second-degree burns and full-thickness third-degree burns of his anterior chest, anterior abdomen, upper right arm, both shoulders and right hand. There is singed nasal hair apparent on physical exam and some minor burns apparent on his face. A Foley catheter is inserted and a small amount of clear urine is obtained. Two IV routes are established for fluid replacement.

38. In conducting the physical examination of Kenny's burns the nurse calculates the extent of body surface area involvement. How would the nurse best assess to see if circulation to the area is intact?
    A. Touch the area to see if Kenny feels pain.
    B. Test injured surfaces for blanching and capillary refill.
    C. Inspection of the burns for eschar formation.
    D. Watch for edema of the affected part.

39. Based on the information given, the nurse would be careful to watch Kenny for immediate signs of which complication?
    A. Inhalation injury
    B. Facial deformities
    C. Sepsis
    D. Renal failure related to formation of myoglobin

40. During the acute phase of Kenny's burn management, the nursing plan indicates a need to administer pain medication by the intravenous route rather than by the intramuscular route. What is the rationale for this decision?
    A. Relieves pain more effectively
    B. Bypasses the impaired peripheral circulation
    C. Prevents further damage to sensitive tissue
    D. Reduces the risk of skin irritation and infection

41. Kenny has normal bowel sounds 24 hours following admission and is placed on a high-caloric, high-protein diet of which he eats very little. Kenny's hydrotherapy is scheduled right after breakfast and before supper. Which one of the following interventions by the nurse would MOST likely increase Kenny's dietary intake?
    A. Show Kenny a feeding tube and explain to him that if he does not eat more the tube will need to be inserted.
    B. Maintain the current meal schedule and stay with Kenny until he eats all of his meal.
    C. Rearrange his meal and hydrotherapy schedule to prevent conflicts.
    D. Insist that Kenny stop snacking between meals.

42. Considering the extent and distribution of Kenny's burns, which one of the following nursing diagnoses would be recognized as having the highest priority for Kenny during the management phase of his illness?
    A. Impaired gas exchange related to inhalation injury
    B. High risk for altered nutrition, less than body requirements related to loss of appetite
    C. Fluid volume deficit related to edema associated with burn injury
    D. High risk infection related to denuded skin, presence of pathogenic organisms, and altered immune response

43. Kenny progressed well with skin grafts and healing and is now ready for discharge. The nurse will know that Kenny's parents understand discharge instructions by which one of the following statements?

A. "Kenny will only need to wear this elastic support bandage for one month."

B. "Kenny will not be able to participate in any sports until the grafts have taken hold firmly."

C. "We will visit the teacher and Kenny's peers before Kenny returns to school to prepare them for his appearance."

D. "We will need to protect Kenny from normal activities until he requires no further surgery."

CHAPTER 30
The Child with Renal Dysfunction

1. Identify the following statements as TRUE or FALSE.

   __F__ The primary responsibility of the kidney is to maintain the composition and volume of the body fluids in excess of body needs.

   __T__ The kidney functions in the production of erythropoietin and thus in the formation of red blood cell production.

   __T__ Renin is secreted by the kidney in response to reduced blood volume, decreased blood pressure or increased secretion of catecholamines.

   __F__ Approximately one-half of the total cardiac output makes up the blood flow to the kidneys.

   __F__ Protein is a normal finding in urine because it is too large a molecule to be reabsorbed in the proximal tubule.

   __T__ Glucose is reabsorbed in the proximal tubule and returned directly to the blood.

   __T__ Because there is a limit to the concentration gradient against which sodium can be transported out, when larger than normal amounts of sodium remain in the tubules, water is obliged to remain with the sodium.

   __T__ An end product of protein metabolism is urea.

   __T__ The newborn is unable to dispose of excess water and solute rapidly or efficiently because glomerular filtration and absorption do not reach adult values until the child is between 1 and 2 years of age.

   __T__ The loop of Henle, the site of urine-concentrating mechanism, is short in the newborn, thus reducing the ability to reabsorb sodium and water and produce a concentrated urine output.

   __T__ Newborn infants are unable to excrete a water load at rates similar to those of older persons.

   __T__ The abnormal or backward urine movement is termed reflux.

2. Jordan is a 2-year-old who has had a clean-catch urinalysis done as part of a diagnostic work-up. Match the following results with the nurse's correct interpretation. (Answers can be used more than once.)

   A. Normal
   B. Abnormal

   __B__ +1 glucose
   __A__ specific gravity 1.020
   __B__ RBC 3-4
   __B__ WBC greater than 10
   __A__ occasional casts
   __A__ trace protein
   __B__ + nitrites

3. Match the following term with its description.

A. bacteriuria
B. efflux
C. reflux
D. glomerular filtration rate
E. creatinine

F. cystitis
G. urethritis
H. pyelonephritis
I. urosepsis
J. vesicoureteral reflux
K. azotemia

L. chronic glomerulonephritis
M. uremia
N. hemodialysis
O. peritoneal dialysis
P. hemofiltration

_C_ backward flow of urine

_F_ inflammation of the bladder

_H_ inflammation of the upper urinary tract and kidneys

_J_ retrograde flow of bladder urine into the ureters

_K_ accumulation of nitrogenous waste within the blood resulting in elevated blood urea nitrogen and creatinine levels

_B_ forward movement of urine from kidney to bladder

_D_ measure of the amount of plasma from which a substance is cleared in one minute

_I_ febrile urinary tract infection coexisting with systemic signs of bacterial illness; blood culture reveals presence of urinary pathogen

_E_ an end product of protein metabolism in muscle

_G_ inflammation of the urethra

_A_ presence of bacteria in the urine

_M_ retention of nitrogenous products produces toxic symptoms

_L_ a variety of different disease processes that may be distinguished from each other by renal biopsy

_O_ The abdominal cavity acts as a semipermeable membrane through which water and solutes of small molecular size move by osmosis and diffusion according to their respective concentrations.

_N_ Blood is circulated outside the body through artificial cellophane membranes that permit a similar passage of water and solutes.

_P_ Blood filtrate is circulated outside the body by hydrostatic pressure exerted across a semipermeable membrane and replaced simultaneously by electrolyte solution.

4. The nurse, in preparing the child for a diagnostic test, explains that which one of the following tests provides direct visualization of the bladder through a small scope?
   (A) Cystoscopy
   B. Voiding cystourethrogram
   C. IVP
   D. Renal biopsy

5. Preprocedural preparation of the child who is scheduled to have a cystourethrography includes:
   A. keeping the child NPO for 8 hours before the test.
   B. assessing for an allergy to iodine.
   C. administering a fleet enema before the exam.
   (D.) preparing the child for catheterization.

6. Which one of the following does NOT predispose the client to urinary tract infections?
   A. The short urethra in the young female
   B. The presence of urinary stasis
   C. Urinary reflux
   (D.) Lowering of urine pH

7. Symptoms of urinary tract infection often observed in children over age two include:
   1. incontinence in a child previously toilet trained.
   2. abdominal pain.
   3. strong or foul odor to the urine.
   4. frequency of urination.
   5. vomiting.

   A. 1, 2, and 3
   B. 3 and 4
   C. 3, 4, and 5
   (D.) 1, 2, 3, and 4

8. The objectives of treatment of children with urinary tract infections include:

   1._____

   2._____

   3._____

   4._____

9. Which symptom suggests pyelonephritis in a 3-year-old child?
   (A.) Flank pain and tenderness
   B. Foul-smelling urine
   C. Dysuria or urgency
   D. Enuresis or daytime incontinence

10. The nurse is requested to obtain a urine specimen from 5-year-old Anne. Which of the following methods is the CORRECT procedure?
    A. Place a urine bag on Anne to collect the next specimen.
    B. Obtain a catheterized specimen.
    C. Encourage Anne to drink large volumes of water in an attempt to obtain a specimen.
    (D.) Obtain a midstream specimen, preferably the first morning specimen.

11. Justin, age 8 years, has been diagnosed with pyelonephritis. The nurse would expect medical management to include:
    A. administration of oral nitrofurantoin.
    B. admission to the hospital with intravenous antibiotics administered for the first 24 hours.
    C. radiographic evaluation before antibiotic therapy.
    (D.) urine cultures repeated every month for 3 months.

12. The nurse is developing a preventive teaching plan for Tracy, a sexually active 16-year-old who was diagnosed with a urinary tract infection. Which one of the following does the nurse include in the plan?
    A. Promotion of perineal hygiene by wiping back to front
    (B.) Avoid constipation
    C. Douche as soon as possible after intercourse to flush out bacteria
    D. Eliminate all carbonated and caffeinic beverages because they irritate the bladder

13. Vesicoureteral reflux is closely associated with which one of the following?
    A. Acute glomerulonephritis
    B. Nephrotic syndrome
    C. Renal scarring and kidney damage
    D. High alkaline content in the urine

14. Which of the following clinical manifestations are associated with acute glomerulonephritis?
    A. Normal blood pressure, generalized edema, oliguria
    B. Periorbital edema, hypertension, dark colored urine
    C. Fatigue, elevated serum lipid levels, elevated serum protein levels
    D. Temperature elevation, circulatory congestion, normal BUN and creatinine serum levels

15. Nursing interventions in caring for the child with acute glomerulonephritis include:
    A. enforced bed rest.
    B. daily weights.
    C. keeping the child NPO.
    D. high sodium diet.

16. Clinical manifestations of nephrotic syndrome include:
    A. hypercholesterolemia, hypoalbuminemia, edema, and proteinuria.
    B. hematuria, hypertension, periorbital edema, flank pain.
    C. oliguria, hypocholesterolemia, and hyperalbuminemia.
    D. hematuria, generalized edema, hypertension and proteinuria.

17. Therapeutic management in nephrotic syndrome includes the administration of prednisone. The nurse teaches which of the following as correct administration guidelines?
    A. Corticosteroid therapy is begun after BUN and serum creatinine elevation.
    B. Prednisone is administered orally in a dosage of 4 mg/kg of body weight.
    C. After the child is free of proteinuria and edema, the daily dose of prednisone is gradually tapered over several weeks to months.
    D. The drug is discontinued as soon as the urine is free from protein.

18. Identify the following statements as TRUE or FALSE
    __F__ Proximal tubular acidosis is caused by the inability of the kidney to establish a normal pH gradient between tubular cells and tubular contents.
    __T__ Primary functions of the distal renal tubules are acidification of urine, potassium secretion, and selective and differential reabsorption of sodium, chloride, and water.
    __T__ Treatment of both proximal and distal disorders consists of administration of sufficient bicarbonate or citrate to balance metabolically produced hydrogen ions and maintain the plasma bicarbonate level within normal range.
    __T__ In nephrogenic diabetes insipidus, the distal tubules and collecting ducts are insensitive to the action of antidiuretic hormone and vasopressin.
    __F__ Nephrogenic diabetes insipidus occurs primarily in females and appears in the newborn period with vomiting, fever, failure to thrive, dehydration and hypernatremia.
    __T__ Hemolytic-uremic syndrome is characterized by acute renal failure, hemolytic anemia, thrombocytopenia.
    __T__ Alport syndrome is a syndrome of chronic hereditary nephritis which consists of hematuria, high-frequency sensorineural deafness, ocular disorders, and chronic renal failure.
    __F__ Transient proteinuria generally means renal disease.

19. Multiple cases of hemolytic uremic syndrome caused by enteric infection of the E. coli 0157:H7 serotype have been traced to:
    1. undercooked meat, especially ground beef
    2. unpasteurized apple juice
    3. alfalfa sprouts

    A. 1
    B. 1 and 2
    C. 1, 2, and 3
    D. 2 and 3

20. Diagnostic evaluation results for hemolytic uremic syndrome would include which of the following findings?
    A. Proteinuria, hematuria, urinary cast, elevated BUN and serum creatinine, low hemoglobin and hematocrit and a high reticulocyte count
    B. High potassium, low sodium, high hemoglobin and hematocrit and proteinuria
    C. High number of urinary cast, low serum BUN and creatinine, decreased sedimentary rates
    D. Urine negative for protein but positive for RBC, normal hemoglobin and hematocrit, and elevated serum BUN and creatinine

21. In evaluation of the child with possible renal trauma, which one of the following are usually indicative of kidney damage?
    A. Flank pain and hematuria
    B. Dysuria, proteinuria, and nausea
    C. Abdominal ascites, nausea, and hematuria
    D. Proteinuria and bladder spasms

22. The MOST frequent cause of prerenal failure in infants and children is:
    A. nephrotoxic agents.
    B. obstructive uropathy.
    C. dehydration related to diarrhea and vomiting.
    D. burn shock.

23. The primary manifestation of acute renal failure is:
    A. edema.
    B. oliguria.
    C. metabolic acidosis.
    D. weight gain and proteinuria.

24. The MOST immediate threat to the life of the child with acute renal failure is:
    A. hyperkalemia.
    B. anemia.
    C. hypertension crisis.
    D. cardiac failure from hypovolemia.

25. Drug therapy utilized in the removal of potassium is:
    A. peritoneal dialysis.
    B. glucose, 50% and insulin.
    C. Kayexalate.
    D. calcium gluconate.

26. The MAJOR nursing task in the care of the infant or child with acute renal failure is:

_____

27. Which one of the following manifestations of chronic renal failure can have the MOST social consequences for the developing child?
   A. Anemia
   B. Growth retardation
   C. Bone demineralization
   D. Septicemia

28. Dietary regulation in the child with chronic renal failure includes:
   A. restriction of protein intake below the recommended daily allowance.
   B. protein in the diet of high biologic value.
   C. restriction of potassium when creatinine clearance falls below 50 ml/min.
   D. vitamin A, E, and K supplements.

29. Three goals for the child with chronic renal failure are:

_____

_____

_____

30. Fill in the blanks in the following statements.
   A. Methods of dialysis for management of renal failure are _____,
   _____ _____, _____ .
   B. _____ is the preferred method for children with life-threatening hyperkalemia.
   C. In peritoneal dialysis, _____ _____ is greater than with hemodialysis.
   D. _____ is not recommended for small children because of the rapid changes in blood volume, systemic blood pressure, and the difficulty of placing vascular access devices.
   E. The major complication associated with peritoneal dialysis is _____.
   F. The nurse can expect to see the child undergoing dialysis to have improved _____ _____ and _____ _____ but not to recover to _____ _____.
   G. Continuous arteriovenous hemofiltration is an ideal form of dialysis for children with _____ _____ from _____ _____.

31. Johnny, age 12, had a renal transplant 5 months ago. He now presents to the hospital outpatient clinic with fever, tenderness over the graft area, decreased urinary output and a slightly elevated blood pressure. The nurse's priority at this time is:
   A. to recognize that Johnny is probably undergoing acute rejection and to notify the physician immediately.
   B. to recognize that this is an episode of increased inflammation within the donor kidney because Johnny has probably been noncompliant with his immunosuppressant drugs. The nurse should educate Johnny regarding drug compliance and notify Johnny's physician when he makes rounds.
   C. to obtain a urine for culture and sensitivity and a blood count to quickly identify Johnny's infection before alerting the physician.
   D. to recognize that Johnny is in chronic rejection and that no present therapy can halt the progressive process.

Critical Thinking • Case Study

Dean, age 3 years, is brought to the clinic by his mother. He has a history of a recent fever of 100.2° F, sore throat and slight cough approximately eight days ago that lasted about three days. Yesterday morning his mother noticed "puffiness around his eyes" when he "got up" and then "swelling of his lower legs and scrotal area." Dean's appetite and activity level have decreased. This morning Dean's mother noticed that Dean's urine was "darker in color" and "seemed to be smaller in volume." Physical examination of Dean reflects a child who does not appear acutely ill, but who is irritable and appears fatigued, with pallor skin color. His blood pressure, pulse, and temperature are within normal limits. He has generalized edema. Laboratory findings of his urine specimen include large amounts of protein and microscopic hematuria. Serum protein levels are very low with elevated lipid levels.

32. Based on the above information, the nurse would suspect that Dean has developed which one of the following conditions?
   A. Acute poststreptococcal glomerulonephritis
   B. Minimal-change nephrotic syndrome
   C. Acute renal failure
   D. Hemolytic-uremic syndrome

33. Dean is diagnosed by the health care provider as having nephrotic syndrome. Identify goals for restoring renal function in Dean.
   1. Urine is protein free.
   2. Edema is resolved.
   3. Fluid and electrolyte balance are restored.
   4. Nutritional needs have returned to a state of positive nitrogen balance.

   A. 1, 2, and 3
   B. 1, 2, and 4
   C. 2 and 3
   D. 1, 2, 3, and 4

34. Which one of the following nursing diagnoses is of LEAST benefit in planning for Dean's care?
   A. Impaired skin integrity related to edema, lowered body defenses
   B. Altered nutrition less than body needs related to decreased appetite
   C. Altered patterns of elimination related to obstruction
   D. Fluid volume excess related to fluid accumulation in tissues and third space

35. Which nursing intervention is appropriate for Dean's nursing diagnosis of impaired skin integrity?
    A. Administer corticosteroids on time with careful monitoring for infections.
    B. Monitor for complications, strict intake and output, daily checks of urine for protein, daily weight, and abdominal girth.
    C. Enforce bed rest during the edema phase of the disease.
    D. Support scrotum on small pillow.

36. Dean has progressed well and is being discharged. What teaching interventions will be necessary to prepare the family for discharge?

    _____

    _____

    _____

37. Darlene, age 15 years, diagnosed with chronic renal failure is being discharged and will need peritoneal dialysis at home. Describe the teaching interventions the nurse would include in the discharge plan.

    _____

    _____

    _____

    _____

38. The nurse has developed the nursing diagnosis of altered nutrition related to restricted diet based on Darlene's diagnosis of chronic renal failure. Discuss expected nursing interventions to be used with this nursing diagnosis.

    _____

    _____

    _____

    _____

CHAPTER 31
The Child with Disturbance of Oxygen and Carbon Dioxide Exchange

1. Matching—Respiratory Tract Structure

A. respiratory tract
B. thoracic cavity
C. mediastinum
D. parietal pleura
E. visceral pleural sac
F. pneumothorax
G. pleural effusion
H. hydrothorax
I. hemothorax

J. empyema
K. barrel chest
L. nasal structures
M. upper airway
N. pharynx
O. larynx
P. glottis
Q. epiglottis
R. cricoid cartilage

S. lower airway
T. trachea
U. carina
V. bronchioles
W. conducting airways
X. terminal respiratory units
Y. alveoli
Z. septa
AA. lung growth

_____G_____ the diseases state in which there is fluid in the space between the visceral and the parietal pleura

_____B_____ encased in the bony framework provided by the ribs, vertebrae, and sternum; consists of three major partitions: the three-lobed lung on the right, the two lobed lung on the left and the space between them—the mediastinum

_____I_____ the disease state in which there is blood in the space between the visceral and the parietal pleura

_____A_____ consists of many complex structures that function under neural and hormonal control with the primary responsibility to distribute air and exchange gases so that cells are supplied with oxygen while carbon dioxide is removed

_____E_____ encases each lung separated by the parietal membrane by only enough fluid to lubricate the surface for painless movement during filling and emptying of the lungs

_____J_____ pyothorax; the disease state in which there is pus in the space between the visceral and the parietal pleura

_____D_____ adheres to the ribs and superior surface of the diaphragm

_____K_____ the condition in severe obstructive lung disease where the anteroposterior measurement approaches the transverse (side to side) measurement

_____C_____ contains the esophagus, trachea, large blood vessels, and the heart; located in the thoracic cavity between the right and left lungs

_____AA_____ affected by numerous pathological conditions; such as, kyphoscoliosis; coxsackievirus, hormone level changes, and biochemical substances

_____L_____ rigid passageways for air that warm and moisten the air, filter impurities, and destroy microorganisms

_____T_____ composed of smooth muscle supported by C-shaped rings of cartilage; ensures an open airway

_____M_____ oronasopharynx, pharynx, larynx and upper part of the trachea; shared by both the respiratory and alimentary tracts; dilates during inspiration; constricts during exhalation

_____X_____ the respiratory generation of bronchioles

_____U_____ the dividing point of the trachea into two primary bronchi

_____N_____ a passageway for the entry and exit of air; plays a role in phonation; helps to produce vowel sounds

_U_ the disease state in which there is serum in the space between the visceral and the parietal pleura

_W_ the nonrespiratory generation of bronchioles

_V_ the part of the respiratory system one generation below the bronchi

_O_ at the upper end of the trachea; constructed of a rigid circular framework of cartilage; contains the epiglottis and the glottis (vocal cords)

_F_ the disease state in which there is air in the space between the visceral and the parietal pleura

_Y_ airsacs; gas exchange occurs through these thin-walled sacs

_P_ vibrates to produce voice sounds; located closer to the head in infancy than in later childhood; very active reflexes in infancy

_Q_ prevents solids or liquids from entering the airway during swallowing; is longer and projects further posteriorly in infants

_Z_ the term for the shared walls of the alveoli

_R_ The narrowest portion of the larynx is located here.

_S_ consists of the lower trachea, mainstem bronchi, segmental bronchi, subsegmental bronchioles, terminal bronchioles, and alveoli

2. Matching—Respiratory Function

A.	respiratory movements	I. surfactant	Q. oxyhemoglobin dissociation curve
B.	ventilation	J. elastic recoil	
C.	~~artificial ventilation~~	K. resistance	R. neural system
D.	~~positive pressure breathing devices~~	L. partial pressures	S. chemical system
E.	~~negative pressure ventilator~~	M. torr	T. neural control
		N. fraction of inspired air	U. proprioceptive vagal impulses
F.	rocking bed		V. central chemoreceptors
G.	compliance	O. oxyhemoglobin	W. peripheral chemoreceptors
H.	alveolar surface tension	P. oxyhemoglobin saturation	X. acid base balance

_H_ one of the major factors determining compliance; lowered by surfactant

_B_ the passage of air in and out of the lungs; results from changes in pressure gradients created by changes in the size of the thoracic cavity

_I_ a lipoprotein at the air-fluid interface that allows alveolar expansion and prevents alveolar collapse

_C_ based on the concept of air moving from higher pressure into the lungs which have a lower pressure

_J_ the tendency of the lungs to return to the resting state after inspiration; a major factor in determining compliance

_N_ FIO_2; the expression used for inspired oxygen; 1.0 indicates 100%; ambient air at 21% is express as 0.21

_A_ first evident at about 20 weeks gestation when amniotic fluid is exchanged in alveoli

_K_ determined primarily by airway size; sources during breathing are: the chest wall, lungs, and flow in the airways; determined by flow rate velocity, gas viscosity, length of the airway and airway diameter

_E_ artificial respiratory device that increases the negative pressure within the thoracic cavity; not effective in infants because of their shorter abdominal length

_O_ the oxygen that is carried by hemoglobin; a large portion of oxygen is transported throughout the body this way

_D_ artificial respiratory devices that increases the pressure entering the air passages

_L_ tensions; expressed in torr

_G_ measure of chest wall and lung dispensability; represents the relative ease with which the chest and lungs expand with increasing volume and then collapse away from the pleural wall with decreasing volume (elastic recoil)

_M_____ millimeters of mercury; partial pressures are expressed in this manner

_P_____ arterial oxygen saturation (SaO$_2$); hemoglobin saturation

_T_____ located in a pneumotaxic center, apneustic center and the medullary respiratory centers

_G_____ artificial respiratory device that lowers the atmospheric pressure around the body

_V_____ located in the medulla; mediate respiratory changes by responding to changes in pH, PCO$_2$, and PO$_2$

_Q_____ the non-linear relationship between the PaO$_2$ and the SaO$_2$

_W_____ located in the great vessels; e.g. the carotid bodies; mediate respiratory changes by responding to changes in pH, PCO$_2$, and PO$_2$

_X_____ the lungs play an important role by acting as a chemical buffer; adjusts pH by eliminating or retaining PCO$_2$, acts within 1-3 minutes

_U_____ lungs stretching transmits a signal to the respiratory center which inhibits further inflation and prevents overdistention—the Hering-Breuer reflex R1421 one of the categories that control respiration; maintains a coordinated, rhythmic respiratory cycle and regulates the depth of respiration

_S_____ neurohumoral system that regulates alveolar ventilation and maintains normal blood gas pressure

3. Matching—Defenses of the Respiratory Tract

A. lymphoid tissues
B. mucous blanket
C. ciliary action
D. cough
E. tracheobronchial dynamics
F. position changes
G. lymphatics
H. humoral defenses

_____ encourage drainage of tracheobronchial passages

_____ tissues that localize and contain organisms to be destroyed by the humoral defense mechanisms

_____ the ability of the tracheobronchial tree to elongate and dilate on inspiration and shorten and narrow on expiration

_____ remove invading organisms; drain the terminal bronchi

_____ explosive force that propels foreign material out of the lower tract

_____ epithelium that secretes a sticky mucus to which airborne organisms adhere

_____ phagocytes, enzymes, and immunoglobulins secreted by the bronchial epithelium

_____ keeps mucus flowing; carries microorganisms and other foreign agents way from the lungs to be coughed or swallowed

4. Matching—Physical Assessment

A. auscultation
B. palpation
C. tachypnea
D. hyperpnea
E. hypopnea

F. retractions
G. nasal flaring
H. head bobbing
I. noisy breathing
J. grunting
K. skin color changes

L. chest pain
M. parietal pleural pain
N. diaphragmatic pleural irritation
O. clubbing
P. cough

____K____ mottling, pallor, cyanosis; significant in the infant; suggest cardiopulmonary disease (except circulatory stasis or cyanosis from a cool environment)

____D____ respirations that are too deep

____E____ respirations that are too shallow

____L____ may be a complaint of older children; may be caused by disease of any of the chest structures

____H____ a sign of dyspnea in the infant who is sleeping or exhausted

____N____ may be referred to the base of the neck posteriorly and anteriorly or to the abdomen

____B____ provides information regarding areas of pain

____P____ may be associated with disorders other than respiratory disease; serves as a protective mechanism; indicates irritation

____F____ sinking in of soft tissues relative to the cartilaginous and bony thorax; noted in some pulmonary disorders

____A____ essential to determine airway patency

____C____ rapid ventilations; observed with anxiety, elevated temperature, severe anemia and metabolic acidosis

____G____ significant finding in an infant; helps reduce resistance and maintain airway patency

____O____ proliferation of tissue at the terminal phalanges; associated with chronic hypoxia; does not reflect disease progression

____I____ frequently associated with hypertrophied adenoidal tissue, choanal obstruction, polyps or foreign body in the nasal passages

____M____ usually localized over the affected area and is aggravated by respiratory movement

____J____ frequently a sign of chest pain, suggests acute pneumonia, pleural involvement, pulmonary edema, or respiratory distress syndrome; increases end-respiratory pressure and prolongs gas exchange

5. Matching—Diagnostic Procedures

A. pulse oximetry
B. functional hemoglobins
C. oxyhemoglobin

D. deoxyhemoglobin
E. transcutaneous monitoring

F. arterial blood gas sampling
G. Allen test

____G____ performed to assess adequacy of collateral circulation

____C____ hemoglobin saturated with O_2

____A____ provides a noninvasive method of determining SaO_2

____E____ a noninvasive method of continually monitoring partial pressure of O_2 in arterial blood; some devices also measure CO_2

____F____ performed on blood from an artery or capillary

____B____ hemoglobin capable of carrying O_2

____D____ hemoglobin that is not saturated with O_2

6. Matching—Respiratory Therapy

A. hypoxemia
B. plastic hood
C. nasal cannula
D. mask
E. oxygen tent
F. atelectasis
G. O_2 induced CO_2 narcosis
H. hand-held nebulizers

I. metered dose inhaler (MDI)
J. spacer device
K. rotohaler/turbuhaler
L. percussion
M. vibration
N. squeezing
O. deep breathing

P. breathing/postural exercises
Q. bag-valve-mask
R. high-frequency ventilation
S. Extracorporeal membrane oxygenation (EMCO)
T. endotracheal airway
U. speaking valves

_____ prongs; the method of oxygen administration used for older infants and children

_____ a method of oxygen administration that may be used for children beyond early infancy; does not require any device to come into direct contact with the face; concentration of oxygen within the tent is difficult to control

__A__ reduced blood oxygenation

_____ a hazard of oxygen therapy; may occur in persons with chronic pulmonary disease; seldom encountered in children except those with cystic fibrosis

_____ a self-contained, hand held device that allows for intermittent delivery of a specified amount of medication

__F__ occurs as a result of the washing out of nitrogen from the alveoli by the high concentrations of oxygen; more likely to occur in persons with low tidal volume and retention of secretions

_____ a method of aerosolizing a medication; using a mask that the child holds over the nose and mouth

__U__ Passy Muir; Kistner, Tucker

_____ holding chamber to coordinate breathing and aerosol delivery

__N__ a maneuver that is useful while the child is in the drainage position; increases the depth of the expiratory effort by brief, firm pressure from the practitioner's hands compressing the side of the chest

_____ hand-operated self-inflating ventilation bag with a mask and a nonreturnable valve to prevent rebreathing

__T__ nasaltracheal, orotracheal, tracheostomy; artificial airway that is usually used in association with artificial ventilation

__M__ used to help move secretions toward the head during exhalation

_____ a new type of metered-dose inhaler that does not require a space device

__O__ encouraged when the child is relaxed and in the desired position of drainage; uses diaphragmatic breathing; may stimulate a cough; incentive spirometers, blow bottles and games with blowing are all techniques that may be used

__S__ a form of cardiopulmonary bypass; provides both pulmonary and cardiac support

_____ a technique that may be used with older motivated children with kyphoscoliosis, cystic fibrosis, asthma, and bronchiectasis

_____ provides information regarding tissue density; the most common technique used in association with postural drainage; the practitioner gently strikes the chest wall with a cupped hand, asis are good candidates

_____ the method of oxygen administration that is best tolerated by infants

__R__ a generic term for devices that use a rapid cycling rate and deliver small tidal volumes with each cycle

_____ a method of oxygen administration that is not usually well tolerated by children

7. Matching—Respiratory Emergency

A. hypercapnea
B. respiratory insufficiency
C. respiratory failure
D. respiratory arrest
E. apnea
F. central apnea
G. obstructive apnea

H. mixed apnea
I. obstructive lung disease
J. restrictive lung disease
K. primary inefficient gas transfer
L. respiratory center depression

M. pulmonary diffusion defects
N. head tilt
O. chin lift
P. jaw thrusts
Q. back blows
R. chest thrusts
S. heimlich maneuver

_____ absence of airflow (or absence of breathing that lasts for more than 15 seconds)

_____ applies in two conditions: 1) when there is increased work of breathing with near normal gas exchange function, and 2) when hypoxemia and acidosis develop secondary to CO_2 retention

_____ absence of air flow in which respiratory efforts are absent

_____ Components of central and obstructive apnea are present.

_____ the cessation of respiration

_____ disease involving increased resistance to airflow

_____ inadequate CO_2 removal

_____ disease involving impaired lung expansion

_____ may be caused by cerebral trauma; intracranial tumors central nervous system infection, tetanus

_____ the inability of the respiratory apparatus to maintain adequate oxygenation of the blood

_____ includes pulmonary edema, fibrosis, embolism

_____ used to relieve foreign body obstruction in infants; involves hand placement on the sternum and chest compressions

_____ absence of air flow in which respiratory efforts are present

_____ used to relieve foreign body obstruction in infants; involves hand placement over the spine between the shoulder blades

_____ accomplished by placing one hand on the victim's forehead and applying firm, backward pressure with the palm

_____ involves a series of nondiaphragmatic abdominal thrusts; recommended for children over 1 year of age

_____ accomplished by placing the fingers of the hand under the bony portion of the lower jaw to lift

_____ insufficient alveolar ventilation from dysfunction of the respiratory control mechanism or a diffusion defect

_____ accomplished by grasping the angle of the victim's lower jaw and lifting with both hands

8. Which one of the following structures of the respiratory system does NOT distribute air?
   A. Bronchioles
   B. Alveoli
   C. Bronchus
   D. Trachea

9. The general shape of the chest at birth is:
   A. relatively round.
   B. flattened from side to side.
   C. flattened from front to back.
   D. the same shape as an adult's.

10. The infant relies primarily on:
    A. mouth breathing.
    B. intercostal muscles for breathing.
    C. diaphragmatic abdominal breathing.
    D. all of the above.

11. Because of the position of the diaphragm in the newborn:
    A. there is additional abdominal distention from gas and fluid in the stomach.
    B. the diaphragm does not contract as forcefully as that of an older infant or child.
    C. diaphragmatic fatigue is uncommon.
    D. lung volume is increased.

12. Which one of the following statements is TRUE in regard to the anatomy of an infant's nasopharyngeal area?
    A. The glottis is located deeper in infants than in older children.
    B. The laryngeal reflexes are weaker in infants than in older children.
    C. The epiglottis is longer and projects more posteriorly in infants than in adults.
    D. The infant and young child are both less susceptible than adults to edema formation in the nasopharyngeal regions.

13. List four anatomical factors that significantly effect the development of respiratory disorders in infants.

    _____ _____

    _____ _____

14. Which one of the following conditions will reduce the number of alveoli?
    A. Maternal heroine use
    B. Increased prolactin
    C. Hyperthyroidism
    D. Kyphoscoliosis

15. As the child grows, chest wall compliance (circle one) INCREASES or DECREASES.

16. As the child grows, elastic recoil of the lungs (circle one) INCREASES or DECREASES.

17. Relaxation of the bronchial smooth muscles occurs in response to:
    A. parasympathetic stimulation.
    B. inhalation of irritating substances.
    C. sympathetic stimulation.
    D. histamine release.

18. Room air consists of:
    A. 7% oxygen.
    B. 21% oxygen
    C. 50% oxygen.
    D. 79% oxygen.

19. A child with anemia tends to be fatigued and breathes more rapidly, because the majority of oxygen is carried through the blood as:
    A. a solute dissolved in the plasma and the water of the red blood cell.
    B. bicarbonate and hydrogen ions.
    C. carbonic acid.
    D. oxyhemoglobin.

20. Retractions are defined as:
    A. the sinking in of soft tissues during the respiratory cycle.
    B. proliferation of the tissue near the terminal phalanges.
    C. increases the end expiratory pressure.
    D. contraction of the sternocleidomastoid muscles.

21. In a child, cough may be absent in the early stages of:
    A. cystic fibrosis.
    B. measles.
    C. pneumonia.
    D. croup.

22. Define the term capacity in relation to lung volume.

    _____

    _____

23. Match the pulmonary function parameter with how it is measured and its significance.

Pulmonary Function	Measurement	Significance
A. Forced Vital Capacity (FVC) (peak flow)	_B_ volume of air remaining in lungs after passive expiration	_C_ allows for aeration of alveoli; increased in hyperinflated lungs of obstructive lung disease
B. Tidal Volume (TV or V_T)	_C_ maximum amount of air that can be expired after maximum inspiration	_B_ information needed to determine rate and depth of artificial ventilation; multiplied by respiratory rate to provide minute volume
C. Functional Residual Volume (FRV); Functional Residual Capacity (FRC)	_A_ amount of air inhaled and exhaled during any respiratory cycle	_A_ reduced in obesity, obstructive airway disease

24. Match the diagnostic test with the information that the test measures.

A. arterial blood gas   _B_   photometric measurement of O_2 saturation (SaO_2)
B. oximetry   _F_   a sequence of pictures each representing a cross
C. transcutaneous CO_2 section or cut through lung tissue at a different
    monitoring   depth
D. radiography   _A_   a sensitive indicator to monitor O_2, CO_2, and pH
E. magnetic resonance   _E_   clearly identifies soft tissues with a two or three
    imaging   dimensional image
F. computerized   _D_   produces images of internal structures of the chest,
    tomography   including air-filled lungs, vascular markings, heart
                                                  and great vessels
                                          _C_   provides a non-invasive, continuous, and reliable
                                                  measurement of arterial carbon dioxide

25. When caring for the infant who is connected to a pulse oximeter, which part of the sensor is placed on the top of the nail when digits are used?
A. The photodetector
B. The microprocessor
C. The light emitting diode (LED)
D. The electrode

26. The nurse performs a precautionary assessment of the collateral circulation when arterial puncture is performed on the child. This test is called the:
A. cover test.
B. Allen test.
C. Miller test.
D. Weber test.

27. Which one of the following arterial blood gas results indicates acidosis?
A. pH of 7.32
B. pH of 7.47
C. pCO_2 of 44 mm Hg
D. O_2 of 75 mm Hg

28. Oxygen delivered to older infants is BEST tolerated when it is administered:
A. directly in the face of the infant under a hood.
B. by a hood that extends to touch the infant's shoulders.
C. by an oxygen tent that does not come into direct contact with the face.
D. by nasal canula or prongs.

29. The oxygen mist tent is a satisfactory means of O_2 administration for children past early infancy who need oxygen, because the oxygen mist tent:
A. comes into direct contact with the face.
B. controls and maintains the oxygen above 50%.
C. does not come into direct contact with the face.
D. keeps the child warm and dry.

30. When caring for the child receiving oxygen via a mist tent, the nurse should:
    A. encourage the child to have a stuffed animal in the tent.
    B. open the tent as little as possible.
    C. open the tent at the bottom of the bed to allow as little oxygen to escape as possible.
    D. keep the child cool because the tent becomes very warm.

31. Oxygen induced CO_2 narcosis is encountered MOST frequently in children with:
    A. prematurity.
    B. asthma.
    C. cystic fibrosis.
    D. congenital heart disease.

32. For a child under the age of 5 who needs intermittent delivery of an aerosolized medication, the nurse should consider using a:
    A. hand held nebulizer.
    B. metered-dose inhaler with a spacer device.
    C. humidified mist tent with low flow oxygen.
    D. metered-dose inhaler without a spacer device.

33. Postural drainage should be performed:
    A. before meals but following other respiratory therapy.
    B. after meals but before other respiratory therapy.
    C. before meals and before other respiratory therapy.
    D. after meals and after other respiratory therapy.

34. Which of the following children would need special modifications of the usual postural drainage techniques?
    A. Infants
    B. Children with head injuries
    C. Children in traction
    D. All of the above

35. Which one of the following techniques of chest physiotherapy has been shown through research to be an effective modality?
    A. Postural drainage with forced expiration
    B. Postural drainage with percussion
    C. Percussion and vibration
    D. All of the above

36. Which one of the following statements about chest percussion is CORRECT?
    A. Making a slapping sound
    B. May be painful
    C. May use a soft circular mask
    D. Performed over the rib cage and diaphragm

37. The BEST method to stimulate deep breathing in children is to:
    A. encourage the child to cover their mouth and suppress their cough.
    B. encourage the child to cough repeatedly.
    C. use games that extend expiratory time and pressure.
    D. leave some balloons at the bedside for the child to blow up.

38. When using the bag-valve-mask devise the nurse should:
    A. use the type without a reservoir.
    B. use the type with a reservoir.
    C. use a low oxygen concentration.
    D. hyperextend the child's neck.

39. Which one of the following urinary output values would indicate a problem for the younger child who weighs 30 kg?
    A. 100 ml from 2 a.m. to 3 a.m.
    B. 100 ml from 2 a.m. to 6 a.m.
    C. 200 ml from 2 a.m. to 4 a.m.
    D. 200 ml from 2 a.m. to 5 a.m.

40. The MOST severe complication that can occur during the intubation procedure is:
    A. infection.
    B. sore throat.
    C. laryngeal stenosis.
    D. hypoxia.

41. Which one of the following vaccuum pressures is acceptable for a child?
    A. 30 mm Hg
    B. 50 mm Hg
    C. 80 mm Hg
    D. 120 mm Hg

42. When suctioning a child's airway the nurse should always:
    A. use intermittent suction.
    B. inject saline into the tube.
    C. insert the catheter until it meets resistance.
    D. use continuous suction.

43. Suctioning obstructs the airway, therefore the suction catheter should remain in the child's airway no longer than:
    A. 3 seconds.
    B. 5 seconds.
    C. 8 seconds.
    D. 10 seconds.

44. Which of the following tracheostomy dressings is unacceptable?
    A. Duoderm CGF
    B. Allevyn dressing
    C. A 4 X 4 gauze pad cut into the needed shape
    D. Hollister Restore

45. After the initial postoperative change, the tracheostomy tube is usually changed:
    A. weekly by the surgeon.
    B. weekly by the nurse/family.
    C. monthly by the surgeon.
    D. monthly by the nurse/family.

46. Describe 3 factors in the home environment that need to be considered when discharging a child with a tracheostomy?

_____

_____

_____

47. A tracheostomy with a speaking valve:
   A. decreases secretions.
   B. decreases the child's sense of taste and smell.
   C. limits gas exchange.
   D. has no effect on the ability to swallow.

48. List at least ten conditions that would predispose a child to respiratory failure.

_____   _____

_____   _____

_____   _____

_____   _____

_____   _____

49. Which one of the following signs is an early subtle indication of hypoxia?
   A. Peripheral cyanosis
   B. Central cyanosis
   C. Hypotension
   D. Mood changes and restlessness

50. Which one of the following strategies is INAPPROPRIATE to use to control O_2 demand of the child with respiratory distress?
   A. Maintain temperature within normal limits
   B. Place the child in the supine position
   C. Control pain
   D. Maintain an ambient room temperature

51. Cardiac arrest in the pediatric population is MOST often a result of:
   A. Atherosclerosis.
   B. Aongenital heart disease.
   C. Prolonged hypoxia.
   D. Undiagnosed cardiac conditions.

52. The FIRST action the nurse should take when discovering a child in an emergency outside the hospital is to:
   A. transport the child to an acute care facility.
   B. determine whether the child is unconscious.
   C. administer rescue breathing.
   D. transport the child by car for help.

53. At what age range would the nurse place the bag-valve-mask over both the mouth and the nose?
    A. Birth to 1 year
    B. One year to 3 years
    C. Birth to 3 years
    D. Birth to 2 years

54. At what age range in an emergency situation should the nurse assess circulation by palpating the carotid pulse?
    A. 2 to 3 years
    B. Birth to 3 years
    C. Birth to 2 years
    D. Birth to 1 year

55. In a child who is conscious and choking the nurse should attempt to relieve the obstruction if the victim:
    A. is making sounds.
    B. has an effective cough.
    C. has stridor.
    D. all of the above.

56. Match the drug used for pediatric emergency care with its use during resuscitation.

    A.   sodium bicarbonate   ___I___ reverses respiratory arrest that is due to excessive opiate administration
    B.   calcium chloride
    C.   bretylium   ___H___ increases cardiac output and heart rate by blocking vagal stimulation in the heart
    D.   adenosine
    E.   dopamine   ___C___ antidysrhythmic that is used if lidocaine is ineffective
    F.   lidocaine
    G.   epinephrine   ___B___ used for hypermagnesemia; needed for normal cardiac contractility
    H.   atropine
    I.   naloxone   ___E___ causes vasoconstriction and increases cardiac output

                                   ___F___ used for ventricular dysrhythmias

                                   ___G___ acts on alpha and beta-adrenergic receptor sites causing contraction especially at the site of the heart, vascular and other smooth muscle

                                   ___D___ administer rapidly; causes a temporary block through the atrioventricular node

                                   ___A___ used to buffer the pH

57. The Heimlich maneuver is recommended for children over the age of:
    A. 4 years.
    B. 3 years.
    C. 2 years.
    D. 1 year.

58. A 14-month-old male child is admitted to the pediatric unit with a respiratory infection. If he has the cough which is characteristic of croup syndromes, the nurse would expect to hear:
    A. paroxysmal cough with an inspiratory "whoop".
    B. a brassy cough.
    C. a very severe cough.
    D. a quiet cough.

59. If the child has no cough at all, the nurse would MOST likely suspect:
    A. cystic fibrosis.
    B. pertussis.
    C. pneumonia.
    D. measles.

60. The child is placed under mist tent at 40% oxygen. Chest physiotherapy and intravenous antibiotics are started. The nurse is monitoring his oxygen saturation with pulse oximetry. The pulse oximeter alarm sounds and the saturation registers at 76%. The nurse should begin the assessment with an evaluation for changes in:
    A. behavior.
    B. skin color.
    C. placement of the oximeter sensor.
    D. hemoglobin.

61. If the child is diagnosed as having pneumonia, which one of the following adjunctive techniques would be of NO value?
    A. Intravenous antibiotics
    B. The mist tent at 40% oxygen
    C. Pulse oximetry
    D. Chest physiotherapy

CHAPTER 32
The Child with Respiratory Dysfunction

1. Terms—Matching—Respiratory Infection

   A. upper respiratory tract
   B. lower respiratory tract
   C. strep throat
   D. acute rheumatic fever (ARF)
   E. acute glomerulonephritis
   F. cefdinir (Omnicef)

   G. Waldeyer tonsillar ring
   H. palatine tonsils
   I. pharyngeal tonsils
   J. lingual tonsils
   K. tubal tonsils
   L. tonsillectomy
   M. adenoidectomy

   N. Epstein-Barr (EB)
   O. heterophil antibody test
   P. spot test (Monospot)
   Q. antigenic shift
   R. antigenic drift
   S. meningitis
   T. cholesteatoma

   _____ the serious sequelae of strep throat; an inflammatory disease of the heart, joints, and central nervous system

   _____ adenoids; located above the palatine tonsils on the posterior wall of the nasopharynx

   _____ an acute kidney infection

   _____ removal of the adenoids recommended for those children in whom hypertrophied adenoids obstruct nasal breathing

   _____ a suppurative intracranial complication of a middle ear or mastoid infection

   _____ the pairs of tonsils that are part of a mass of lymphoid tissue that encircles the nasal and oral pharynx

   _____ consists of the bronchi and bronchioles (the reactive portion on the airway with smooth muscle and the ability to constrict), and the alveoli

   _____ faucial tonsils; located on either side of the oropharynx, behind and below the pillars of the fauces; the surface of these tonsils is usually visible during oral examination; removed during tonsillectomy

   _____ a slide test of high specificity for the diagnosis of infectious mononucleosis

   _____ consists primarily of the nose and pharynx; upper airway

   _____ removal of the palatine tonsils; indicated for massive hypertrophy that results in difficulty breathing or eating

   _____ 5 days of treatment with this drug has been shown to be safe and effective therapy for streptococcal pharygitis

   _____ major changes in viruses that occur at intervals of years (usually 5 to 10)

   _____ a virus; the principal cause of infectious mononucleosis

   _____ group A ß-hemolytic streptococcus (ABHS) infection of the upper airway

   _____ one of the least common but most potentially dangerous sequelae of otitis media with effusion (OME); the formation of a ketatinized epithelial cell that forms scales within the middle ear space; erodes all of the structures it encounters especially bone

   _____ located at the base of the tongue; found near the posterior nasopharyngeal opening of the eustachian tubes; not a part of the Waldeyer tonsillar ring

   _____ minor variations in viruses that occur almost annually

   _____ determines the extent to which the patient's serum will agglutinate sheep red blood cells; a titer of 1:160 is diagnostic of infectious mononucleosis; rapid, sensitive, inexpensive and easy to perform

2. Croup Syndromes and Other Respiratory Infections

A. croup
B. racemic epinephrine
C. tracheobronchitis
D. respiratory syncytial virus (RSV)
E. Ribavirin
F. RespiGam

G. meningism
H. tubercle
I. miliary TB
J. TB infection
K. TB disease
L. purified protein derivative (PPD)

M. multiple puncture tests (MPT's)
N. positive reaction TB skin test
O. negative reaction TB skin Test
P. BCG

_____O_____ usually means the child has never been infected with the organism

_____ responsible for at least 50% of children admitted for bronchiolitis

_____ produces limited immunity to TB; vaccine containing bovine bacilli with reduced virulence

_____ nebulized epinephrine; used in children with stridor at rest, retractions, or difficulty breathing

_____ meningeal symptoms

_____A_____ a symptom complex characterized by hoarseness, a resonant cough described as "barking" or "brassy", inspiratory stridor, and respiratory distress from swelling in the region of the larynx

_____ formed by epithelial cells surrounding and encapsulating multiplying bacilli in an attempt to wall off the invading organisms

_____ an antiviral agent; may be used to treat RSV

_____ used widely; standard dose is 5 tuberculin units in 0.1 ml of solution, injected inradermally; Mantoux test

_____ widespread dissemination of the tubercle bacillus to near and distant sites

_____N_____ person has been infected; does not confirm the presence of active disease

_____ respiratory syncytial virus immune globulin; has been used prophylactically to prevent RSV in high-risk infants

_____ the inflammation of the large airways, which is frequently associated with an upper respiratory infection; primary cause: viral agents

_____J_____ manifested by a positive skin test; symptomatic

_____ Tine test; limited in their usefulness

_____K_____ positive chest radiograph, positive sputum culture and signs of the disease are present

3. Non Infectious Irritants

A. aspiration pneumonia
B. carbon monoxide (CO)

C. carboxyhemoglobin (COHb)

D. hyperbacric oxygen chamber

_____ forms when carbon monoxide enters the bloodstream and binds with hemoglobin

_____ a colorless odorless gas with an affinity for hemoglobin 200 to 250 times greater than that of oxygen

_____ therapy for smoke toxicity that facilitates the breakdown of the carboxyhemoglobin bond and improves oxygen delivery to the tissues

_____ occurs when food, secretions, inert material, volatile compounds, or liquids enter the lung and causes inflammation and a chemical pneumonitis

4. Long-Term Respiratory Dysfunction

A. seasonal allergic rhinitis
B. house dust mites
C. cockroach
D. long-term control medications
E. quick-relief medications
F. nebulization
G. exercise-induced bronchospasm
H. written action plan
I. Peak expiratory flow meters
J. spacers
K. cystic fibrosis
L. meconium ileus
M. distal intestinal obstruction syndrome
N. prolapse of the rectum
O. chest physiotherapy
P. Flutter Mucus Clearance Device
Q. ThAIRapy vest
R. dormase alfa
S. lung transplantation

_____O_____ used daily to prevent infection and to maintain pulmonary hygiene in children with cystic fibrosis

_____ a method of medication administration in which the medication is mixed with saline and changed into an aerosol with a compressed air machine

_____I_____ used by the child with asthma at home to monitor their personal best values

_____ hay fever

_____J_____ holding chamber; devices that attach to a metered dose inhaler and hold medication long enough for the patient to inhale slowly

_____ an important allergen in children with asthma; most common allergen in inner-city environments

_____K_____ the protein product that is located on the long arm of chromosome 7; indicator of cystic fibrosis

_____ rescue medications; used to treat acute symptoms and exacerbations of asthma

_____ allergen identified most often in children allergic to inhalants

_____ should be given to all children with asthma to use in the event of an exacerbation

_____ the earliest postnatal manifestation of cystic fibrosis; occurs in 7% to 10% of newborns with the disease; thick, putty-like tenacious mucilaginous meconium blocks the lumen of the small intestine usually at or near the ileocecal valve which gives rise to signs of intestinal obstruction

_____ provides a high-frequency chest wall oscillation to help loosen secretions

_____ small, handheld plastic pipe with a stainless-steel ball on the inside that facilitates removal of mucus

_____ caused by a loss of heat and/or water from the lungs because of hyperventilation of air that is cooler and dryer than that of the respiratory tract

_____ the most common gastrointestinal complication associated with cystic fibrosis; occurs most often in infancy and early childhood and is related to large bulky stools and lack of supportive fat pads around the rectum

_____ preventor medications; used to achieve and maintain control of inflammation in asthma

_____ a final therapeutic option for a few end-stage cystic fibrosis patients

_____ name given to a partial or complete intestinal obstruction that occurs in some children with cystic fibrosis

_____ recombinant human deoxyribonuclease; (Pulmozyme); an aerosolized medication that decreases the viscosity of mucus

5. The largest percentage of respiratory infections in children are caused by:
   A. pneumococci.
   B. viruses.
   C. streptococci.
   D. *Haemophilus influenza.*

6. The MOST likely reason that the respiratory infection rate increases drastically in the age range from 3 to 6 month is that the:
   A. infant's exposure to pathogens is greatly increased during this time.
   B. viral agents that are mild in older children are extremely severe in infants.
   C. maternal antibodies have disappeared and the infant's own antibody production is immature.
   D. diameter of the airways is smaller in the infant than in the older child.

7. Which one of the following situations is LEAST likely to be associated with a febrile seizure?
   A. Fever in a 2-year-old child.
   B. A family history of febrile seizures.
   C. Fever in an 8-year-old child.
   D. All of the above

8. The primary concern of the nurse when giving tips for how to increase humidity in the home of a child with a respiratory infection should be to be sure the child has:
   A. a steam vaporizer.
   B. a warm humidification source.
   C. a humidification source that is safe.
   D. a cool humidification source.

9. Which one of the following options would be the BEST choice for the child with a respiratory disorder who needs bedrest, but is not cooperating?
   A. Be sure the mother takes the advise seriously.
   B. Allow the child to play quietly on the floor.
   C. Insist that the child play quietly in bed.
   D. Allow the child to cry until he/she stays in bed.

10. For children who are having difficulty breathing through their noses because of a stuffy nose, the nurse should recommend:
    A. dextromethorphan nose drops.
    B. phenylephrine nose drops.
    C. dextromethorphan cough squares.
    D. steroid nose drops.

11. Children with nasopharyngitis may be treated with:
    A. decongestants.
    B. antihistamines.
    C. expectorants.
    D. all of the above.

12. The BEST technique to use to prevent spread of nasopharyngitis is:
    A. prompt immunization.
    B. to avoid contact with infected persons.
    C. mist vaporization.
    D. to assure adequate fluid intake.

13. Group A beta-hemolytic streptococci infection is usually a:
    A. serious infection of the upper airway.
    B. common cause of pharyngitis in children over the age of 15 years.
    C. brief illness that leaves the child at risk for serious sequelae.
    D. disease of the heart, lungs, joints, and central nervous system.

14. The American Academy of Pediatrics recommends that health care providers base their diagnosis of group A beta-hemolytic streptococcus on:
    A. antibody responses.
    B. antistreptolysin O responses.
    C. complete blood count.
    D. throat culture.

15. Which one of the following strategies should the nurse recommend for the prevention of streptococcal disease?
    A. Children with streptococcal infection should not return to school until after 48 hours of antibiotic therapy.
    B. Children with streptococcal infection should discard their toothbrush and replace it with a new one after 24 hours of antibiotic therapy.
    C. Children with streptococcal infection should not return to school until 36 hours of antibiotic therapy.
    D. Children with streptococcal infection should discard their toothbrush and replace it with a new one as soon as the streptococcus is identified.

16. Offensive mouth odor, persistent dry cough and a voice with a muffled nasal quality are commonly the result of:
    A. tonsillectomy.
    B. adenoidectomy.
    C. mouth breathing.
    D. otitis media.

17. An adenoidectomy would be CONTRAINDICATED in a child:
    A. with recurrent otitis media.
    B. with malignancy.
    C. with thrombocytopenia.
    D. under the age of three years.

18. In the postoperative period following a tonsillectomy the child should:
    A. be placed in Trendelenburg position.
    B. be encouraged to cough and deep breath.
    C. be suctioned vigorously to clear the airway.
    D. rest in bed the rest of the day after the surgery.

19. Pain medication for the child in the postoperative period following a tonsillectomy should be administered:
    A. orally at regular intervals.
    B. orally as needed.
    C. rectally or intravenously at regular intervals.
    D. rectally or intravenously as needed.

20. Which one of the following foods is MOST appropriate to offer first to an alert child who is in the postoperative period following a tonsillectomy?
    A. Ice cream
    B. Red gelatin
    C. Flavored ice pops
    D. All of the above are appropriate.

21. Which one of the following signs is an early indication of hemorrhage in a child who has had a tonsillectomy?
    A. Frequent swallowing
    B. Decreasing blood pressure
    C. Restlessness
    D. All of the above

22. Which one of the following findings is almost always present in an adolescent with infectious mononucleosis?
    A. Skin rash
    B. Otitis media
    C. Hepatic involvement
    D. Failure to thrive

23. Diagnosis of infectious mononucleosis is established when the:
    A. leukocyte count is elevated.
    B. leukocyte count is depressed.
    C. antibody testing is positive.
    D. antibody testing is negative.

24. Infectious mononucleosis is usually a:
    A. disease complicated with pneumonitis and anemia.
    B. self limiting disease.
    C. disabling disease.
    D. difficult and prolonged disease.

25. Clinical manifestations of influenza would usually include all of the following EXCEPT:
    A. nausea and vomiting.
    B. fever and chills.
    C. sore throat and dry mucous membranes.
    D. photophobia and myalgia.

26. The infant is predisposed to developing otitis media because the eustachian tubes:
    A. lie in a relatively horizontal plane.
    B. have a limited amount of lymphoid tissue.
    C. are long and narrow.
    D. are underdeveloped.

27. List at least 5 complications of otitis media.

_____   _____

_____   _____

_____

28. The clinical manifestations of otitis media include:
    A. purulent discharge in the external auditory canal.
    B. clear discharge in the external auditory canal.
    C. enlarged axillary lymph nodes.
    D. enlarged cervical lymph nodes.

29. An abnormal otoscopic exam would reveal:
    A. visible landmarks.
    B. a light reflex.
    C. dull gray tympanic membrane.
    D. mobile tympanic membrane.

30. Which one of the following antibiotics would most likely be prescribed for uncomplicated otitis media?
    A. Tetracycline
    B. Amoxacillin
    C. Gentamicin
    D. Methicillin

31. To help alleviate the discomfort and fever of otitis media the nurse may administer:
    A. acetaminophen or ibuprofen.
    B. antihistamines and decongestants.
    C. analgesic ear drops.
    D. all of the above.

32. Recurrent otitis media in high-risk infants may be managed therapeutically by:
    A. tonsillectomy.
    B. steroids.
    C. polyvalent pneumococcal polysaccharide vaccine.
    D. immune globulin with antibodies.

33. Children with tympanostomy tubes should:
    A. never swim without earplugs.
    B. keep bath water out of the ear.
    C. notify the physician immediately if a grommet appears.
    D. never allow any water to enter their ears.

34. Which one of the following techniques would be CONTRAINDICATED for the nurse to recommend to parents to prevent recurrent otitis externa?
    A. Administer a combination of vinegar and alcohol after swimming.
    B. Allow the child to swim every day.
    C. Dry the ear canal after swimming with a cotton swab.
    D. Use a hair dryer on low heat at 1-2 feet for 30 seconds several times a day.

35. Most children with croup syndromes:
    A. require hospitalization.
    B. will need to be intubated.
    C. can be cared for at home.
    D. are over 6 years old.

36. Which one of the following croup syndromes is potentially life threatening?
    A. Spasmodic croup
    B. Laryngotracheobronchitis
    C. Acute spasmodic laryngitis
    D. Epiglottitis

37. The nurse should suspect epiglottitis if the child has:
    A. cough, sore throat and agitation.
    B. cough, drooling and retractions.
    C. absence of cough, drooling and agitation.
    D. absence of cough, hoarseness and retractions.

38. In the child who is suspected to have epiglottitis the nurse should:
    A. have intubation equipment available.
    B. prepare to immunize the child for *Haemophilus influenza.*
    C. obtain a throat culture.
    D. all of the above.

39. Since the advent of immunization for *Haemophilus influenza,* there has been a decrease in the incidence of:
    A. laryngotracheobronchitis.
    B. epiglottitis.
    C. Reye's syndrome.
    D. croup syndrome.

40. Which one of the following children is most likely to be hospitalized for treatment of croup?
    A. A 2-year-old child whose croupy cough worsens at night
    B. A 5-year-old child whose croupy cough worsens at night
    C. A 2-year-old child using the accessory muscles to breath
    D. A child with inspiratory stridor during the physical exam

41. Which one of the following choices includes the primary therapeutic regimens for croup?
    A. Vigilant assessment, racemic epinephrine and corticosteroids
    B. Vigilant assessment, racemic epinephrine and antibiotics
    C. Intubation, racemic epinephrine and corticosteroids
    D. Intubation, racemic epinephrine and corticosteroids

42. Which one of the following conditions is MOST likely to require intubation?
    A. Acute spasmodic laryngitis
    B. Bacterial tracheitis
    C. Acute laryngotracheobronchitis
    D. Acute laryngitis

43. Respiratory syncytial virus is:
    A. an uncommon virus that usually causes severe bronchiolitis.
    B. an uncommon virus that usually does not require hospitalization.
    C. a common virus that usually causes severe bronchiolitis.
    D. a common virus that usually does not require hospitalization.

44. In the infant who is admitted with possible respiratory syncytial virus, the nurse would expect the lab to perform:
    A. the ELISA antibody test on nasal secretions.
    B. a viral culture of the stool.
    C. a bacterial culture of nasal secretions.
    D. an anaerobic culture of the blood.

45. Nurses caring for a child with respiratory syncitial virus should:
    A. have a skin test applied every six months.
    B. wear gloves and gowns when entering the room.
    C. turn off the aerosol machine before opening the tent.
    D. not take care of other children with respiratory syncitial virus at the same time.

46. Match the age of the child with the most common cause of pneumonia in that age group.

    A. *Haemophilus influenza*   _____ over 5 years of age
    B. *Streptococcus*   _____ 3 months to 5 years old
       pneumonia
                                    _____ under 3 months
    C. *Mycoplasma pneumonia*

47. Closed chest drainage is most likely to be used when pneumonia is caused by which of the following organisms?
    A. *Haemophilus influenzae*
    B. *Mycoplasma pneumoniae*
    C. *Streptococcus pneumoniae*
    D. *Staphylococcal pneumoniae*

48. Describe 4 nursing measures to use to care for the child with pneumonia.

    _____

    _____

    _____

49. In an 8-month-old infant admitted to the hospital with pertussis, the nurse should particularly assess the:
    A. living conditions of the infant.
    B. labor and delivery history of the mother.
    C. immunization status of the infant.
    D. alcohol and drug intake of the mother.

50. The BEST test to screen for tuberculosis is the:
    A. chest x-ray.
    B. purified protein derivative (PPD) test.
    C. sputum culture.
    D. multipuncture tests (MPT) like the tine test.

51. The recommended treatment for the child who has active tuberculosis includes:
    A. isoniazid.
    B. rifampin.
    C. pyrazinamide.
    D. all of the above.

52. Which one of the following Mantoux Test results would be considered positive?
    A. Induration 5 mm in a 3-year-old child with HIV
    B. Induration 2 mm in a 5-year-old child without TB contacts
    C. Induration 7 mm in an 8-year-old child without any risk factors
    D. All of the above

53. The usual site of bronchial obstruction is the:
    A. left bronchus because it is shorter and straighter.
    B. left bronchus because it is longer and angled.
    C. right bronchus because it is shorter and straighter.
    D. right bronchus because it is longer and angled.

54. The DEFINITIVE DIAGNOSIS of airway foreign bodies in the trachea and larynx requires:
    A. radiographic examination.
    B. fluoroscopic examination.
    C. bronchoscopic examination.
    D. ultrasonographic examination.

55. Parents may be taught to deal with aspiration of a foreign body in an infant under 12 months old by using:
    A. back blows and chest thrusts.
    B. back blows only.
    C. the Heimlich maneuver only.
    D. a blind finger sweep.

56. The child who has ingested lighter fluid usually receives:
    A. the same treatment as a child who has hepatitis.
    B. medication to induce vomiting.
    C. the same treatment as a child who has pneumonia.
    D. activated charcoal.

57. List 5 strategies that may be used to manage Adult Respiratory Distress Syndrome in children.

    _____   _____

    _____   _____

    _____

58. Deaths from fires are most often a result of:
    A. full thickness burns over 50% of the body.
    B. full thickness burns to the chest and neck.
    C. noxious substances from incomplete combustion.
    D. injuries sustained in escape attempts.

59. Treatment of smoke toxicity with a COHb level of 10% would most likely consist of:
    A. humidified O_2 at 70%.
    B. humidified O_2 at 100%.
    C. intubation.
    D. use of a hyperbaric oxygen chamber.

60. The biochemical marker for environmental smoke exposure is called _____.

61. List at least five physical findings commonly seen in the child with allergic rhinitis.

    _____   _____

    _____   _____

    _____

62. Which one of the following children is MOST LIKELY suffering from allergy rather than a cold?
    A. A two-year-old with fever and runny nose
    B. An adolescent with itchy eyes, constant sneezing without fever
    C. A two-year-old with sporadic sneezing and a runny nose
    D. An adolescent with sporadic sneezing and a runny nose

63. The severity of asthma in a child with daily asthmatic symptoms would be classified as:
    A. mild intermittent.
    B. mild persistent.
    C. moderate persistent.
    D. severe persistent.

Critical Thinking • Case Study

Jason Wilson who is 8 years old is admitted to the pediatric unit with a diagnosis of reactive airway disease. This is his first hospitalization for this disorder. Both of Jason's parents smoke cigarettes, but they try to smoke outdoors. Jason usually does quite well. His asthma tends to increase in severity during the winter months. This year he has had several colds and his asthma has flared up each time. This time, however, he is quite uncomfortable. He has wheezes in all lung fields.

64. Which one of the following questions would be important for the nurse to ask Jason's mother?
    A. "What brings you to the hospital?"
    B. "What is your ethnic background?"
    C. "Do you have any history of asthma in your family?"
    D. "Was your pregnancy and delivery uneventful?"

65. Mrs. Wilson wants the nurse to explain exactly what reactive airway disease is. She says she has been told many times, but it is always when Jason is in so much distress that she is not sure that she hears it correctly. The nurse would respond knowing that:
    A. asthma is caused by a certain inflammatory mediator.
    B. the one mechanism responsible for the obstructive symptoms of asthma is excess mucous secretion.
    C. the one mechanism responsible for the obstructive symptoms of asthma is spasm of the smooth muscle of the bronchi.
    D. most theories do not explain all types and causes of asthma.

66. In general Jason does not have difficulty with any food or emotional triggers for asthma. An asthmatic episode for Jason starts with itching all over the upper part of his back. He is usually quite irritable and very restless. He complains of headache, chest tightness, and feeling tired. He usually will cough and sweat and sit up right with his shoulders in a hunched over position. Today he has no fever and he is in the tripod position. His skin is sweaty. Based on this information the nurse would decide that Jason is:
    A. severely ill.
    B. moderately ill.
    C. mildly ill.
    D. not ill at all.

67. Jason's younger sister Tanya is an infant. Tanya's disease is much worse than Jason's. Mrs. Wilson states that she often has movements of her chest muscles which look like she is working very hard to breath, but that her respiratory rate does not change. When this is happening Tanya is not breathing a long breath out like Jason. These differences between Jason and Tanya are confusing to Mrs. Wilson and she asks the nurse for advice about what to do when this happens to Tanya. The nurse's response is based on the knowledge that:
    A. dyspnea is much more difficult to evaluate in an infant than in a young child.
    B. infants and young children's bodies respond to the asthmatic episode the same way.
    C. boys tend to have a more severe disease of asthma than girls.
    D. dyspnea is much more difficult to evaluate in a young child than in an infant.

68. The nurse examines Jason and finds that he has hyperresonance on percussion. His breath sounds are coarse and loud with sonorous crackles throughout the lung fields. Expiration is prolonged. There is generalized inspiratory and expiratory wheezing. Based on these findings the nurse suspects that there is:
    A. minimal obstruction.
    B. significant obstruction.
    C. imminent ventilatory failure.
    D. an extrathoracic obstruction.

69. The nurse determines that Jason's peak expiratory flow rate is in the yellow zone. The nurse recognizes that this test result indicates that Jason's asthma control is about:
    A. 80% of his personal best and that his routine treatment plan can be followed.
    B. 50% of his personal best and that he needs an increase in his usual therapy.
    C. 50% of his personal best and he needs immediate bronchodilators.
    D. less than 50% of his personal best and that he need immediate bronchodilators.

70. Jason's test results are back from the lab. The white blood cell count is 11,200/mm^3. The eosinophils are 728/mm^3. The chest x-ray shows hyperexpansion of the airways. The nurse knows that these findings:
   A. support the diagnosis of pneumonia without an episode of asthma.
   B. support the diagnosis of asthma complicated with pneumonia.
   C. do not support the diagnosis of an acute episode of asthma or pneumonia.
   D. support the diagnosis of an acute episode of asthma without pneumonia.

71. The physician orders albuterol via inhaler for Jason. Mrs. Wilson is very concerned, because she says that Jason usually receives theophylline intravenously. The nurse's response is based on the fact that:
   A. Jason's asthma episode is probably not as severe as usual.
   B. Jason's physician must be using information that is out of date.
   C. theophylline is a third line drug that is a weak bronchodilator and not considered as effective as nebulized beta agonists.
   D. theophylline is a third line drug because it has been shown to adversely affect school performance.

72. Jason's physician has ordered a corticosteroid via aerosol in addition to the albuterol. Which medication should the nurse administer first?
   A. Albuterol
   B. The corticosteroid

73. When preparing for discharge, the nurse would MOST likely plan to teach the Wilson family to:
   A. keep the humidity at home above 50%.
   B. vacuum the carpets at least twice weekly.
   C. treat carpets with a 3% tannic acid solution.
   D. launder sheets/blankets regularly in cold water.

74. Jason uses aerosolized steroids at home; therefore he should be taught to rinse his mouth thoroughly with water:
   A. before each treatment to increase absorption.
   B. after each treatment to minimize the risk of oral candidiasis.
   C. before each treatment to minimize the adverse effects of the drug.
   D. after each treatment to increase absorption.

75. Based on the nurse's assessment, a care plan is developed. Which one of the following nursing diagnoses would be LEAST likely to appear on Jason's care plan?
   A. Activity intolerance related to imbalance between oxygen supply and demand
   B. Ineffective airway clearance related to allergenic response and inflammation in the bronchial tree
   C. High risk for infection related to the presence of infective organisms
   D. Altered family process related to a chronic illness

76. Which one of the following principles should be a part of Jason's home self-management program?
   A. Individuals must learn not to abuse their medications so that they will not become addicted.
   B. It is easy to treat an asthmatic episode as long as the child knows the symptoms.
   C. Although quite uncommon, asthma is very treatable.
   D. Children with asthma are usually able to participate in the same activities as non-asthmatic children.

Andrea MacAuley is an 8-year-old with cystic fibrosis. She is in the fifth percentile for both height and weight. This failure to thrive persists even though she has a voracious appetite. She has been managed at home most recently for about six months without the need for hospitalization. She is admitted today with blood tinged sputum. The sputum culture obtained two days ago is positive for pseudomonas The nurse hears crackles in both lungs and she has significant clubbing of her fingers with a capillary refill time of greater than 5 seconds.

77. Based on the information presented in Andrea MacAuley's case study, the nurse suspects that Andrea's:
   A. condition is improving and she will soon return to home care.
   B. condition is progressively worsening.
   C. condition is worse, but intravenous antibiotic therapy will correct the problem.
   D. family has been non-compliant causing this set back.

78. The admission orders included an order for gentamicin at a dose that the nurse calculated to be higher than usual for a child of Andrea's size. This dose may be high due to the fact that:
   A. the physician used Andrea's age rather than her size to determine the dose.
   B. the pharmacy has made an error.
   C. children with cystic fibrosis metabolize antibiotics rapidly.
   D. children with cystic fibrosis metabolize antibiotics slowly.

79. Which one of the following strategies would most likely be CONTRAINDICATED for Andrea to use?
   A. Forced expiration
   B. Aerobic exercise
   C. Chest physiotherapy
   D. High flow oxygen therapy

80. The blood tinged sputum progresses to an amount greater than 300 cc. per day. The nurse recognizes that increased tendency to bleed may be a result of
   A. iron deficiency anemia.
   B. vitamin K deficiency.
   C. thrombocytopenia.
   D. vitamin D deficiency.

81. At the present time, family support for Andrea will most likely include strategies to help her family cope with all of the following issues EXCEPT:
   A. pregnancy and genetic counseling.
   B. relief from the continual routine with respite care.
   C. dealing with a chronic illness and anticipatory grieving.
   D. abnormal psychological adjustment and dysfunctional family patterns.

82. Andrea takes 7 pancreatic enzyme capsules about 30 minutes before each meal. She usually has 2 to 3 bowel movements per day. Which one of the following statements is CORRECT in regard to Andrea's pancreatic enzyme dosage?
   A. The dosage is adequate.
   B. The dosage should always be fewer than 5 capsules.
   C. The dosage should be 7 to 10 capsules.
   D. The dosage is adequate, but she should take it between meals.

CHAPTER 33
The Child with Gastrointestinal Dysfunction

1. Which one of the following is NOT a function of the GI system?
   A. Process and absorb nutrients necessary to support growth and development
   B. Maintain thermoregulatory functions *(circled)*
   C. Perform excretory functions
   D. Maintain fluid and electrolyte balance

2. Identify the following as TRUE or FALSE.

   __F__ At birth the term infant has the ability to move food particles from the front of the mouth to the back of the mouth.

   __T__ The infant has no voluntary control of swallowing for the first 3 months.

   __T__ The chewing function is facilitated by eruption of the primary teeth.

   __T__ The primary purpose of saliva in the newborn is to moisten the mouth and throat.

3. Fill in the blanks in the following statements.
   A. Three processes, _____, _____, and _____, are
      necessary to convert nutrients into forms that can be utilized by the body.
   B. Chemical digestion involves five general types of GI secretions: _____,
      _____, _____ _____, _____,
      and _____ _____ _____.
   C. The ___small___ ___intestine___ is the principal absorption site in the GI system.

4. What are the five MOST important basic nursing assessments included in a thorough GI
   assessment?

   _____I + O_____   _____abd exam_____

   _____Ht_____   _____urine + stool tests_____

   _____Wt_____

5. The nurse is preparing Dottie, age 7, for an upper GI endoscopy. Which one of the following
   does the nurse recognize as NOT being an appropriate preparation for this test?
   A. Bowel cleansing with magnesium citrate or Golytely *(circled)*
   B. NPO for 8 hours before the procedure
   C. Dottie will need to be given sedation before the procedure is begun.
   D. The nurse will need to explain to Dottie in advance about the procedure by use of pictures
      or play with dolls and demonstration.

6. Match the term with its description.

A. pica
B. failure to thrive
C. regurgitation
D. projectile vomiting
E. encopresis

F. hematemesis
G. hematochezia
H. melena
I. dysphagia
J. hemoccult test

K. stool for O & P (ova and parasites)
L. meconium
M. peristalsis
N. steatorrhea
O. obstipation

___N___ appearance of ingested fat in the feces

___J___ detects presence of blood in the stool

___F___ vomiting of bright red blood as a result of bleeding in the upper GI tract or from swallowed blood from the upper respiratory tract

___G___ passage of bright red blood from the rectum

___H___ passage of dark-colored "tarry" stools

___M___ wavelike movements that squeeze food along the entire length of the alimentary tract

___A___ eating disorder in which there is compulsive eating of both food and nonfood substances

___L___ thick greenish-black secretions normally expelled from the intestine shortly after birth

___O___ having long intervals between bowel movements

___D___ accompanied by vigorous peristaltic waves

___E___ outflow of incontinent stool causing soiling

___B___ deceleration from normal pattern of growth or below the 5th percentile

___I___ difficulty swallowing

___K___ aids in the diagnosis of parasitic infections

___C___ a backward flowing as from the return of gastric contents into the mouth

7. Pica should be considered in which of the following children presenting to the health clinic?
   A. 7-year-old with nausea and vomiting for the past 3 days
   B. 4-year-old with history of celiac disease presenting with anemia and abdominal pain
   C. 2-year-old who is still on the bottle and presents with anemia
   D. 4-month-old who presents with crying, irritability and reddish colored stools

8. Lance, a 2-year-old, has been brought to the clinic because his parents are afraid he has swallowed a small button battery from his father's watch that he was playing with. The nurse recognizes which one of the following as the MOST appropriate nursing action at this time?
   A. Reassure the parents that Lance has probably not swallowed the battery because he has no symptoms, is playing in the exam room and his lung fields are clear.
   B. Explain to the parents that Lance will probably be allowed to normally pass the battery through the GI system because Lance has been able to eat and drink normally since the event.
   C. Start immediate teaching of Lance's parents on how to assess Lance's environment for hazardous objects, and how to assess Lance's toys and other items he might play with for safety.
   D. Explain to Lance's parents that x-ray examination will be conducted, and the battery will most probably need to be removed to prevent local damage.

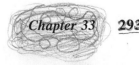

9. John, age 16, asks the nurse why he has to have an endoscopy exam to determine if he has helicobacter pylori. "Why can't they just do the blood test?" Formulate a correct response to this question.

_____

_____

_____

10. The nurse is counseling the mother of 12-month-old Brian on methods to prevent constipation. Which one of the following methods would be CONTRAINDICATED for Brian?
   A. Add bran to Brian's cereal.
   B. Increase Brian's intake of water.
   C. Add prunes to Brian's diet.
   D. Add popcorn to Brian's diet.

11. Sally, age 5, is being started on bowel habit retraining program for chronic constipation. Instructions to the family should include which one of the following?
   A. Decrease the water and increase the milk in Sally's diet.
   B. Establish a regular toilet time twice a day after meals when Sally will sit on the toilet for 5 to 10 minutes.
   C. Withhold Sally's play time with her friend Julie if she does not have a daily bowel movement.
   D. Have Sally sit on the toilet each day until she has a bowel movement.

12. To confirm the diagnosis of Hirschsprung disease, the nurse prepares the child for which one of the following tests?
   A. Barium enema
   B. Upper GI series
   C. Rectal biopsy
   D. Esophagoscopy

13. The nurse would expect to see what clinical manifestations in the child diagnosed with Hirschsprung disease?
   A. History of bloody diarrhea, fever, and vomiting
   B. Irritability, severe abdominal cramps, fecal soiling
   C. Decreased hemoglobin, increased serum lipids, and positive stool for O & P (ova and parasites)
   D. History of constipation, abdominal distention, and palpable fecal mass

14. Explain the defects present in congenital aganglionic megacolon.

_____

_____

_____

15. The nurse would expect postoperative care for the child with Hirschsprung disease (megacolon) to include which of the following?
    1. nothing by mouth until return of bowel sounds
    2. measuring intake and output, including NG tube
    3. colostomy care
    4. monitoring intravenous fluids
    5. daily saline enemas
    6. explaining to the parents and child that the colostomy is permanent and encouraging them to assume care before discharge

    A. 1, 2, 3, and 4
    B. 2, 3, and 5
    C. 1, 2, 3, 4, and 6
    D. 1, 2, 4, and 5

16. The passive transfer of gastric contents into the esophagus is termed:
    A. esophageal atresia.
    B. Meckel diverticulum.
    C. gastritis.
    D. gastroesophageal reflux.

17. The most common clinical manifestation of GER is __emesis__.

18. The nurse instructs the parents of a 4-month-old with gastroesophageal reflux to include which one of the following in the infant's care?
    A. Stop breast-feeding since breast milk is too thin and easily leads to reflux.
    B. Place the infant in either the flat prone or head-elevated prone position following feeding and at night.
    C. Increase the infant's intake of fruit or citrus juices.
    D. Try to increase feeding volume right before bedtime because this is the time when the stomach is more able to retain foods.

19. The child presenting with irritable bowel syndrome is MOST likely to represent which one of the following?
    A. History of colic with feeding difficulties and a family history of bowel problems
    B. Alternating patterns of constipation and bloody diarrhea with little flatulence
    C. History of parasitic infections, poor nutrition and low abdominal pain
    D. History of colic, laxative abuse, and growth retardation

20. Which one of the following would alert the nurse to possible peritonitis from a ruptured appendix in a child suspected of having appendicitis?
    A. Colicky abdominal pain with guarding of the abdomen
    B. Periumbilical pain that progresses to the lower right quadrant of the abdomen with an elevated WBC
    C. Low-grade fever of 100.6° F with the child having difficulty walking and assuming a side lying position with the knees flexed toward the chest
    D. Temperature of 103° F, absent bowel sounds and sudden relief from abdominal pain

21. What is the most intense site of pain in ~~appendicitis~~ called?

_____McBurney point_____

Where is this site located?

_____

What is the term used to describe pain elicited by light percussion around the perimeter of the abdomen that indicates the presence of peritoneal irritation?

_____

22. The MOST common clinical manifestations expected with Meckel diverticulum include which of the following?
    A. Fever, vomiting, and constipation
    B. Weight loss, hypotension, obstruction
    C. Painless rectal bleeding, abdominal pain or intestinal obstruction
    D. Abdominal pain, bloody diarrhea, and foul-smelling stool

23. A common feature of inflammatory bowel diseases is:
    A. growth abnormalities.
    B. chronic constipation.
    C. obstruction.
    D. burning epigastric pain.

24. Describe the pathophysiologic differences between Crohn's disease and ulcerative colitis.

_____

_____

_____

25. Nursing considerations for the adolescent with inflammatory bowel disease include:
    A. assisting the adolescent to cope with feelings of being different from peers and negative self-esteem.
    B. encouraging three large meals a day of high-protein, high-caloric foods.
    C. stopping drug therapy with remission of symptoms.
    D. elimination of all high-fiber foods from the diet.

26. Billy, age 14, has an ulcer involving the mucosa of the stomach that has resulted from prolonged use of nonsteroidal antiinflammatory agents. The BEST term to describe the ulcer Billy has is:
    A. duodenal ulcer caused by secondary factors.
    B. duodenal ulcer caused by primary factors.
    C. gastric ulcer caused by secondary factors.
    D. gastric ulcer caused by primary factors.

27. Which one of the following is NOT thought to contribute to peptic ulcer disease?
    A. Helicobacter pylori
    B. Alcohol and smoking
    C. Caffeine-containing beverages and spicy foods
    D. Psychologic factors such as stressful life events

28. Common therapeutic management of peptic ulcer disease includes which one of the following?
    A. Corticosteroids
    B. Cimetidine or ranitidine
    C. Acetaminophen
    D. Sulfasalazine and sucralfate

29. Justin, age 1 month, is brought to the clinic by his mother. The nurse suspects pyloric stenosis. Which one of the following symptoms would support this theory?
    A. Diarrhea
    B. Projectile vomiting
    C. Fever and dehydration
    D. Abdominal distention

30. Preoperatively, the nursing plan for suspected pyloric obstruction should include which of the following?
    1. observation for dehydration
    2. keep body temperature below 100 degrees F
    3. parental support and reassurance
    4. observation for coughing and gagging after feeding
    5. observation of quality of stool

    A. 1, 2, 3, 4, and 5
    B. 1, 3, and 4
    C. 3, 4, and 5
    D. 1 and 3

31. Postoperative feedings for the infant having undergone a pyloromyotomy include:
    A. keeping NPO for the first 24 hours then introduction of normal formula.
    B. glucose feedings beginning 4 to 6 hours after surgery and continuing for the first 72 hours.
    C. small, frequent feedings of glucose beginning 4 to 6 hours after surgery.
    D. thickened formula feeding within 24 hours after surgery.

32. An invagination of one portion of the intestine into another is called:
    A. intussusception.
    B. pyloric stenosis.
    C. tracheoesophageal fistula.
    D. Hirschsprung disease.

33. Al, age 5 months, is suspected of having intussusception. What clinical manifestations would he MOST likely have?
    A. Crying with abdominal exam, vomiting, currant jelly appearing stools
    B. Fever, diarrhea, vomiting and lowered WBC
    C. Weight gain, constipation, and refusal to eat
    D. Abdominal distention, periodic pain, hypotension

34. The use of barium as the contrast agent to reduce intussusceptions is being replaced in favor of water-soluble contrast and air pressure. Explain why.

    _____

    _____

35. Al's intussusception is reduced without surgery. The nurse should expect care for Al after the reduction to include:
    A. administration of antibiotics.
    B. enema administration to remove remaining stool.
    C. observation of stools.
    D. rectal temperatures every 4 hours.

36. Symptoms in celiac disease include stools that are:
    A. watery, pale, and with an offensive odor.
    B. currant-jelly appearing.
    C. small, frothy, and dark green.
    D. constipated, white, with ammonia smell.

37. The MOST important therapeutic management for the child with celiac disease is:
    A. eliminating corn, rice, and millet from the diet.
    B. adding iron, folic acid, and fat-soluble vitamins to the diet.
    C. eliminating wheat, rye, barley and oats from the diet.
    D. educating the child's parents about the short-term effects of the disease and the necessity of reading all food labels for content until the disease is in remission.

38. The prognosis for children with short bowel syndrome has improved as a result of:
    A. dietary supplemental Vitamin B_{12} additions.
    B. improvement in surgical procedures to correct the defect.
    C. improved home care availability.
    D. total parenteral nutrition and enteral feeding.

39. Jerry, a 4-year-old, is brought to the emergency room by his parents, who say he vomited a large amount of bright red blood. Jerry is pale, cool to the touch, with an increased respiratory and heart rate. The nurse expects priority care at this time to include:
    A. administration of intravenous fluids, usually normal saline or lactated ringers.
    B. stool testing for blood by hemocult.
    C. insertion of an NG tube for iced water lavage.
    D. preparation for tracheostomy.

40. Match the viral hepatitis type with the description. (Types may be used more than once.)

A. hepatitis A	C. hepatitis C	E. hepatitis E
B. hepatitis B	D. hepatitis D	F. hepatitis G

    __A__ most common form of acute viral hepatitis

    __A__ immunity by two inactivated vaccines given 6-12 months apart

    __E__ non A, non B with transmission through the fecal-oral route or with contaminated water

    __A__ spread directly and indirectly by the fecal-oral route

    __D__ occurs with children already infected with hepatitis B

    __C__ primary cause of post-transfusion hepatitis; often becomes a chronic condition and can cause cirrhosis

    __G__ incubation period 14 to 180 days; average 50 days

    __B__ universal vaccination recommended for all newborns

    __F__ virus is an RNA virus with a structure similar to that of HCV; is blood-borne, and high-risk groups include individuals infected with HCV

41. Sandy, age 2, is brought to the clinic by her mother because a fellow day school toddler has been diagnosed with hepatitis A. Sandy's mother is concerned that Sandy might develop the disease. Which one of the following serum laboratory tests would indicate to the nurse that Sandy has immunity to hepatitis A?
    A. anti-HAV IgG
    B. anti-HAV IgM
    C. HAsAg
    D. HAcAg

42. Sandy's testing reflects that she has not had hepatitis A. Because her exposure to hepatitis A has occurred within the last two weeks, the nurse would expect the physician to order which one of the following for prophylactic administration?
    A. hepatitis B immune globulin (HBIG)
    B. HBV vaccine
    C. standard immune globulin (IG)
    D. HAV vaccine

43. What are the four major goals of management for viral hepatitis?

    _____   _____

    _____   _____

44. Which one of the following would NOT be expected in the child diagnosed with cirrhosis?
    A. Hepatospenomegaly
    B. Elevated liver function tests
    C. Decreased ammonia levels
    D. Ascites

Critical Thinking • Case Study

Danny, age 17, is a junior in high school. He comes to the clinic with complaints of right lower abdominal pain, and slight fever.

45. What questions should be included in the history of present illness if appendicitis is suspected?

    _____

    _____

    _____

46. Danny should be advised to avoid which of the following until seen by the physician?
    A. All activity
    B. All laxatives
    C. Ice to the abdomen
    D. All of the above

47. Danny is admitted to the hospital with a diagnosis of acute appendicitis. The nurse should institute which one of the following independent nursing actions?
    A. Allow clear liquids only.
    B. Start intravenous fluids with antibiotics.
    C. Insert a nasogastric tube and connect to suction.
    D. Monitor closely for progression of symptoms.

48. What laboratory blood evaluation and results would the nurse expect to see in a patient with acute appendicitis?

    _____

    _____

49. Danny is now two hours postoperative. During surgery, Danny's appendix was found to have ruptured before surgery. A priority nursing diagnosis at this time would be:
    A. high risk for spread of infection related to rupture.
    B. pain related to inflamed appendix.
    C. altered growth and development related to hospital care.
    D. anxiety related to knowledge deficit regarding disease.

50. The MOST critical outcome for Danny after surgery is:
    A. peritonitis has resolved as evidenced by no fever, lack of elevated WBC, and the wound is clean and healing.
    B. pain is relieved as evidenced by no verbalization of pain, and Danny is resting quietly.
    C. Danny and his family demonstrate understanding of hospitalization.
    D. Danny is able to express feelings and concerns.

CHAPTER 34
The Child with Cardiovascular Dysfunction

1. General Cardiac Terms

A.	congenital heart defects	F.	pericardium
B.	acquired cardiac disorders	G.	pericardial space
		H.	pericardial fluid
C.	mediastinum	I.	atria
D.	myocardium	J.	ventricles
E.	endocardium	K.	valves

L. tricuspid valve
M. mitral valve
N. atrioventricular (AV) valves
O. chordae tendineae
P. semilunar valves

_____ structures located in the pulmonary artery (pulmonic valve) and the aorta (aortic valve) that prevent back flow of blood

_____ a few drops of serous fluid that is found normally between the two layers of membrane that cover the heart

_____ located between left atrium and the left ventricle; prevents flow from the right ventricle back into the left ventricle

_____ the two bottom chambers of the interior of the heart

_____ a double walled membrane that forms a covering for the heart

_____ the muscular tissue that forms the main mass of the heart

_____ disease processes or abnormalities that occur after birth; can be seen in the normal heart or in the presence of congenital heart defects

_____ prevent back flow in the heart

_____ anatomic abnormalities present at birth that result in abnormal cardiac function

_____ located between the right atrium and the right ventricle; prevents flow from the right ventricle back into the right ventricle

_____ a thin layer of endothelial tissue that lines the inner surface of the myocardium

_____ the two upper chambers of the interior of the heart

_____ the space between the two pleural cavities

_____ term used to describe both the mitral valve and the tricuspid valve together

_____ cord-like structures that attach atrioventricular valves to the heart muscle

_____ the slight space between the two layers of membrane that cover the heart

2. Embryologic Development Terms

A. endocardial cushions   E. truncus arteriosus   J. membranous septum
B. 5 week structures   F. atrial septum   K. ductus venousus
C. bulbus cordis   G. foramen ovale   L. ductus arteriousus
D. sinus venosus   H. venticular septum   M. coronary arteries
   I. muscular septum   N. coronary veins

_____ develops into the inferior and superior vena cava

_____ the vessel that allows blood to travel directly to the inferior vena cava prior to birth

_____ embryologic internal bulges that eventually merge to divide the heart chambers

_____ the structure that permits blood to be shunted to the descending aorta from the pulmonary artery prior to birth

_____ eventually helps to form the outflow tracts of the ventricles

_____ develops out of an intricate growth of the endocardial cushions, conal cushions, and conotruncal septum

_____ collect blood and return it directly to the right atrium or through the coronary sinus which drains into the right atrium

_____ divides into the pulmonary artery and aorta, and gives rise to the aortic arch

_____ Time when the beginnings of the common atrium, common ventricle and bulbus cordis, sinus venosus, and truncus arteriosus form

_____ develops from the joining of the muscular and membranous ventricular sept during the fourth to eight weeks of embryologic growth

_____ a temporary flap opening that is formed from the overlapping of the septum primum and the septum secundum before they fuse

_____ develops when the right and left ventricular chambers fuse

_____ supply the heart muscle with its blood supply; arise above the aortic valve

_____ formed by the growth of septum primum and septum secundum at about the fourth week of fetal growth

3. Wave Forms

A. P wave   C. QRS complex   E. Q-T interval
B. P-R interval   D. T wave   F. ST segment

_____ represents ventricular repolarization

_____ represents the spread of the impulse over the atria (atrial depolarization). The sinus node's electrical activity is not represented in the ECG.

_____ represents ventricular depolarization and repolarization. This interval varies with heart rate; the faster the rate, the shorter the Q-T interval. In children this interval is normally shorter than in adults.

_____ represents the time that elapses from the beginning of atrial depolarization to the beginning of ventricular depolarization.

_____ represents the time that the ventricles are in absolute refractory period, the period between ventricular depolarization and repolarizaton

_____ represents ventricular depolarization; actually composed of three separate waves that result from the currents generated when the ventricles depolarize before their contraction

4. Conduction System and Physiology

A. cardiac cycle
B. systole
C. diastole
D. cardiac output
E. stroke volume
F. preload
G. afterload
H. systemic vascular resistance
I. pulmonary vascular resistance
J. contractility
K. Starling law
L. tachycardia
M. bradycardia
N. tachypnea

_____ the efficiency of myocardial fiber shortening; the ability of the cardiac muscle to act as an efficient pump

_____ the amount of blood ejected by the heart in any one contraction

_____ slow heart rate

_____ composed of sequential contraction and relaxation of both the atria and the ventricles

_____ fast heart rate

_____ the volume of blood ejected by the heart in 1 minute

_____ refers to the resistance against which the ventricles must pump when ejecting blood; blood pressure gives some indication of this resistance

_____ contraction of both the atria and ventricles

_____ the resistance of the pulmonary circulation

_____ relaxation of both the atria and the ventricles

_____ the volume of blood returning to the heart; the circulation blood volume

_____ the principle that demonstrates that an increase in ventricular end-diastolic volume somewhat increases stroke volume

_____ resistance of the systemic circulation

_____ fast respiratory rate

5. Congenital Heart Disease

A. left to right shunt
B. acyanotic-cyanotic defects
C. hemodynamic characteristics
D. cor pulmonale
E. right sided failure
F. left sided failure
G. cardiac reserve

_____ dysfunction that results in increased end diastolic pressure with lung congestion and pulmonary edema

_____ term for congestive heart failure resulting from obstructive lung diseases such as cystic fibrosis or bronchopulmonary dysplasia

_____ traditional categories of congenital heart defects that divide defects based on a physical characteristic; problematic because of the complexity of the many defects and the variability of their clinical manifestations

_____ dysfunction that results in systemic venous hypertension that in turn causes hepatomegaly and edema

_____ the directional flow from an area of higher pressure to one of lower pressure in congenital heart disease

_____ the compensatory mechanisms that initially try to meet the body's demand for increased cardiac output including hypertrophy and dilation of the cardiac muscle, as well as stimulation of the sympathetic nervous system

_____ a useful classification system for congenital heart defects that uses movements involved in circulation of blood

6. Tests of Cardiac Function

A. chest radiograph
B. electrocardiography (ECG/EKG)
C. Holter monitor
D. echocardiography
E. transthoracic echocardiography
F. M-Mode echocardiography
G. two dimensional echocardiography
H. doppler echocardiography
I. fetal echocardiography
J. transesophageal echocardiography
K. cardiac catheterization
L. hemodynamics
M. angiography
N. biopsy
O. electophysiology
P. exercise stress test
Q. right side cardiac catheterization
R. left sided cardiac catheterization
S. interventional cardiac catheterization
T. diagnostic electophysiologic catheterization

_____ use catheters with tiny electrodes that record the heart's electrical impulses directly from the conduction system to evaluate and treat dysrhythmias

_____ venous; diagnostic catheterization of the venous side in which the catheter is introduced from a vein into the right atrium

_____ type of echocardiography that uses real time, cross sectional views of heart; used to identify cardiac structures and cardiac anatomy

_____ type of echocardiography that obtains a one dimensional graphic view; used to estimate ventricular size and function

_____ measures pressures and oxygen saturations in heart chambers

_____ graphic measure of the electrical activity of the heart

_____ type of echocardiography that images the fetal heart in utero

_____ use of contrast material to illuminate heart structures and blood flow patterns

_____ use of high frequency sound waves obtained by a transducer to produce an image of cardiac structures

_____ type of echocardiography that uses a transducer placed in the esophagus behind the heart to obtain images of the posterior heart structures in patients with poor images from the chest approach

_____ employs a special catheter with electrodes to record electrical activity from within heart used to diagnose rhythm disturbances

_____ an alternative to surgery for some congenital heart defects

_____ use of special catheter to remove tiny samples of heart muscle for microscopic evaluation; used for assessing infection, inflammation or muscle dysfunction disorders; also used to evaluate for rejection following heart transplant

_____ provides information about heart size and pulmonary blood flow

_____ type of echocardiography done with transducer on chest

_____ type of echocardiography that identifies blood flow patterns and pressure gradients across structures

_____ arterial; diagnostic catheterization of the arterial side in which the catheter is threaded retrograde into the aorta, or from a right sided approach to the left atrium by means of a septal puncture, or through an existing septal opening

_____ 24 hour continuous ECG recording used to assess dysrhythmias

_____ imaging study using radiopaque catheters placed in a peripheral blood vessel and advanced into heart to measure pressures and oxygen levels in heart chambers and visualize heart structures and blood flow patterns

_____ monitoring of heart rate, blood pressure, ECG, and oxygen consumption at rest and during progressive exercise on a treadmill or bicycle

7. Clinical Manifestation of Congenital Heart Disease

A. gallop rhythm
B. diaphoresis
C. poor perfusion
D. mild cyanosis
E. dyspnea
F. costal retractions

G. pulmonary edema
H. orthopnea
I. wheezing
J. cough
K. hoarseness
L. gasping/grunting respirations

M. developmental delays
N. hepatomegaly
O. edema
P. weight gain
Q. ascites/pleural effusions
R. distended veins

_____ dyspnea in the recumbent position

_____ manifested by cold extremities, weak pulses, slow capillary refill, low BP, and mottled skin

_____ a late sign of heart failure

_____ extra heart sounds S_3 and S_4 resulting from ventricular dilation and excess preload

_____ occurs as the pliable chest wall in the infant is drawn inward during attempts to ventilate the non compliant lungs

_____ results from poor weight gain and activity intolerance

_____ occurs when the pulmonary capillary pressure exceeds the plasma osmotic pressure and fluid is forced into the interstitial space

_____ caused by mucosal swelling and irritation of the bronchial mucosa

_____ result from a consistently elevated central venous pressure; venous return is slow; difficult to detect in the short, fat neck of infants; usually observed only in older children

_____ occurs from pooling of blood in the portal circulation and transudation of fluid into the hepatic tissues

_____ results from impaired gas exchange and is relieved with oxygen administration

_____ caused by edema of the bronchial mucosa from obstruction to airflow

_____ forms from sodium and water retention that causes systemic vascular pressure to rise

_____ caused by pressure from edema on the laryngeal nerve

_____ caused by decrease in the distensibility of the lungs; initially may be evident only on exertion; in infants may be accompanied by flaring nares

_____ the earliest sign of edema

_____ often seen during exertion when myocardial function is impaired; in children especially noted on the head

_____ later signs of gross fluid accumulation

8. Congestive Heart Failure—Therapeutic Management

A. digoxin (Lanoxin)
B. angiotensin converting enzyme (ACE) inhibitors

C. captopril/enalapril
D. furosemide (Lasix)

E. spironolactone (Aldactone)

_____ blocks action of aldosterone to produce diuresis; allows retention of potassium

_____ causes vasodilation that decreases pulmonary and systemic vascular resistance, decreased blood pressure, a reduction in afterload and decreased right and left atrial pressures

_____ blocks reabsorption of sodium and water to produce diuresis

_____ used because of its rapid onset and decreased risk of toxicity; increases the force of contraction (positive inotropic effect), decreases the heart rate (negative chronotropic effect), slows the conduction of impulses through the AV note (negative dromotropic effect), and indirectly enhances diuresis

_____ ACE inhibitors that are frequently used in pediatrics

9. Hypoxemia

A. right to left shunting
B. Eisenmenger complex
C. polycythemia
D. clubbing
E. squatting
F. blue spells/tet spells/ hypercyanotic spells
G. cerebrovascular accidents (CVAs)
H. bacterial endocarditis
I. shunt
J. modified Blalock-Taussig shunt

_____ uses a Gore-Tex or Impra tube graft to create a communication between the subclavian artery and the pulmonary artery to increase blood flow to the lungs; the preferred palliative treatment for severely hypoxemic newborns

_____ may occur in any child whose heart defect includes obstruction to pulmonary blood flow and communication between the ventricles; acute cyanotic episode with hyperpneia

_____ an increased number of red blood cells

_____ a palliative surgical procedure that serves the same purpose as the ductus arteriosus; increases blood flow to the lungs through a systemic artery-to-pulmonary artery connection

_____ results from severe obstruction to pulmonary blood flow; desaturated venous blood enters the system circulation without passing through the lungs and cyanosis is present; Tetralogy of Fallot is the most common cause of this type of obstruction

_____ strokes; occurs in about 2% of the children with hypoxia

_____ a thickening and flattening of the tips of the fingers and toes; thought to occur because of chronic tissue hypoxemia and polycythemia

_____ increased risk of this disorder in children who are cyanotic especially those who have systemic to pulmonary shunts

_____ a syndrome in which a left-to-right shunt becomes a right-to-left shunt because of a progressive increase in pulmonary vascular resistance

_____ characteristically seen in children with unrepaired Tetralogy of Fallot; an unconscious attempt to relieve chronic hypoxia; reduces the return of venous blood from the lower extremities and increases systemic vascular resistance

10. Acquired Disorders

A. rheumatic heart disease
B. Aschoff bodies
C. carditis
D. polyarthritis
E. erythema marginatum; subcutaneous nodules
F. subcutaneous nodules
G. chorea/Sydenham chorea
H. antistreptolysin-O (ASLO) titer
I. ectasia
J. hypertension
K. primary hypertension
L. secondary hypertension
M. severe hypertension
N. hyperlipidemia
O. hypercholesterolemia
P. atherosclerosis
Q. coronary artery disease
R. cholesterol
S. triglycerides
T. chylomicrons
U. very low density lipoproteins
V. low density lipoprotein
W. high density lipoproteins
X. population approach
Y. individualized approach
Z. Step one diet
AA. Step two diet
BB. cholestyramine/ colestipol
CC. niacin/nicotinic acid
DD. dilated cardiomyopathy
EE. hypertrophic cardiomyopathy
FF. restrictive cardiomyopathy

_____ dietary restrictions that include a saturated fatty acid intake of 7% of the calories and a cholesterol intake of less than 200 mg /day

_____ fatty plaques on the arteries

_____ measures the concentration of antibodies formed in the blood against a product that is present in streptococcal infection in children

_____ primary cause of morbidity and mortality in the adult population

_____ formed in rheumatic heart disease; inflammatory, hemorrhagic, bullous lesions; causes swelling, fragmentation and alterations in the connective tissue

_____ rare in children; describes a restriction to ventricular filling caused by endocardial or myocardial disease or both; characterized by diastolic dysfunction and absence of ventricular dilation or hypertrophy

_____ dilation

_____ major cardiac manifestation of rheumatic fever; involves the endocardium, pericardium, and myocardium

_____ a fat-like steroid alcohol; part of the lipoprotein complex in plasma that is essential for cellular metabolism

_____ essential hypertension; no identifiable cause

_____ caused by edema, inflammation, and effusions in joint tissue; reversible; migratory; favors large joints such as knees, elbows, hips, shoulders and wrists; usually accompany the acute febrile period in rheumatic fever

_____ characterized by an increase in heart muscle mass without an increase in cavity size usually occurring in the left ventricle and associated with abnormal diastolic filling; idiopathic hypertrophic subaortic stenosis is a subgroup

_____ contain low concentrations of triglycerides, high levels of cholesterol, and moderate levels of protein; high levels are a strong risk factor in cardiovascular disease

_____ small non tender swellings that persist indefinitely after the onset of rheumatic fever and gradually resolve with no resulting damage

_____ characterized by ventricular dilation and greatly decreased contractility resulting in symptoms of congestive heart failure

___A___ a poorly understood autoimmune reaction to group A beta-hemolytic streptococcal pharyngitis; self limited disease that involves the joint, skin, brain, serous surface, and heart; cardiac valve damage is the most serious consequence

_____ St. Vitus dance; characterized by sudden, aimless, irregular movements of the extremities; involuntary facial grimaces, speech disturbances, emotional lability and muscle weakness that can be profound in rheumatic fever; exaggerated by anxiety and attempts at deliberate fine motor activity and is relieved by rest, especially sleep

_____ a general term for excessive lipids

_____ decreases total cholesterol and LDL levels and increases HDL cholesterol; generally administered to older children who do not tolerate resin binding agents well

_____ contains very low concentrations of triglycerides, relatively little cholesterol, and high levels of protein; thought to protect against cardiovascular disease

_____ natural fats synthesized from carbohydrates

_____ the consistent elevation of blood pressure beyond values considered the upper limits of normal

_____ a distinct erythematous macule with a clear center and wavy well demarcated border; transitory nonpruritic rash found most often on the trunk and proximal portion of the extremities in rheumatic fever

_____ produced in the intestine in response to the intake of dietary fat; principal transporter of dietary fat

_____ subsequent to an identifiable cause of hypertension; significant hypertension; a blood pressure that is consistently between the 95th and 99th percentile for age and sex

_____ a blood pressure persistently at or above the 99th percentile for age and sex

_____ drugs recommended for the treatment of severe hypercholesterolemia

_____ an approach to controlling hypercholesterolemia that is based on selective screening

_____ refers to excessive cholesterol in the blood

_____ a diet that has the same nutrient intake as for the general population (i.e., less than 10% of total calories from saturated fatty acids, no more than 30% of calories from total fat, less than 300 mg/day of cholesterol and adequate calories to support growth and development and to reach or maintain desirable body weight

_____ contains high concentrations of triglycerides, moderate concentrations of cholesterol, and little protein

_____ aims to lower the average levels of blood cholesterol among all American children through population wide changes in nutrient intake and eating patterns

11. Defects

A. median sternotomy
B. lateral thoracotomy
C. intraarterial monitoring
D. intracardiac monitoring
E. low cardiac output syndrome
F. dysrhythmias
G. cardiac tamponade
H. paradoxical pulse pressure
I. cerebral edema/brain damage
J. seizure

_____ decreased peripheral perfusion; symptoms are similar to the signs of shock

_____ seen in approximately 10% of infants who require the use of cardiopulmonary bypass; may be focal or generalized

_____ compression of the heart by blood and other effusion (clots) in the pericardial sac

_____ a type of incision that is made in heart surgery where the sternum is split

_____ characteristic sign of compression of the heart; systolic pressure drops during inspiration because of accumulated blood compressing the heart; results in drop in cardiac output

_____ can result from electrolyte imbalance, especially hypokalemia and surgical intervention to the septum or myocardium

_____ almost always used following open-heart surgery to measure blood pressure; more reliable than indirect blood pressure readings and provides continuous rather than intermittent monitoring

_____ may occur during open-heart surgery; thought to be result of tissue ischemia or emboli; evidence is assessed by checking reflexes in both extremities, pupil size, equality and reaction to light and accommodation, and child's orientation to environment

_____ provides data on cardiac function and output; allows assessment of pressures inside the cardiac chambers giving information about blood volume, cardiac output, ventricular function, pulmonary artery pressures and responses to drug therapy

_____ a type of incision that is made in heart surgery which extends from the midaxillary line to the scapula

12. Cardiac Dysrhythmias

A. bradydysrhythmias
B. tachydysrhythmias
C. conduction disturbances
D. complete atrioventricular block (AV block)
E. sinus bradycardia
F. junctional/nodal rhythms
G. sinus tachycardia
H. supraventicular tachycardia
I. AV blocks
J. premature contractions
K. electophysiologic cardiac catheterization
L. transesophageal recording
M. vagal maneuvers
N. transesophageal atrial overdrive pacing
O. synchronized cardioversion
P. pacemaker
Q. pulse generator
R. lead
S. epicardial leads
T. orthotopic heart transplantation
U. heterotopic heart transplantation

_____ applying ice to the face, massaging the carotid artery on one side of the neck only or having the child perform a valsalva maneuver; used to treat supraventricular tachycardia

_____ the most common bradydysrhythmia in children

_____ leaving the recipient's own heart in place and implanting a new heart to a act as and additional pump or 'piggyback" heart; rarely used in children

_____ one of the most common dysrhythmias found in children; a rapid regular heart rate of 200 to 300 beats per minute

_____ abnormally slow rates

_____ most often related to edema around the conduction system and resolve without treatment

_____ implant made of a pulse generator and the lead

_____ can occur from an atrial ventricular or junctional focus; significant depending on the degree of compromise and the presence or absence of underlying congenital heart disease

_____ composed of a battery and the electronic circuitry

_____ allow for identification of the conduction disturbance and immediate investigation of drugs that may control the dysrhythmia; selective induction of the dysrhythmia and treatment under observation

_____ irregular heart rates

_____ accomplished through placement of a protected lead into the esophagus behind the left atrium of the heart; the lead is then attached to a stimulator capable of pacing at a very rapid rate to interrupt the tachydysrhythmia

_____ an insulated flexible wire that conducts electrical impulses

_____ abnormally rapid rates

_____ an electrode catheter is passed into the esophagus and when in position at a point proximal to the heart is used to simulate and record dysrhythmias

_____ may be due to the influence of the autonomic nervous system or in response to hypoxia and hypotension

_____ the timed delivery of a preset amount of energy through the chest all in an attempt to reestablish an organized rhythm

_____ a wire directly attached to the heart that conducts impulses

_____ common in the postoperative patient; impulse for these rhythms originates further down the conduction system in the AV node rather than the sinoatrial node

_____ removing the recipient's own heart and implanting a new heart from a donor

_____ usually secondary to fever, anxiety, pain, anemia, dehydration or any factor that requires an increased cardiac output

13. The embryologic development of the heart results in a heart beat by the:
    A. fourth week.
    B. fifth week.
    C. sixth week.
    D. eighth week.

14. During the embryologic development of the lower heart, chambers are formed from:
    A. a common ventricle.
    B. the sinus venosus.
    C. a common atrium.
    D. the truncus arteriosus.

15. The process of the formation of the heart's atrial septum results in a temporary flap called the:
    A. truncus arteriosus.
    B. foramen ovale.
    C. sinus venosus.
    D. ductus venosus.

16. In fetal circulation the ductus venosus bypasses the:
    A. heart.
    B. lungs.
    C. liver.
    D. placenta.

17. In fetal circulation the majority of the most oxygenated blood is pumped through the:
    A. foramen ovale.
    B. lungs.
    C. liver.
    D. coronary sinus.

18. When obtaining a history from the parents of a infant suspected to have altered cardiac function, the nurse would expect to hear:
    A. specific concerns related to palpitations the infant is having.
    B. vague nonspecific complaints such as feeding difficulties.
    C. specific concerns about the infant's shortness of breath.
    D. all of the above.

19. A history of which disease in the mother during pregnancy is an important clue to the diagnosis of congenital heart disease?
    A. Rheumatoid arthritis
    B. Rheumatic fever
    C. Streptococcal infection
    D. Rubella

20. Coarctation of the aorta should be suspected when:
    A. the blood pressure in the arms is different from the blood pressure in the legs.
    B. the blood pressure in the right arm is different from the blood pressure in the left arm.
    C. apical pulse is greater than the radial pulse.
    D. point of maximum impulse is shifted to the left.

21. Which one of the following descriptions of heart sounds would be considered normal in a young child?
    A. Splitting of S_1
    B. Splitting of S_2

22. The standard pediatric electrocardiogram has:
    A. 6 leads.
    B. 12 leads.
    C. 15 leads.
    D. 18 leads.

23. The test that requires intravenous sedation and has been used increasingly in recent years to confirm the diagnosis of a congenital heart defect without a cardiac catheterization is the:
    A. electrocardiogram.
    B. echocardiagram.
    C. transesophageal echocardiagram.
    D. two dimensional echocardiagram.

24. In children, the usual approach to the left ventricle of the heart in a cardiac catheterization is through the:
    A. left side of the heart.
    B. right side of the heart.

25. List at least 5 of the most significant complications following a cardiac catheterization in an infant or young child.

    _____   _____

    _____   _____

    _____

26. If bleeding occurs at the insertion site after a cardiac catheterization, the nurse should apply:
    A. warmth to the unaffected extremity.
    B. pressure one inch below the insertion site.
    C. warmth to the affected extremity.
    D. pressure one inch above the insertion site.

27. When children develop congestive heart failure from a congenital heart defect, the failure is usually:
    A. right-sided only.
    B. left-sided only.
    C. cor pulmonale.
    D. both right- and left-sided.

28. Which one of the following heart rates would be considered tachycardia in an infant?
    A. A resting heart rate of 120 beats per minute
    B. A crying heart rate of 200 beats per minute
    C. A resting heart rate of 160 beats per minute
    D. A crying heart rate of 180 beats per minute

29. Labored breathing in an infant may be identified by:
   A. inability to feed.
   B. circumoral cyanosis.
   C. costal retractions.
   D. all of the above.

30. Developmental delays in the infant with congestive heart failure are MOST pronounced in the:
   A. fine motor areas.
   B. gross motor areas.
   C. social skill areas.
   D. cognitive areas.

31. Evaluation of the infant for edema is different from the older child in that:
   A. weight is not reliable as an early sign.
   B. pedal edema will be most pronounced in the newborn.
   C. edema is usually generalized and difficult to detect.
   D. distended neck veins are the most reliable sign.

32. In the child taking digoxin, electrocardiographic signs that the drug is having the intended effect are:
   A. prolonged PR interval and slowed ventricular rate.
   B. shortened PR interval and slowed ventricular rate.
   C. prolonged PR interval and faster ventricular rate.
   D. shortened PR interval and faster ventricular rate.

33. The two main angiostensin-converting enzyme (ACE) inhibitors MOST commonly used for children with congestive heart failure are:
   A. digoxin and captopril.
   B. enalapril and captopril.
   C. enalapril and furosemide.
   D. spironolactone and captopril.

34. The electrolyte that is usually depleted with diuretic therapy is:
   A. sodium.
   B. chloride.
   C. potassium.
   D. magnesium.

35. The nutritional needs of the infant with congestive heart failure are usually:
   A. the same as an adult's.
   B. less than a healthy infant's.
   C. the same as a healthy infant's.
   D. greater than a healthy infant's.

36. The calories are usually increased for an infant with congestive heart failure by:
   A. increasing the number of feedings.
   B. introducing solids into the diet.
   C. increasing the density of the formula.
   D. gavage feeding.

37. Which one of the following clinical manifestations is a sign of chronic hypoxemia?
    A. Squatting
    B. Polycythemia
    C. Clubbing
    D. All of the above

38. Prostaglandin is administered to the newborn with a congenital heart defect to:
    A. close the patent ductus arteriosus.
    B. keep the ductus arteriosus open.
    C. keep the foramen ovale open.
    D. close the foramen ovale.

39. Dehydration must be prevented in children who are hypoxemic because the dehydration places the child at risk for:
    A. infection.
    B. cerebral vascular accident.
    C. fever.
    D. air embolism.

40. It would be considered unusual if the parents of a child with a congenital heart defect felt:
    A. self-confident with their parenting abilities.
    B. exhausted and discouraged.
    C. they could not leave their child with anyone.
    D. a fear that the child might die.

41. Match the type of defect with the specific disorder. (Defects may be used more than once.)

    A. defects with decreased pulmonary blood flow
    B. mixed defects
    C. defects with increased pulmonary blood flow
    D. obstructive defects

    _____ patent ductus arteriosus
    _____ coarctation of the aorta
    _____ ventricular septal defect
    _____ subvalvular aortic stenosis
    _____ hypoplastic left heart syndrome
    _____ atrioventricular canal defect
    _____ pulmonic stenosis
    ___A___ Tetralogy of Fallot
    _____ aortic stenosis
    _____ tricuspid atresia
    _____ valvular aortic stenosis
    _____ truncus arteriosus
    _____ atrial septal defect
    _____ transposition of the great vessels

42. Which one of the following defects has the BEST prognosis?
    A. Tetralogy of Fallot
    B. Ventricular septal defect
    C. Atrial septal defect
    D. Hypoplastic left heart syndrome

43. Which of the following defects has the WORST prognosis?
    A. Tetralogy of Fallot
    B. Atrial ventricular canal defect
    C. Transposition of the great vessels
    D. Hypoplastic left heart syndrome

44. Which one of the following sets of assessment findings are the MOST frequent clinical manifestations of congenital heart disorders in an infant or child?
    A. Decreased cardiac output and low blood pressure
    B. Congestive heart failure and murmurs
    C. Increased blood pressure and pulse
    D. All of the above

45. Surgical intervention is always necessary in the first year of life when an infant is born with:
    A. atrial septal defect.
    B. ventricular septal defect.
    C. transposition of the great vessels.
    D. patent ductus arteriosus.

46. The BEST approach for the nurse to use in regard to discipline for the child with a congenital defect is to:
    A. provide the parents with anticipatory guidance.
    B. teach the parents to overcompensate.
    C. help the parents focus on the child's defect.
    D. teach the parents to use benevolent overreaction.

47. Parents of the child with a congenital heart disorder are usually interested primarily in information about the:
    A. anatomy and physiology of the heart.
    B. pathophysiology and morbidity of the disorder.
    C. prognosis and surgical correction of the disorder.
    D. all of the above.

48. Parents of the child with a congenital heart defect should know the signs of congestive heart failure, which include:
    A. poor feeding.
    B. sudden weight gain.
    C. increased efforts to breathe.
    D. all of the above.

49. List at least three major categories that should be included in a teaching plan for parents of a child with a congenital heart disorder.

_____

_____

_____

50. A visit to the intensive care unit prior to open heart surgery should take place:
    A. several days before the surgery.
    B. at a busy time with a lot to see and hear.
    C. the day before surgery.
    D. several weeks before the surgery.

51. Children who will undergo cardiac surgery should be informed about:
    A. the location of the intravenous lines.
    B. the pain at the intravenous insertion sites.
    C. the need to lie still at all times after surgery.
    D. all of the above.

52. Which one of the following patterns is indicative of infection in the postoperative period following cardiac surgery?
    A. Temperature of 38.6° C (101.5° F) 72 hours after surgery
    B. Temperature of 37.7° C (100° F) 36 hours after surgery
    C. Hypothermia in the early postoperative period
    D. All of the above

53. Following cardiac surgery in a child, congestive heart failure would be suspected if the central venous pressure catheter (CVP) readings begin to:
    A. fall with a rise in blood pressure.
    B. rise with a rise in blood pressure.
    C. fall with a fall in blood pressure.
    D. rise with a fall in blood pressure.

54. While suctioning an infant after cardiac surgery, the nurse should:
    A. hyperoxygenate before suctioning.
    B. suction for no more than five seconds.
    C. provide supplemental O_2.
    D. all of the above.

55. List five observations the nurse should be making while suctioning an infant after cardiac surgery.

    _____ _____

    _____ _____

    _____

56. Which one of the following reasons is NOT a common reason for chest tube drainage in the child following cardiac surgery?
    A. Removal of secretions
    B. Removal of air
    C. Prevention of pneumothorax
    D. Removal of an empyema

57. Which one of the following strategies is NOT acceptable to include in the care of the child prior to removing chest tube(s) after cardiac surgery?
    A. Explain that the removal is uncomfortable but not painful.
    B. Administer intravenous fentanyl.
    C. Administer intravenous morphine sulfate.
    D. Use a topical anesthetic on the site.

58. The MOST painful part of cardiac surgery for the child is usually the:
    A. thoracotomy incision site
    B. graft site on the leg.
    C. sternotomy incision site.
    D. intravenous insertion sites.

59. An infant who weighs 7 kg has just returned to the intensive care unit following cardiac surgery. The chest tube has drained 30 cc in the past hour. In this situation, what is the FIRST action for the nurse to take?
    A. Notify the surgeon.
    B. Identify any other signs of hemorrhage.
    C. Suction the patient.
    D. Identify any other signs of renal failure.

60. An infant who weighs 7 kg has just returned to the intensive care unit following cardiac surgery. The urine output has been 20 ml in the past hour. In this situation, what is the FIRST action for the nurse to take?
    A. Notify the surgeon.
    B. Identify any other signs of hypervolemia.
    C. Suction the patient.
    D. Identify any other signs of renal failure.

61. Following cardiac surgery, fluid intake calculations for a child would include:
    A. intravenous fluids.
    B. arterial and CVP line flushes.
    C. fluid used to dilute medications.
    D. all of the above.

62. Following cardiac surgery, fluid output calculations in a child would include:
    A. nasogastric secretions.
    B. blood drawn for analysis.
    C. chest tube drainage.
    D. all of the above.

63. One of the factors that increases blood volume in open-heart surgery in children is the postoperative:
    A. reabsorption of potassium.
    B. secretion of antidiuretic hormone.
    C. inhibition of aldosterone.
    D. diffusion of fluid into the interstitial spaces.

64. One of the strategies the nurse can use to progressively increase a child's activity in the postoperative period after cardiac surgery is to plan:
    A. to expect some degree of dyspnea.
    B. to ambulate on the first day.
    C. to ambulate after analgesic medication.
    D. all of the above.

65. List at least 5 complications of cardiac surgery in children.

    _____   _____

    _____   _____

    _____

66. Techniques to provide emotional support to the child and family following cardiac surgery include:
    A. realizing that some procedures are too difficult for the child to perform.
    B. encouraging the child to keep being brave.
    C. reassuring the parents that a child's anger or rejection of them is normal.
    D. all of the above.

67. Which one of the following patients with bacterial endocarditis (BE) is at highest risk for mortality?
    A. A 15-year-old with BE caused by a bacteria which is susceptible to ampicillin
    B. A 2-month-old infant with no cardiac problems
    C. A 5-year-old child with BE following a mitral valve replacement
    D. A 9-year-old with BE and aortic stenosis

68. One of the MOST important factors in preventing bacterial endocarditis is:
    A. administration of prophylactic antibiotic therapy.
    B. surgical repair of the defect.
    C. administration of prostaglandin to correct patent ductus arteriosus.
    D. administration of antibiotics after dental work.

69. One of the MOST common findings on physical examination of the child with acute rheumatic heart disease is:
    A. a systolic murmur.
    B. pleural friction rub.
    C. an ejection click.
    D. a split S_2.

70. The test that provides the MOST reliable evidence of recent streptococcal infection is the:
    A. throat culture.
    B. Mantoux test.
    C. elevation of liver enzymes.
    D. antistreptolysin-O test

71. Children who have been treated for rheumatic fever:
    A. do not need additional prophylaxis against bacterial endocarditis.
    B. are immune to rheumatic fever for the rest of their lives.
    C. will have transitory manifestations of chorea for the rest of their lives.
    D. may need antibiotic therapy for years.

72. The peak age for the incidence of Kawasaki disease is in the:
   A. infant age group.
   B. toddler age group.
   C. school-age group.
   D. adolescent age group.

73. Which one of the following doses of aspirin would be considered adequate for the initial treatment of Kawasaki disease for a child who weighs 20 kg?
   A. 80 mg every 6 hours
   B. 100 mg every 6 hours
   C. 500 mg every 6 hours
   D. 2000 mg every 6 hours

74. Kawasaki disease is treated with:
   A. aspirin and gamma globulin.
   B. aspirin and cryoprecipitate.
   C. meperidine hydrochloride and gamma globulin.
   D. meperidine hydrochloride and cryoprecipitate.

75. Because of the drug used for long term therapy, children with Kawasaki disease are at risk for:
   A. chicken pox.
   B. influenza.
   C. Reye syndrome.
   D. myocardial infarction.

76. Most cases of hypertension in children are a result of:
   A. essential hypertension.
   B. secondary hypertension.
   C. primary hypertension.
   D. congenital heart defects.

77. Most children with essential hypertension that is resistant to nonpharmocologic intervention are managed with:
   A. diuretics.
   B. ACE inhibitors.
   C. beta blockers.
   D. any of the above.

78. The nurse's role in relation to hypertension may include:
   A. routine accurate assessment of blood pressure in infants and children.
   B. providing information.
   C. follow-up of the child with hypertension.
   D. all of the above.

79. Elevated cholesterol in childhood:
   A. can predict the long-term risk of heart disease for the individual.
   B. can predict the risk of hypertension in adulthood.
   C. is a major predictor of the adult cholesterol level.
   D. is usually symptomatic.

80. The National Cholesterol Education Program recommends screening for cholesterol in:
    A. children over 5 years of age.
    B. children with a family history of premature cardiovascular disease.
    C. children with congenital heart disease.
    D. all children.

81. The MOST common kind of cardiomyopathy found in children is:
    A. dilated cardiomyopathy.
    B. hypertrophic cardiomyopathy.
    C. restrictive cardiomyopathy.
    D. secondary cardiomyopathy.

82. The heart transplant procedure that is used MOST often in children is the
    A. heterotopic heart transplantation.
    B. orthotopic heart transplantation.

83. Which one of the following dysrhythmias would be included on a list of dysrhythmias commonly seen in children?
    A. Ventricular tachycardia
    B. Asystole
    C. Supraventricular tachycardia
    D. All of the above

Critical Thinking • Case Study

Pauline Smith is a 3-year-old child admitted for repair of an atrial septal defect. Her parents have known about the defect since her birth. She has had numerous respiratory infections with occasional episodes of congestive heart failure in the past year. Pauline has taken digoxin and furosemide in the past, but currently takes only vitamins with iron. Her parents state that they are anxious to have the surgery over with, so that they can treat Pauline like the other children. They have 3 other children who are all older than Pauline.

84. On admission Pauline is afebrile and playful and has no signs of congestive heart failure. As part of the admission process the nurse would want to be sure to have a baseline assessment of Pauline's:
    A. sucking and swallowing abilities.
    B. reading ability.
    C. exercise tolerance level.
    D. all of the above.

85. When developing a nursing care plan for Pauline's admission for the surgical repair of the atrial septal defect, the nurse would MOST likely have identified a nursing diagnosis of:
    A. altered family process.
    B. impaired skin integrity.

86. One of the BEST ways for the nurse to provide emotional support for Pauline and her family in the stressful postoperative period is to:
    A. facilitate a swift transfer out of ICU.
    B. expect courage and bravery from Pauline.
    C. limit Pauline's expression of anger toward her parents.
    D. praise Pauline for her efforts to cooperate.

CHAPTER 35
The Child with Hematologic or Immunologic Dysfunction

1. Identify the following statements as TRUE or FALSE.

    __F__ The major physiologic component of red cells is erythropoietin.

    __F__ A complete blood count with differential describes the components of blood known as platelets.

    __F__ A child with a suspected bacterial infection would have a differential count that shows a shift to the left with more mature cells present.

    __T__ Erythrocytes supply oxygen and remove CO_2 from cells.

    __T__ The mature RBC has no nucleus.

    __T__ Reticulocytes indicate active RBC production.

    __T__ The regulator of erythrocyte production is tissue oxygenation and renal production of erythropoietin.

    __f__ The regulatory mechanism for the production of erythrocytes is their circulating numbers.

    __T__ The absolute neutrophil count reflects the body's ability to handle bacterial infection.

    __f__ Monocytes and lymphocytes are granulocytes.

    __T__ In the child with increased numbers of eosinophils, the nurse should suspect allergies or parasite infection.

    __f__ Monocytosis is more evident in acute inflammation.

    __T__ The hematocrit is approximately three times the hemoglobin content.

    __f__ The mean corpuscular hemoglobin is the average volume of a single RBC.

    __T__ Mean corpuscular hemoglobin concentration is the average concentration of hemoglobin in a single cell.

    __x__ Bands are immature neutrophils, and they increase in number during bacterial infections.

2. The nurse would expect laboratory results for the patient with chronic blood loss to include:
   A. high iron levels.
   B. macrocytic and hyperchromic erythrocytes.
   C. microcytic and hypochromic erythrocytes.
   D. normocytic and normochromic erthrocytes.

3. What are the four basic causes of anemia?

   _____ _____

   _____ _____

4. What is the basic physiologic defect caused by anemia?

   _____

   _____

5. Match the term with its description.

A. normocytes
B. macrocytes
C. microcytes
D. sperocytes
E. poikilocytes
F. drepanocytes
G. normochromic
H. hypochromic
I. hemolysis
J. MCHC
K. MCV
L. hemostasis

_____ indicates the average volume or size of a single RBC
_____ reduced amount of hemoglobin concentration
_____ sickle-shaped cells
_____ indicates the average concentration of Hgb in the RBC
_____ process that stops bleeding when a blood vessel is injured
_____ excessive destruction of red blood cells
_____ larger than normal cell size
_____ smaller than normal cell size
_____ normal cell size
_____ sufficient or normal hemoglobin concentration
_____ globular-shaped cells
_____ irregular-shaped cells

6. When the hemoglobin level falls sufficiently to produce clinical manifestations of anemia, the patient experiences:
   A. cyanosis.
   B. tissue hypoxia.
   C. nausea and vomiting.
   D. feelings of anxiety.

7. Which of the following does the nurse expect to include in the care plan of a patient with anemia?
   1. prepare the child for laboratory tests
   2. observe for complications of therapy
   3. decrease tissue oxygen needs
   4. implement safety precautions

   A. 1 and 4
   B. 1, 2, 3, and 4
   C. 2 and 3
   D. 1 and 2

8. The nurse is scheduled to administer 100 cc of packed red blood cells to 3-year-old Amy. Which one of the following is NOT a correct guideline when administering the blood?
   A. Take vital signs before administration.
   B. Infuse the blood through an appropriate filter.
   C. Administer 50 cc of the blood within the first few minutes to detect for possible reactions before proceeding with the remainder of the infusion.
   D. Start the blood within 30 minutes of its arrival from the blood bank or return it to the blood bank.

9. Lucas, age 7 years, is receiving a transfusion of packed red blood cells. After 45 minutes, he begins to have chills, fever, a sensation of tightness in his chest, and headache. The priority action of the nurse is to:
   A. stop the transfusion and administer acetaminophen.
   B. stop the transfusion and notify the practitioner.
   C. slow the transfusion rate until the symptoms subside.
   D. slow the transfusion and send a sample of the patient's blood and urine to the laboratory.

10. At birth the normal full-term newborn has maternal stores of iron sufficient to last how long?
    A. The first 5 to 6 months of life
    B. The first 2 to 3 months of life
    C. The first 8 months of life
    D. Less than 1 month of life

11. Which one of the following laboratory values is diagnostic of anemia caused by inadequate intake or absorption of iron?
    A. Elevated TIBC and reduced SIC
    B. Reduced TIBC and SIC
    C. Elevated TIBC and SIC
    D. Reduced TIBC and elevated SIC

12. Angie, age 11 months, is brought into the clinic by her mother for a routine check-up. On physical exam, the nurse observes that Angie appears chubby, that her skin looks pale, almost porcelain-like, and that Angie has poor muscle development. Based on these observations, which one of the following questions is MOST important for the nurse to include when completing Angie's history?
    A. "Did you have any complications during pregnancy or delivery of Angie?"
    B. "Tell me about what you are currently feeding Angie."
    C. "Has Angie had any recent infections or high fevers?"
    D. "Have you noticed if Angie is having difficulty with her movements or advancing in her growth and development abilities?"

13. The nurse is instructing a new mother in how to prevent iron deficiency anemia in her new premature infant when she takes her home. The mother intends to breast-feed. Which one of the following statements reflects a need for further education of the new mother?
    A. "I will only use breast milk or formula as a source of milk for my baby until she is at least 12 months old."
    B. "My baby will need to have iron supplements introduced when she is 2 months old."
    C. "As my baby is able to tolerate other foods, such as cereal, I should limit her formula intake to about 1 L/day to encourage intake of iron-rich cereals."
    D. "I will need to add iron supplements to my baby's diet when she is 6 months old."

14. When teaching the parents of 4-year-old Tony how to administer the iron supplement ordered for his iron deficiency, the nurse includes which one of the following in the teaching plan?
    A. Give the iron twice daily in divided doses with orange juice.
    B. Give the iron twice daily with milk.
    C. Administer the oral liquid iron preparation with the use of a syringe or medicine dropper directly into each side of the mouth in the cheek areas.
    D. Make sure parents have at least 3-months supply of the iron preparation on hand so that they will not run out.

15. On a return clinical visit after Tony has been taking the iron supplement, his mother tells the nurse that Tony's stools are now greenish black in color and she is concerned. What would your response be?

_____

_____

16. Hereditary spherocytosis (HS) is:
    A. transmitted as an autosomal recessive disease.
    B. a hemolytic disorder that does not involve an abnormality of hemoglobin.
    C. rarely evident until the infant is 4-6 months of age.
    D. usually resolved when additional folic acid supplements are administered.

17. Sally and David Brown are returning with Jason, their 6-week-old infant, for a routine newborn exam. Sally is a carrier for sickle cell anemia; David is not. What are the chances that Jason was born with sickle cell anemia?
    A. 25% chance
    B. 50% chance
    C. 75% chance
    D. 0% chance

18. Infants are often not diagnosed with sickle cell anemia until they are one year of age. Why?
    A. Usually there are no symptoms until after age one year.
    B. High intake of fluids from formulas prevent sickle cell crises during this age.
    C. the presence of fetal hemoglobin during the first year of life.
    D. compensation by increased hemoglobin and hemocrit amounts during this period.

19. Under conditions of _____, _____, _____, and
    _____ _____, the relatively insoluble HbS changes its molecular structure to filamentous crystals that cause distortion of the cell membrane to a sickle-shaped RBC.

20. Bruce, age 12 years, is admitted to your unit with a diagnosis of sickle cell crisis. Which one of the following activities is MOST likely to have precipitated this episode?
    A. Attending the football game with his friends
    B. Going camping and hiking in the mountains with his friends
    C. Going to the beach and surfing with his friends
    D. Staying indoors and reading for several hours

21. Pat is a 5-year-old being admitted because of diminished RBC production triggered by a viral infection. What type of sickle cell crisis is she MOST likely experiencing?
    A. Vaso-occlusive crisis
    B. Splenic sequestration crisis
    C. Aplastic crisis
    D. Hyperhemolytic crisis

22. Therapeutic management of sickle cell crisis generally includes which one of the following?
    A. Long-term oxygen use to enable the oxygen to reach the sickled RBCs
    B. Decrease in fluids to increase hemoconcentration
    C. Diet high in iron to decrease anemia
    D. Bed rest to minimize energy expenditure

23. In controlling pain related to vaso-occlusive sickle cell crisis, which one of the following can the nurse expect to be included in the plan of care?
   A. Administration of long-term oxygen
   B. Application of cold compresses to the area
   C. Meperidine (Demerol) to be titrated and administered to a therapeutic level
   D. Adding codeine to acetaminophen or ibuprofen if neither one of these is effective in relieving the pain alone

24. In planning for a child's discharge after a sickle cell crisis, the nurse recognizes which one of the following as a critical factor to include in the teaching plan?
   A. Ingestion of large quantities of liquids to promote adequate hydration
   B. Rigorous exercise schedule to promote muscle strength
   C. A high caloric diet to improve nutrition
   D. At least 12 hours of sleep per night

25. Norma, age 2 years, is to begin therapy for beta-thalassemia. Which one of the following would be appropriate for the nurse to include in the educational session held with the parents?
   A. Norma will need frequent blood transfusions to keep her Hgb level above 12 g/dl.
   B. Large doses of vitamin C will be needed throughout the disease.
   C. Chelation therapy is delayed until after 6 years of age to promote normal physical development.
   D. To minimize the effect of iron overload, deferoxamine (Desferal), an iron-chelating agent, will be given intravenously or subcutaneously.

26. A diagnostic evaluation used to distinguish the type and severity of the various thalassemias is:
   A. hemoglobin electrophoresis.
   B. Sickledex.
   C. stained blood smear.
   D. microscopic exam of RBC.

27. What are the two etiologies of aplastic anemia?

   _____   _____

28. A. Definite diagnosis of aplastic anemia is determined by:

   _____

   B. Acquired aplastic anemia presents with clinical manifestations of _____,
   _____, and _____ _____ _____.

   C. Two main approaches aimed at restoring function to the marrow in aplastic anemia are:

   _____   _____

29. Danny is scheduled to receive antithymocyte globulin (ATG) for treatment of his aplastic anemia. Based on knowledge about this therapy, which one of the following does the nurse recognize as TRUE?
   A. ATG is administered intramuscularly every 3-4 weeks.
   B. ATG is administered intravenously in a peripheral vein.
   C. All reactions to ATG will occur within the first hour of administration and include skin rash and fever.
   D. ATG suppresses T-cell-dependent autoimmune responses but does not cause bone marrow suppression.

30. Match the term with its description.

A. bleeding time

B. prothrombin time (PT)

C. partial thromboplastin time (PTT)

D. thromboplastin generation test (TGT)

E. fibrinogen level

F. hemophilia A

G. hemophilia B

_____ allows for determination of specific factor deficiencies, especially factors VIII and IX

_____ directly measures fibrinogen level in blood

_____ function depends on platelet aggregation and vasoconstriction

_____ measures factors necessary for prothrombin conversion to thrombin and fibrogen

_____ measures the activity of thromboplastin and specific for factor deficiencies except factor VII

_____ factor IX deficiency

_____ factor VIII deficiency

31. When discussing hemophilia with the parents of a child recently diagnosed with this disease, the nurse tells the parents that:
    1. hemophilia is an x-linked disorder in which the mother is the carrier of the illness but is not affected by it.
    2. hemophilia is a recessive disorder carried by either the mother or the father.
    3. all of the daughters of the parents will be carriers.
    4. each of their sons has a 50% chance of being affected and each of their daughters has a 50% chance of being a carrier.

    A. 1 and 4
    B. 2 and 3
    C. 1 and 3
    D. 2 and 4

32. Which one of the following is the MOST frequent form of internal bleeding in the child with hemophilia?
    A. Hemarthrosis
    B. Epistaxis
    C. Intracranial hemorrhage
    D. Gastrointestinal tract hemorrhage

33. Which one of the following is no longer recommended for use in treating factor VIII deficiency because the risk of hepatitis or HIV cannot be safely eliminated?
    A. Factor VIII concentrate
    B. Cryoprecipitate
    C. DDAVP (1-deamino-8-D-arginine vasopressin)
    D. Epsilon aminocaproic acid (Amicar, EACA)

34. Donald, age 5 and previously diagnosed with hemophilia A, is being admitted with bleeding into the joints. The nurse knows that which of the following is CONTRAINDICATED in the plan of care for Donald?
   1. ice packs to the affected area
   2. application of a splint or sling to the area
   3. administration of corticosteroids
   4. administration of aspirin, indocin or butazolidin
   5. passive range-of-motion exercises
   6. active range-of-motion exercises
   7. teaching Donald how to administer AHF to himself

   A. 1, 3, and 6
   B. 2, 3, 4, and 6
   C. 1, 5, and 7
   D. 4, 5, and 7

35. Which one of the following statements about von Willebrand disease is TRUE?
   A. The characteristic clinical feature is an increased tendency toward bleeding from mucous membranes.
   B. It affects females but not males.
   C. It will be unsafe for the female affected with the disease to have children because of hemorrhage.
   D. It is an inherited autosomal recessive disease.

36. An acquired hemorrhagic disorder characterized by excessive destruction of platelets and a discoloration caused by petechiae beneath the skin is called _____ _____ _____.

37. Which one of the following does the nurse recognize as TRUE when administering anti-D antibody for idiopathic thrombocytopenic purpura?
   A. The platelet count will increase immediately after administration.
   B. Eligible patients include those with lupus.
   C. Bone marrow examination to first rule out leukemia is necessary before administration.
   D. Premedicate the patient with acetaminophen before medication is infused.

38. In severe cases of disseminated intravascular coagulation, treatment may include the administration of heparin. What is the rationale for this therapy?
   A. Inhibit thrombin formation
   B. Decrease the platelet count
   C. Increase the bleeding time
   D. All of the above

39. The MOST common manifestations of chronic benign neutropenia are _____ _____ and _____ _____ .

40. What are the four characterizations of Henoch-Schonlein Purpura?

   _____ _____

   _____ _____

41. In children, HIV is likely to be transmitted by which of the following methods?
    A. Exposure in utero to an infected mother or an infected mother may transmit the virus in breast-milk
    B. Received infected blood products by transfusion before 1985
    C. Adolescents engaged in high-risk behaviors (sexual or IV drugs)
    D. All of the above

42. What are the seven MOST common clinical manifestations of HIV infection in children?

    _____   _____

    _____   _____

    _____   _____

    _____

43. Goals of therapy for HIV infection in children are:

    _____   _____

    _____   _____

44. Identify the following as TRUE or FALSE.
    _____ Combinations of antiretroviral drugs are more likely to delay the emergence of drug resistance in the treatment of HIV than is single drug therapy.
    _____ Pneumoncystis carinii pneumonia is the most common opportunistic infection of children infected with HIV.
    _____ Prophylaxis antibiotic therapy is rarely recommended for children with HIV until after the age of 1 year.
    _____ The ELISA and Western blot immunoassay tests are not accurate in infants because these tests may be positive up to the age of 18-months because of maternal antibodies.
    _____ Developmental delay in children with AIDS includes receptive language delays rather than expressive language delays.

45. Immunization needs of the child with HIV infection includes which one of the following?
    A. Delay of all immunizations until the child has the HIV infection under control
    B. Withholding pneumococcal and influenza vaccines
    C. Using inactivated poliovirus (IPV) rather than oral poliovirus (OPV)
    D. Administration of varicella vaccine at the age of 12 months

46. Nursing strategies, to improve the growth and development of the child with HIV infection, include which one of the following?
    A. Provide high-fat and high-calorie meals and snacks to meet body requirements for growth.
    B. Provide only those foods that the child feels like eating.
    C. Fortify foods with nutritional supplements to maximize quality of intake.
    D. Weigh the child and measure height and muscle mass on a daily basis.

47. Nursing strategies to improve school and peer interactions of the child with HIV infection would BEST include which one of the following?
   A. Encouraging the child to have one best friend to whom he/she relates.
   B. Assisting the child in identifying personal strengths to facilitate coping.
   C. Telling the child that the hospitalization will not contribute to isolation from peers and allowing the child's friends to send letters.
   D. Discouraging the child's parents from allowing school friends to visit the child at home recuperating because rest is especially important to the HIV-infected child.

48. Early clinical manifestations of severe combined immunodeficiency include:
   A. failure to thrive.
   B. delayed developmental milestone achievement.
   C. feeding problems.
   D. susceptibility to infections.

49. The only definitive treatment for SCID is _____ _____ _____.

50. In Wiskott-Aldrich syndrome, the MOST notable effect of the disease at birth is which one of the following?
   A. Bleeding
   B. Infection
   C. Eczema
   D. Malignancy

51. What are the three abnormalities associated with Wiskott-Aldrich syndrome?

_____

_____

_____

Critical Thinking • Case Study

Mary, age 9, has sickle cell anemia. She is admitted to the hospital with knee and back pain and is diagnosed as being in vaso-occlusive crisis.

52. The nurse, in developing a plan of care for Mary, formulated a diagnosis of pain. The nurse understands that Mary's pain is related to which one of the following?
   A. Pooling of large amounts of blood in the liver and spleen
   B. Shorter life span of the RBC's and the fact that the bone marrow cannot produce enough RBC's
   C. Tissue anoxia brought on by sickle cells occluding blood vessels
   D. RBC destruction related to a viral infection or transfusion reaction

53. Describe interventions that the nurse can include in the plan of care to control pain during this vaso-occlusive crisis to prevent undermedicating.

_____

_____

54. The nurse is developing an educational plan about sickle cell anemia for Mary and her parents. In order to prevent recurrence of this type of crisis, which one of the following is MOST important to include in the educational session?
    A. Explaining the signs of dehydration
    B. Explaining that frequent rest periods are required when the child is in a low-oxygen atmosphere
    C. Explaining that the child should avoid injury to joints to decrease sickling of blood cells
    D. Explaining the importance of avoiding infection by routine immunization and protection from known sources of infection

55. Evaluation of Mary's progress is best based on which one of the following observations?
    A. Mary's verbalization that she no longer has pain or need for pain medication
    B. Mary's ability to perform active range-of-motion exercises
    C. Mary's desire to drink the required level of fluids for hydration
    D. Mary's verbalization of how to prevent future sickle cell crisis

56. Cindy is a 12-month-old being treated for HIV infection. Describe nursing interventions to prevent the spread of the disease to others.

    _____

    _____

    _____

    _____

57. In preparing a nursing care plan for Cindy, expected goals would be:

    _____

    _____

    _____

    _____

    _____

    _____

CHAPTER 36
The Child with Cancer

1. Etiology and Diagnosis

   A. truly cured child
   B. biologic cure
   C. oncogenes
   D. retroviruses
   E. carcinogenic
   F. classification
   G. staging
   H. bone marrow test
   I. aspiration
   J. biopsy

   _____ refers to the biologic characteristics of the tumor

   _____ obtaining a piece of tissue through a special type of needle

   _____ a child who is not just free of disease, but who is developmentally commensurate with age and well adjusted despite the experience of having cancer

   _____ used to determine the extent of bone marrow involvement by malignant cells

   _____ not an absolute term; the complete eradication of all cancer cells

   _____ obtaining a sample through a large or fine-bore needle

   _____ genes having the potential to transform normal cells into malignant ones

   _____ RNA tumor viruses; have the ability to translate RNA back to DNA

   _____ refers to the extent of the disease at the time of diagnosis

   _____ capable of producing cancer

2. Modes of Therapy and Complications of Therapy

   A. clinical trials
   B. protocol
   C. alkylating agents
   D. antimetabolites
   E. plant alkaloids
   F. antitumor
   G. hormones
   H. lethal damage
   I. sublethal damage
   J. total body irradiation (TBI)
   K. monoclonal antibody
   L. mono
   M. clone
   N. human leukocyte antigen (HLA) system complex
   O. Haplotype
   P. graft-vs-host disease (GVHD)
   Q. allogenic BMT
   R. umbilical cord blood stem cell transplantation
   S. autologous BMTs
   T. Peripheral stem cell transplants (PSCTs)
   U. acute tumor lysis syndrome
   V. hyperleukocytosis
   W. obstruction
   X. superior vena cava syndrome
   Y. overwhelming infections

   _____ genes inherited as a single unit

   _____ antibiotics are natural products that interfere with cell division by reacting with DNA in such a way as to prevent further replication of DNA and transcription of RNA

   _____ autologous transplant; stem cells are first stimulated to grow, then collected and filtered from whole blood; whole blood is then returned to the patient; very small children have received these transplants without problems

   _____ the system used to select a suitable donor

   _____ the name given to the formalized treatment plan that is derived from clinical trials

   _____ adrenal and gonadal are used; have antineoplastic properties; the precise mechanism of action is unclear; may bind with DNA to alter the transcription process

   _____ resemble essential metabolic elements needed for cell growth but are sufficiently altered in molecular structure to inhibit further synthesis of DNA and/or RNA

   _____ refers to the death of the cell

_____ comparative evaluations of different types of treatment; may involve any aspect of cancer care; frequently concerned with evaluating investigational drugs

_____ damage refers to injured cells that may subsequently be repaired

_____ replace a hydrogen atom of a molecule by an alkyl group; irreversible; causes unbalanced growth of unaffected cell constituents so that the cell eventually dies; similar action as irradiation

_____ associated with the most severe reactions and is employed to prepare the immune system for bone marrow transplantation

_____ arrests cells in metaphase by binding to microtubular protein needed for spindle formation

_____ antibodies that recognize a single specific antigen

_____ the bone marrow donor's marrow may contain antigens not matched to the recipient's antigens which begin attacking body cells

_____ a new source of hematopoeitic stem cells for use in children with cancer; allows for partially matched unrelated transplants to be successful; lowers risk of GVHD related problems

_____ life threatening condition; peripheral white blood cell count greater than 100,000/mm^3; can lead to capillary obstruction, microinfarction and organ dysfunction

_____ also means one

_____ compression of the mediastinal structures leading to airway compromise and potentially to respiratory failure

_____ exact duplicate

_____ caused by space occupying lesions such as Hodgkin disease and non-Hodgkin lymphoma structures

_____ involves the matching of a histocompatable donor with the recipient

_____ may constitute an emergency situation; can result in complications such as disseminated intravascular coagulation (DIC), hemorrhage, thrombocytopenia and leukocytosis may occur

_____ uses the patient's own marrow that was collected from disease-free tissue, frozen and sometimes treated to remove malignant cells; has been used to treat neuroblastoma, Hodgkin disease, non-Hodgkin lymphoma, rhabdomyosarcoma, Ewing sarcoma and Wilms tumor

_____ life threatening condition caused by the rapid release of intracellular metabolites during the initial treatment of malignancies such as Burkitt and T cell lymphomas and acute leukemia; leads to hyperuricemia, hypocalcemia, hyperphosphatemia and hyperkalemia

3. Signs and Symptoms

A. pain	C. skin	E. abdominal mass
B. fever	D. anemia	F. swollen lymph glands
		G. white reflection

_____ classic sign of retinoblastoma; cat's eye reflex or leukokoria

_____ common finding in children; if enlarged and firm for more than a week may indicate a serious disease

_____ typical finding in children with Wilms tumor and neuroblastoma

_____ caused by the replacement of normal cells with malignant cells in the bone marrow

_____ may show signs of low platelet count; ecchymosis; petechiae

_____ a frequent occurrence caused by numerous illness other than cancer; with cancer usually caused by infection secondary to the malignant process

_____ may be an early or late initial sign of cancer

4. Nursing Care

A. absolute neutrophil count
B. colony-stimulating factors
C. granulocyte colony stimulating factor
D. postirradiation somnolence
E. mood changes

_____ Neupogen; directs granulocyte development and can decrease the duration of neutropenia following immunosuppressive therapy

_____ may be experienced shortly after beginning steroid therapy; range from feelings of well-being and euphoria to depression and irritability

_____ if lower than 500/mm^3 there is a risk for infection and major complications

_____ a neurologic syndrome that may develop 5 to 8 weeks after central nervous system irradiation; characterized by somnolence with or without fever, anorexia, and nausea and vomiting; may be an early indicator of long-term neurologic sequelae after cranial irradiation

_____ a family of glycoprotein hormones that regulate the reproduction, maturation and function of blood cells; used as a supportive measure to prevent the side effects caused by low blood counts

5. Selected Cancers

A. acute lymphoid leukemia (ALL)
B. induction
C. intensification
D. central nervous system prophylactic therapy
E. maintenance
F. Ann Arbor Staging Classification
G. lymphangiogram
H. Sternberg-Reed cell

I. involved field radiation
J. extended field radiation
K. total nodal irradiation
L. Burkitt lymphoma
M. brain tumors
N. neuroblastoma
O. infra tentorial
P. supra tentorial
Q. astrocytes
R. astrocytomas

S. sterotactic surgery
T. lasers
U. brain mapping
V. phantom limb pain
W. somatic mutations
X. germinal mutations
Y. cobalt plaque applicators
Z. light coagulation
AA. cryotherapy

_____ vaporize tumor tissue

_____ consolidation therapy; the phase of leukemia treatment which decreases the tumor burden

_____ the phase of leukemia therapy which serves to maintain the remission of the disease

_____ determines the precise location of critical brain areas that are avoided during surgery

_____ involves the intradermal injection of a contrast material for visualization of the lymphatic vessels; used to determine the presence of disease in various lymph node regions

_____ lymphatic lymphocytic, lymphoblastic and lymphoblastoid leukemia; terms stem and blast cell leukemia also refer to this type of leukemia

_____ the phase of leukemic therapy that prevents leukemic cells from invading the central nervous system

_____ the phase of leukemia treatment which achieves a complete remission or disappearance of leukemic cells

_____ children with stage I Hodgkin disease are candidates for this treatment

_____ a staging system to classify Hodgkins disease

_____ the entire axial lymph node system is irradiated; usually combined with chemotherapy;

_____ a type of cancer that is rare in the United States; endemic in parts of Africa; a rapidly growing neoplasm that is most commonly seen as a mass in the jaw, abdomen or orbit

_____ a giant cell with a dark staining nucleolus; considered diagnostic of Hodgkin's, but may occur in mononucleosis

_____ the most common solid tumors that occur in children; second only to leukemia as a form of cancer

_____ indicated for stage II or stage III Hodgkin disease; involved areas and the adjacent nodes are irradiated

_____ the most common malignant tumors of infancy and are second only to brain tumors as the type of solid malignancy seen during the first 10 years

_____ may develop following amputation; characterized by sensations such as tingling, itching, and more frequently pain felt in the amputated limb; amitriptyline may decrease the pain

_____ below the tentorium cerebelli

_____ those retinoblastomas occurring in the general body cells as opposed to the germ cells or gametes; sporadic, nonhereditary events; result in unilateral retinoblastoma tumors

_____ within the anterior two thirds of the brain mainly the cerebrum

_____ passed to future generations; bilateral retinoblastomas are considered hereditary; 15% of unilateral disease may be hereditary; transmitted as an autosomal dominant trait

_____ cells that form most of the supportive tissue for the neurons

_____ surgical implantation of a cobalt-60 applicator on the sclera until the maximum radiation dose has been delivered to the tumor

_____ the most common glial tumor

_____ freezing the tumor; destroys the microcirculation to the tumor and the cells themselves through microcrystal formation

_____ involves the use of CT and MRI in conjunction with other special computer techniques to reconstruct the tumor in three dimensions

_____ use of a laser beam to destroy retinal blood vessels that supply nutrition to the tumor

6. The cancer that occurs with the most frequency in children is:
   A. lymphoma.
   B. neuroblastoma.
   C. leukemia.
   D. melanoma.

7. Which one of the following carcinogenic agents has been definitely implicated in the development of childhood cancer?
   A. Low doses of radiation
   B. Excessive sun exposure
   C. Exposure to cigarette smoke
   D. Intramuscular vitamin K at birth

8. Which one of the following assessment findings is MOST likely to be seen in a child with leukemia?
   A. Weakness of the eye muscle
   B. Bruising, nosebleeds, paleness and fatigue
   C. Wheezing and shortness of breath
   D. Abdominal swelling

9. When a clinical trial is used to evaluate an aspect of childhood cancer care, the parents can expect that treatment the child receives will always be:
   A. better than the current treatment usually used.
   B. an evaluation of an investigational drug.
   C. intermittent intravenous infusion of drugs.
   D. at least as good as the best possible treatment presently known.

10. The use of clinical trials and protocols for cancer treatment in the past 20 years has resulted in an increased use of:
    A. intermittent intravenous therapy.
    B. continuous intravenous therapy.
    C. lower doses of single-drug therapy.
    D. prolonged duration of maintenance therapy.

11. Which one of the following complications occurs in almost half of the patients receiving chemotherapeutic agents for cancer?
    A. Extravasation
    B. Cystitis
    C. Hypersensitivity
    D. Neurotoxicity

12. Match the type of chemotherapeutic agent with the side effect/nursing consideration that MOST pertain to that type of drug.

    A. alkylating agents   _____ neurotoxicity
    B. antimetabolits   _____ renal toxicity or hemorrhagic cystitis
    C. plant alkaloids   _____ usually no short term acute toxicity
    D. hormones   _____ mucosal ulceration/stomatitis
    E. enzymes   _____ allergic reactions

13. Bone marrow transplant is the MOST likely treatment to be used when the child:
    A. is unlikely to be cured by other means.
    B. has acute leukemia.
    C. has chronic leukemia.
    D. has a compatible donor in his/her family.

14. Name 4 types of early side effects of radiation therapy and describe one nursing intervention for each type.

    _____ _____

    _____ _____

    _____ _____

    _____ _____

15. A major benefit of using umbilical cord blood for stem cell transplantation is:
    A. stem cells are found in low frequency in newborns.
    B. umbilical cord blood is relatively immunodeficient.
    C. there is a lower risk for acute tumor lysis syndrome.
    D. all of the above.

16. List 5 cardinal symptoms of cancer in children.

_____   _____

_____   _____

_____

17. The family of glycoprotein hormones that regulate the function of blood cells is called

_____.

18. A child who is anemic from myelosuppression should:
    A. strictly limit activities.
    B. regulate his/her own activity with adult supervision.
    C. receive transfusions until the hemoglobin level reaches 12.
    D. receive chemotherapy until the hemoglobin level reaches 10.

19. The nursing intervention that would be MOST helpful to use for the child who has stomatitis from cancer chemotherapy would be:
    A. an anesthetic preparation without alcohol.
    B. viscous xylocaine.
    C. lemon glycerin swabs.
    D. a mild sedative.

20. Describe 3 strategies the nurse can use to prevent sterile hemorrhagic cystitis.

_____

_____

_____

21. Children who develop moon face from steroids used to treat cancer take on an appearance of:
    A. an anorexic, undernourished child.
    B. a malnourished child with a swollen abdomen.
    C. an over weight, but undernourished child.
    D. a well nourished healthy child.

22. The child who receives a bone marrow transplant will require:
    A. meticulous skin care.
    B. multiple peripheral sites for intravenous therapy.
    C. less chemotherapy prior to the transplant.
    D. a room with laminar air flow.

23. After a bone marrow aspiration is performed on a child, the nurse should:
    A. apply an adhesive bandage.
    B. place the child in Trendelenburg position.
    C. ask the child to remain in the supine position.
    D. apply a pressure bandage.

24. Dental care for a child whose platelet count is 32,000/mm^3 and granulocyte count is 450/mm^3 should include daily:
   A. tooth brushing with flossing.
   B. tooth brushing without flossing.
   C. flossing without tooth brushing.
   D. wiping with moistened sponges.

25. The siblings and household contacts of an immunocompromised child should NOT receive:
   A. any vaccines.
   B. any live attenuated vaccines.
   C. the routine poliovirus vaccine.
   D. live measles mumps and rubella (MMR) vaccine.

26. Currently the term *acute* is used in the classification of the leukemias to imply that:
   A. there is an increased number of abnormal mature cells present in the bone marrow.
   B. the course of the disease progresses slowly.
   C. the course of the disease involves rapid deterioration.
   D. there is an increased number of immature blast cells present in the bone marrow.

27. Name the 3 main consequences of bone marrow dysfunction and list their causes.

   _____ _____

   _____ _____

   _____ _____

28. Staging the child with leukemia by using initial white blood cell count, the patient's age, sex and the histologic type of the disease are used to:
   A. determine potential chemotherapy side effects.
   B. estimate long term survival.
   C. make a definitive diagnosis.
   D. determine whether metastases have occurred.

29. The child who receives reinduction therapy for a relapse in their cancer is likely to experience:
   A. more severe alopecia than during their first chemotherapy experience.
   B. thinning of the hair, but full enough to make a wig unnecessary.
   C. hair regrowth that is thinner, straighter and darker than before.
   D. complete baldness, requiring some protection from the cold and sun.

30. Which one of the following children with acute lymphoid leukemia has the BEST prognosis?
   A. A 1-year-old girl with a leukocyte count of 30,000/mm^3
   B. A 6-year-old boy with a leukocyte count of 120,000/mm^3
   C. A 6-year-old boy with a leukocyte count of 30,000/mm^3
   D. A 1-year-old girl with a leukocyte count of 120,000/mm^3

31. To attempt to prevent central nervous system invasion of malignant cells, children with leukemia usually receive prophylactic:
   A. cranial/spinal irradiation.
   B. intravenous steroid therapy.
   C. intrathecal chemotherapy.
   D. intravenous methotrexate and cytarabine.

32. The fact that 95% of children with acute lymphoid leukemia will achieve an initial remission should be interpreted as:
   A. the percentage of children who will live 5 years or longer.
   B. an estimate that applies to children treated with the most successful protocols since diagnosis.
   C. the number to use only for the low-risk group of children.
   D. the estimate that may be used to determine the probability of a cure.

33. Hodgkin disease increases in incidence in children:
   A. under the age of 5 years.
   B. between the ages of 5 and 10 years.
   C. between the ages of 11 and 14 years.
   D. between the ages of 15 and 19 years.

34. Using present treatment protocols, prognosis for Hodgkin disease may be estimated with:
   A. the Ann Arbor Staging Classification.
   B. histologic staging.
   C. degree of tumor burden.
   D. initial leukocyte count.

35. A child with Hodgkin disease who has lesions in both the left and the right supraclavicular area, the mediastinum and in the lungs would be classified as:
   A. Stage I.
   B. Stage II.
   C. Stage III.
   D. Stage IV.

36. The Sternberg-Reed cell is a significant finding, because it:
   A. is absent in all diseases other than Hodgkin disease.
   B. is absent in all diseases other than the lymphomas.
   C. eliminates the need for laparotomy to determine the stage of the disease.
   D. is absent in all lymphomas other than Hodgkin disease.

37. The child who is scheduled for a lymphangiography examination should be told:
   A. to restrict his/her activity to quiet play after the test.
   B. the test will take about 2 hours.
   C. the test often takes 4-5 hours.
   D. to take nothing by mouth for at least 8 hours before the test.

38. Burkitt lymphoma is a type of:
   A. Hodgkin disease.
   B. non-Hodgkin lymphoma.
   C. acute myleocytic leukemia.
   D. neuroblastoma.

39. The early signs and symptoms of brain tumor in the infant:
    A. are similar to those of a young child's.
    B. may be undetectable while the sutures are open.
    C. will be demonstrated as vomiting after feedings.
    D. will be demonstrated as headache and vomiting.

40. Match the major brain tumors of childhood with their corresponding characteristics.

    A.   medulloblastoma   _____ poor prognosis, because tumor is located in vital
    B.   cerebral astrocytoma   brain centers
    C.   low grade astrocytoma   _____ the most common pediatric brain tumor; infiltrates
    D.   ependymoma   brain parenchyma without distinct boundaries
    E.   brainstem glioma   _____ usually invades the ventricles and obstructs the
                                           cerebrospinal fluid flow
                                   _____ slow-growing tumor (if low grade); has a 70%–90%
                                           likelihood of cure (without residual tumor post
                                           operatively)
                                   _____ fast-growing, highly malignant tumor with a high
                                           risk of recurrence

41. Which one of the following surgical techniques involves the use of computerized tomography
    and magnetic resonance imaging during the surgery?
    A. Sclerotherapy
    B. Microsurgery
    C. Laser surgery
    D. Stereotactic surgery

42. Which one of the following tumors has a poor prognosis especially in infants and young
    children?
    A. Hodgkin disease
    B. Osteosarcoma
    C. Ewing sarcoma
    D. Brain tumor

43. Describe 3 strategies the nurse can use to help prepare the child for shaving the hair prior to
    surgery to remove a brain tumor.

    _____

    _____

    _____

44. If a child vomits in the postoperative period following surgery for a brain tumor, it may
    predispose the child to:
    A. incisional rupture.
    B. increased intracranial pressure.
    C. aspiration.
    D. all of the above.

45. Which one of the following signs is MOST abnormal in the child who had surgery for a brain tumor 24 hours ago?
    A. The child is comatose.
    B. There is serous sanguinous drainage on the dressing.
    C. There is colorless drainage on the dressing.
    D. There is decreased muscle strength.

46. Neuroblastoma is often classified as a silent tumor because:
    A. diagnosis is not usually made until after metastasis.
    B. the primary site is intracranial.
    C. the primary site is the bone marrow.
    D. diagnosis is made based on the location of the primary site.

47. The peak age for the appearance of bone tumors is:
    A. 5 to 9 years of age.
    B. 10 to 14 years of age.
    C. 15 to 19 years of age.
    D. 20 to 24 years of age.

48. The most common bone cancer in children has a peak incidence at the age of:
    A. birth to 4 years.
    B. 4 years to 8 years.
    C. 8 years to 10 years.
    D. over eleven years.

49. Treatment for Ewing sarcoma would usually include:
    A. radiation alone.
    B. radiation and chemotherapy.
    C. amputation and chemotherapy.
    D. chemotherapy alone.

50. Wilms tumor in children is treated with:
    A. chemotherapy and radiation based on clinical stage and histologic pattern.
    B. surgery and radiation based on clinical stage and histologic pattern.
    C. surgery, chemotherapy, and radiation based on clinical stage and histologic pattern.
    D. surgery alone.

51. Rhabdomyosarcoma is a:
    A. malignant bone neoplasm.
    B. nonmalignant soft tissue tumor.
    C. nonmalignant solid tumor.
    D. malignant solid tumor of the soft tissue.

52. With a multimodal approach to treatment, five year survival rates for rhabdomyosarcoma have improved to:
    A. 15%.
    B. 35%.
    C. 50%.
    D. 65%.

53. Bilateral malignant retinoblastoma is almost always considered to be transmitted by:
    A. an autosomal dominant trait.
    B. a somatic mutation.
    C. a chromosomal aberration.
    D. an autosomal recessive trait.

54. Instructions for the parents of a child who has an eye enucleation performed should be based on the fact that:
    A. there will be a cavity in the skull where the eye was.
    B. the child's face may be edematous and ecchymotic.
    C. the eyelids will be open and the surgical site will be sunken.
    D. all of the above.

55. A nodule discovered on an adolescent male's testicle should be evaluated because a tumor in this location:
    A. usually causes infertility.
    B. in this age group is usually malignant.
    C. has usually metastasized by the time of discovery.
    D. could not be felt using testicular self exam.

56. Which one of the following children would be most likely to develop malignancies as a result of their cancer treatment?
    A. A 18-year-old who receives radiation for treatment of Hodgkin disease
    B. A 2-year-old who receives interthecal chemotherapy
    C. A 4-year-old who receives radiation for treatment of leukemia
    D. A 15-year-old who receives interthecal chemotherapy

Critical Thinking • Case Study

Cory Henderson is a 6-year-old child who is diagnosed with acute lymphoid leukemia. She receives chemotherapy regularly. Her parents are divorced and she is an only child. She lives with her mother, and rarely sees her father.

Cory attends first grade when she can. She had little difficulty with school before her diagnosis, but lately she has had trouble keeping up with the activities, because she is so tired.

57. Today Cory arrives at the chemotherapy clinic for her regular medication regimen. A complete blood count shows that her white blood count is lower than expected. The BEST nursing diagnosis for the nurse to use for Cory today based on the above information would be:
    A. altered family process related to the therapy.
    B. high risk for hemorrhagic cystitis related to white cell proliferation.
    C. high risk for infection related to depressed body defenses.
    D. altered mucous membranes related to administration of chemotherapy.

58. Cory's mother tells the nurse that she has noticed that after the chemotherapy, Cory's appetite is usually quite poor. She knows that nutrition is essential, so she is trying everything to get Cory to eat even during those times when she is nauseated after the chemotherapy. Strategies the nurse might suggest would include:
   A. gargle with viscous xylocaine to relieve pain.
   B. permit only nutritious snacks.
   C. establish regular meal times.
   D. offer small snacks frequently.

59. To plan for the body image disturbance related to loss of hair, moon face, and debilitation, which of the following actions by Cory's mother would be considered MOST beneficial?
   A. Emphasize the benefits of the therapy.
   B. Encourage Cory to select a wig to wear.
   C. Suggest that Cory keep her hair long for as long as possible.
   D. All of the above

60. Which one of the following expected outcomes would be appropriate for the nurse to measure Cory's mother's progress toward coping with the possibility of her child's death?
   A. Cory's mother frequently talks to the staff about her fear of living without her daughter.
   B. Cory's mother is able to verbalize an understanding of the procedures and tests that have been performed.
   C. Cory's mother is able to provide the care at home that is needed.
   D. Cory's mother complies with the suggestions the nurses make.

CHAPTER 37
The Child with Cerebral Dysfunction

1. General Terms

A. central nervous system
B. peripheral nervous system
C. autonomic nervous system
D. meninges
E. dura mater
F. epidural space
G. falx cerebri
H. falx cerebeli
I. tentorium
J. tentorial hiatus
K. arachnoid membrane
L. subdural area
M. pia mater
N. subarachnoid space
O. arachnoid trabeculae
P. longitudinal fissure
Q. corpus callosum
R. basal ganglia
S. brainstem
T. autoregulation

_____ cerebral nuclei; situated deeply within each hemisphere and on each side of the midline; serve as vital sorting areas for messages passing to and from the hemispheres

_____ the large gap through which the brainstem passes; the site of herniation in untreated intracranial pressure

_____ the part of the nervous system that is composed of the sympathetic and parasympathetic systems, which provide automatic control of vital functions

_____ a potential space that normally contains only enough fluid to prevent adhesion between the arachnoid and the dura mater

_____ a double layered membrane that serves as the outer meningeal layer and the inner periosteum of the cranial bones

_____ located between the pia mater and the arachnoid membrane; filled with cerebrospinal fluid which acts as a protective cushion for the brain tissue

_____ a segment of the sheet of dura which separates the cerebral hemispheres

_____ connected to the hemispheres by thick bunches of nerve fibers; all nerve fibers traverse through this structure as they pass from the hemispheres to the cerebellum and the spinal cord; extends from the base of the hemispheres through the foramen magnum, where it is continuous with the spinal cord

_____ a segment of the sheet of dura which separates the cerebellar hemispheres

_____ the part of the nervous system that is composed of the cranial nerves that arise from or travel to the brainstem and the spinal nerves that travel to or from the spinal cord and which may be motor (efferent) or sensory (afferent)

_____ a segment of dura that separates the cerebellum from the occipital lobe of the cerebrum; a tent-like structure

_____ separates the outer meningeal layer and the inner periosteum of the cranial bones

_____ the middle meningeal layer; a delicate, avascular, weblike structure that loosely surrounds the brain

_____ the innermost covering layer of the brain; a delicate transparent membrane that unlike other coverings adheres closely to the outer surface of the brain conforming to the folds (gyri) and furrows (sulci)

_____ the unique ability of the cerebral arterial vessels to change their diameter in response to fluctuating cerebral perfusion pressure

_____ fibrous filaments which provide protection by helping to anchor the brain

_____ the membranes that cover and protect the brain; the dura mater, arachnoid membranes, and pia mater

_____ separates the upper part of the two large cerebral hemispheres that occupy the anterior and medial fossae of the skull

_____ the part of the nervous system that is composed of two cerebral hemispheres, the brainstem, the cerebellum, and the spinal cord

_____ the largest fiber bundle in the brain; joins the central part of the cerebral hemispheres; interconnects cortical areas of the right and left hemispheres

2. Evaluation of Neurological Status

A. neurological physical examination
B. cranial nerve involvement
C. level of development
D. alertness
E. cognitive power
F. unconsciousness
G. coma
H. comatose state
I. Glasgow Coma Scale
J. brain death
K. reproducible
L. pulse/respiration/blood pressure
M. autonomic activity
N. body temperature
O. corneal reflex
P. doll's head maneuver
Q. caloric test
R. papilledema
S. decorticate posturing
T. decerebrate posturing

_____ indicated by abnormal eye movements, an inability to suck or swallow, lip smacking, asymmetric contraction of facial muscles, and yawning

_____ an arousal-waking state that includes the ability to respond to stimuli; an aspect of consciousness

_____ includes observation of the size and shape of the head, spontaneous activity and postural reflex activity and sensory responses, symmetry of movement

_____ depressed cerebral function; the inability to respond to sensory stimuli and have subjective experiences

_____ provide information regarding the adequacy of circulation and the possible underlying cause of altered consciousness

_____ the aspect of consciousness that includes the ability to process stimuli and produce verbal and motor responsiveness

_____ the continuum of diminished alertness as a result of pathologic conditions

_____ provides essential information about neurologic function; developmental tests are used to determine this element of the neurologic assessment

_____ often elevated in head injury; sometimes extreme and unresponsive to therapeutic measures

_____ consists of a three part assessment; created to meet a clinical need of experienced nurses for objective criteria for the consciousness level; the most popular scale that attempts to standardize the description and interpretation of depressed consciousness

__I__ a sign of increased intracranial pressure observed in the eyes

_____ the total cessation of brainstem and cortical brain function

_____ a sign of dysfunction at the level of the midbrain; characterized by rigid extension and pronation of the arms and legs

_____ most intensively disturbed in deep coma and in brainstem lesions

_____ blinking of the eyelids when the cornea is touched with a wisp of cotton; used to test the integrity of the ophthalmic division of cranial nerve

_____ the fashion in which neurologic examination should be documented; enables the comparison of baseline, previous, and current findings; allows the observer to detect subtle changes in the neurologic status that might not otherwise be evident

_____ the child's head is rotated quickly to one side and then the other; normally the eyes will move in the direction opposite the head rotation

_____ a state of unconsciousness from which the patient cannot be aroused, even with powerful stimuli

_____ oculovestibular response; elicited by irrigating the external auditory canal with ice water; causes movement of the eyes toward the side of the stimulation

_____ seen with severe dysfunction of the cerebral cortex; includes adduction of the arms and shoulders; arms flexed on the chest; wrists flexed; hands fisted; lower extremities extended and adducted

3. Terms—Head Injury

A.	acceleration/deceleration	H. concussion
B.	deformation	I. contusion/laceration
C.	coup	J. linear fractures
D.	contrecoup	K. depressed fractures
E.	shearing stresses	L. compound fractures
F.	localized injuries	M. basilar fracture
G.	generalized injuries	N. diastatic fracture

O. acute subdural hematoma
P. chronic subdural hematoma
Q. postconcussion syndrome
R. posttraumatic seizures
S. structural complications

_____ a fracture in which the bone is locally broken, usually into several irregular fragments that are pushed inward, causing pressure on the brain

_____ bruising at the point of impact

_____ physical forces that act on the head when the stationary head receives a blow; the circumstances responsible for most head injuries; when the head receives a blow

_____ a common sequella to brain injury; common in children under 1 year of age; occurs within minutes to an hour after a head injury; the child sweats, becomes pale, irritable, sleepy, and may vomit

__L__ caused by hemorrhage; associated with contusions or lacerations and develops within minutes or hours of injury

_____ involve the basilar portion of the frontal, ethmoid, sphenoid, temporal, or occipital bones

_____ actual bruising and tearing of cerebral tissue

_____ an effect of brain movement that is caused by unequal movement or different rates of acceleration at various levels of the brain; may tear small arteries; the most serious effects are often in the area of the brainstem

__N__ distortion and cavitation that occur as the brain changes shape in response to the force transmitted from impact to the brain

_____ occur in a number of children who survive a head injury; more common in children than in adults; more likely to occur with severe head injury; usually occur within the first few days after injury; associated with long-term epilepsy when they occur within a few seconds of the trauma

_____ traumatic separation of the cranial sutures

_____ a head injury in which the force is spent on a local area of both the skull and underlying tissue

_____ bruising at a distance from the point of impact

__M__ a head injury in which the force is transmitted to the entire skull causing widespread movement, distortion, and damage

_____ occur as a result of head injuries include hydrocephalus and motor deficits

__K__ the most common head injury; a transient and reversible neuronal dysfunction with instantaneous loss of awareness and responsiveness from trauma to the head that persists for a relatively short time

_____ consists of a skin laceration that extends to the site of the bony fracture

_____ comprise about 75% of childhood skull fractures

_____ caused by hemorrhage; associated with contusions or lacerations, symptoms are delayed; more commonly seen in children with open fontanels and sutures

4. Intracranial Infections

A. meningitis
B. encephalitis
C. myelitis
D. bacterial meningitis

E. viral meningitis
F. tuberculous meningitis
G. *Haemophilus influenzae* meningitis

H. meningococcal sepsis
I. Waterhouse-Fredericksen syndrome
J. hydrophobia

_____ the sudden severe and fulminating onset of meningococcemia

_____ inflammatory process that affects the brain

_____ the term used to describe the symptoms of rabies; severe spasm of respiratory muscles resulting in apnea, cyanosis, and anoxia

_____ pyogenic inflamation caused by pus forming organisms especially the meningococcus, pneumococcus and influenza bacillus

_____ inflammatory process that affects the spinal cord

_____ aseptic meningitis

_____ has decreased in incidence since the use of conjugate vaccines in 1990

_____ inflammatory process that affects the meninges

_____ meningococcemia; one of the most dramatic and serious complications associated with meningococcal infection

_____ meningitis caused by the tuberculin bacillus

5. Match the structure of the brain with its corresponding function.

A. parietal lobes
B. temporal lobes
C. cerebrum
D. thalamus

E. mesencephalon (midbrain)
F. medulla
G. cerebellum
H. frontal lobes

I. occipital lobe
J. diencephalon
K. hypothalamus
L. pons

_____ receive/interpret stimuli for the all of the senses

_____ contains the vasomotor cranial nerves

_____ contains pneumotaxic center and controls respiration

_____ necessary for coordination and balance

_____ vital control center of involuntary functions (temperature regulation)

_____ center for consciousness, thought, memory, sensory input and motor activity

_____ receives stimuli for vision and spatial orientation

_____ connects the forebrain to the hindbrain

_____ a major relay station for sensory impulses to the cerebral cortex

_____ controls motor activity, social interaction and abstract thinking

_____ contains fibers that compose the reticular activation system

_____ important for interpretation of sensation

6. Cerebral blood flow, oxygen consumption and brain growth are all:
A. less in adults than in children.
B. greater in adults than in children.
C. greater in adults than in infants.
D. less in infants than in children.

7. Seizures

A. idiopathic seizures
B. acquired seizures
C. epileptogenic focus
D. ictal state
E. postictal state
F. simple partial seizures with motor signs
G. aversive seizure
H. Rolandic (sylvian) seizure
I. Jacksonian march
J. simple partial seizures with sensory signs

K. partial seizures
L. generalized seizures
M. unclassified epileptic seizures
N. psychomotor seizures
O. aura
P. deja vu
Q. impaired consciousness
R. automatism
S. tonic phase
T. clonic phase

U. status epilepticus
V. drop attacks
W. infantile spasms
X. Salaam seizure
Y. Lennox-Gastaut syndrome
Z. idiopathic Lennox-Gastaut syndrome
AA. symptomatic Lennox-Gastaut syndrome
BB. resective surgery
CC. callosotomy
DD. multiple subpial transection

___B___ occur as a result of brain injury during prenatal, perinatal, or postnatal periods; may be caused by trauma, hypoxia, infections, exogenous or endogenous toxins, and a variety of other factors

_____ simple motor seizure; consists of orderly, sequential progression of clonic movements that begin in a foot, hand, or face and, as electric impulses spread from the irritable focus to contiguous regions of the cortex, move body parts activated by these cerebral regions

___A___ cause is unknown; there is a higher incidence of seizures among relatives of these children

___K___ formerly called focal seizures; limited to a particular local area of the brain

_____ a period of the seizure where there is a rolling of the eyes upward and immediate loss of consciousness

_____ a feeling of familiarity in a strange environment

___M___ all seizures that cannot be classified

___F___ arise from the area of the brain that controls muscle movement

___H___ tonic-clonic movements involving the face, salivation and arrested speech; most common during sleep

_____ Horizontal fibers of the motor cortex are divided to reduce seizures; vertical fibers are spared to allow for function.

_____ a group of hyperexcitable cells that initiate the spontaneous electric discharge that produces a seizure

_____ the period during the time the seizure is occurring

_____ the period following a seizure

___J___ characterized by various sensations, including numbness, tingling, prickling, parasthesia, or pain that originates in one area and spreads to other parts of the body

___L___ seizures that involve both hemispheres of the brain

___N___ partial seizures with complex symptoms

_____ a characteristic of the complex partial seizure; repeated activities without purpose and carried out in a dreamy state such as smacking, chewing, drooling, or swallowing

_____ the period in the seizure where there are intense jerking movements as the trunk and extremities undergo rhythmic contraction and relaxation

_____ atonic seizures; manifested as a sudden, momentary loss of muscle tone

___G___ a common motor seizure in children; the eye(s) and head turn away from the side of the focus

_____ a rare disorder that has an onset within the first 6 to 8 months of life; also know as infantile myoclonus, West syndrome

_____ separation of the connections between the two hemispheres of the brain; used to treat some generalized seizures

_____ a characteristic of the complex partial seizure; child may appear dazed and confused and be unable to respond when spoken to or to follow instruction

_____ also known as jackknife seizures; observed as a sudden, brief, symmetric, muscular contractions by which the head is flexed, the arms extended, and the legs drawn up; the seizure observed in infantile spasms

_____ the focal area of the seizure activity is excised with the expectation that serious deficits will not be produced and that existing deficits will not be increased

_____ a seizure that lasts 30 minutes or longer or a series of seizures at intervals too brief to allow the child to regain consciousness between each seizure; requires emergency intervention

_____ also called cryptogenic Lennox-Gastaut syndrome; appears in children with normal psychomotor development and no history of epilepsy or evidence of brain damage; may occur after infectious illness, vaccination, or febrile episodes

_____ Lennox-Gastaut syndrome with a history of encephalopathy and mental retardation or epilepsy; poorer prognosis than in the cryptogenic type

_____ sensation or sensory phenomenon that reflects the complicated connections and integrative functions of that area of the brain

_____ a syndrome that develops in about 30% of children with infantile spasms

8. The blood-brain barrier in an infant is:
   A. less permeable than in the adult.
   B. impermeable to protein.
   C. impermeable to glucose.
   D. permeable to large molecules.

9. Which one of the following signs is used to evaluate increased intracranial pressure in the infant but not in the older child?
   A. Projectile vomiting
   B. Headache
   C. Non-pulsating fontanel
   D. Pulsating fontanel

10. Which of the following indicators is BEST to use to determine the depth of the comatose state?
    A. Motor activity
    B. Level of consciousness
    C. Reflexes
    D. Vital signs

11. Define the term _persistent vegetative state_.

_____

_____

12. The guidelines for establishing brain death in children:
    A. differ from age to age.
    B. are the same as in the adult.
    C. all require an observation period of at least seven days.
    D. all require an observation period of at least 48 hours.

13. Which one of the following neurologic conditions may be associated with hypothermia?
    A. Intracranial bleeding
    B. Barbituate ingestion
    C. Heat stroke
    D. Serious infection

14. A child in a very deep comatose state would exhibit:
    A. hyperkinetic activity.
    B. purposeless plucking movements.
    C. few spontaneous movements.
    D. combative behavior.

15. After a seizure in a child over 3 years of age, the Babinski reflex often:
    A. remains positive.
    B. changes from positive to negative.
    C. changes from negative to positive.
    D. remains negative.

16. Which one of the following reflex patterns would be considered MOST healthy in young infants?
    A. Negative Moro reflex and a positive tonic neck reflex
    B. Negative Moro reflex and a negative tonic neck reflex
    C. Positive Moro reflex and a positive tonic neck reflex
    D. Positive Moro reflex and a negative tonic neck reflex

17. Which one of the following tests should NOT be used if the patient has an increase in intracranial pressure?
    A. Lumbar puncture
    B. Subdural tap
    C. Computed tomography
    D. Digital subtraction angiography

18. The diagnostic procedure that is usually noninvasive and permits visualization of the neurologic structures using radio frequency emissions from elements is called:
    A. digital subtraction angiography.
    B. positron emission tomography.
    C. magnetic resonance imaging.
    D. computed tomography scan.

19. Which one of the following factors is likely to have the greatest impact on the outcome and recovery of the unconscious child?
    A. Gradual reduction in intracranial pressure
    B. The level of nursing care and observation skills
    C. The emotional response of the parents
    D. The level of discomfort the child experiences

20. Which one of the following nursing observations would usually indicate pain in a comatose child?
    A. increased flaccidity
    B. increased oxygen saturation
    C. decreased blood pressure
    D. increased agitation

21. Intracranial pressure monitoring has been found to be useful in pediatric critical care to:
    A. determine the outcome of a pediatric neurologic injury.
    B. evaluate children with Glasgow Coma Scale scores under seven.
    C. give an indication of the severity of the neurologic insult in the initial evaluation of a child.
    D. all of the above.

22. Which one of the following activities has been shown to increase intracranial pressure?
    A. Using earplugs to eliminate noise
    B. Range-of-motion exercises
    C. Suctioning
    D. Osmotherapy

23. Which one of the following medications would be BEST to use intravenously to treat seizures?
    A. Fosphenytoin (Cerebyx)
    B. Phenytoin (Dilantin)
    C. Midazolam (Versed)
    D. Dexamethozone (Decadron)

24. If a child is permanently unconscious, it would be INAPPROPRIATE for the nurse to:
    A. permit the parents to bring a child's favorite toy.
    B. provide guidance and clarify information that the physician has already given.
    C. suggest the parents plan for periodic relief from the continual care of their child.
    D. use reflexive muscle contractions as a sign of hope for recovery.

25. Because of the ability of the cranium to expand, very young children may tolerate which one of the following neurological conditions better than an adult?
    A. Cerebral edema
    B. Hypoxic brain damage
    C. Cerebral edema
    D. Subdural hemorrhage

26. Head injury that causes the brain to be forced though the tentorial opening is usually referred to as:
    A. contrecoup.
    B. concussion
    C. uncal herniation
    D. deformation

27. Which one of the following symptoms would NOT be considered a hallmark of concussion in a child?
    A. Alteration of mental status
    B. Amnesia
    C. Loss of consciousness
    D. Confusion

28. Epidural hemorrhage is less common in children under 2 years of age than in adults because:
    A. the middle meningeal artery is embedded in the bone surface of the skull until approximately 2 years of age.
    B. fractures are less likely to lacerate the middle meningeal artery in children under 2 years of age.
    C. separation of the dura from bleeding is more likely to occur in children than in adults.
    D. there is an increased tendency for the skull to fracture in children under 2 years of age.

29. Which one of the following features is indicative of a subdural hematoma?
    A. Retinal hemorrhages
    B. Low morbidity
    C. High mortality
    D. Older child

30. The goal in the management of a child with a head injury is to:
    A. eliminate ischemic brain damage.
    B. eliminate original primary insult.
    C. care for the secondary brain injuries.
    D. all of the above.

31. Which one of the following interventions would NOT be considered part of the emergency treatment of a child with a head injury?
    A. Administer analgesics.
    B. Check pupil reaction to light.
    C. Stabilize the neck and spine.
    D. Check level of consciousness

32. Which one of the following clinical manifestations indicates a progression from minor injury to severe head injury?
    A. Confusion
    B. Mounting agitation
    C. An episode of vomiting
    D. Pallor

33. Compared to adults after craniocerebral trauma, children usually have a:
    A. lower incidence of psychological disturbances.
    B. higher mortality rate.
    C. less favorable prognosis.
    D. higher incidence of psychological disturbances.

34. Family support for the child who has suffered head injury includes all of the following EXCEPT to encourage the parents to:
    A. hold and cuddle the child.
    B. bring familiar belongings into the child's room.
    C. make a tape recording of familiar voices/sounds.
    D. search for clues that the child is recovering.

35. Identify 3 factors that contribute to accident risk in children.

    _____   _____

    _____

36. Which one of the following age groups has a higher resistance to asphyxia and anoxia from submersion in water?
    A. Toddler
    B. Preschool
    C. School-age
    D. Adolescent

37. Which of the following would NOT be considered a predictor of outcome in near-drowning victims?
    A. Cardiac rhythm
    B. Degree of acidosis upon admission
    C. Response of the pupils to light
    D. Length of time the child was submerged

38. The etiology of bacterial meningitis has changed in recent years due to the:
    A. increased surveillance of tuberculosis.
    B. increased awareness of rubella vaccines.
    C. routine use of *H. influenzae* type B vaccine.
    D. routine use of Hepatitis B vaccine.

39. The MOST common mode of transmission for bacterial meningitis is:
    A. vascular dissemination of a respiratory tract infection.
    B. direct implantation from an invasive procedure.
    C. direct extension from an infection in the mastoid sinuses.
    D. direct extension from an infection in the nasal sinuses.

40. A child who is ill and develops a purpuric or petechial rash may possibly have developed:
    A. aseptic meningitis.
    B. Waterhouse-Fredericksen syndrome.
    C. citobacter diversus meningitis.
    D. herpes simplex encephalitis.

41. Secondary problems from bacterial meningitis are MOST likely to occur in the:
    A. child with meningococcal meningitis.
    B. infant under 2 months of age.
    C. infant over 2 months of age.
    D. child with *H. influenzae* type B meningitis.

42. Which one of the following types of meningitis is self-limiting and least serious?
   A. Meningococcal meningitis
   B. Tuberculous meningitis
   C. *H. influenzae* meningitis
   D. Nonbacterial (aseptic) meningitis

43. Which one of the following types of encephalitis occurs in children one-third of the time?
   A. Herpes simplex
   B. Measles
   C. Mumps
   D. Rubella

44. Which of the following domestic animals should be the target of a community rabies vaccination program?
   A. Dogs
   B. Hamsters
   C. Cats
   D. Parakeets

45. For the postexposure treatment of rabies, the World Health Organization recommends:
   A. mass immunization using human rabies immune globulin.
   B. administration of human diploid cell rabies vaccine according to schedule for 3 months after the exposure.
   C. mass immunization using human diploid cell rabies vaccine.
   D. administration of human rabies immune globulin 90 days after the exposure.

46. The link between aspirin and Reye Syndrome:
   A. is firmly established.
   B. is a cause-and-effect relationship.
   C. has alerted the public to the hazard of drugs.
   D. all of the above.

47. Symptoms that are similar to those of Reye syndrome have occurred during viral illnesses when the child was given an:
   A. antiemetic drug.
   B. analgesic drug.
   C. antiepileptic drug.
   D. antiarrhythmic drug.

48. The drug that reduces the chance that the HIV-infected pregnant mother will infect her infant is called:
   A. valproate.
   B. zidovudine.
   C. nitrazepam.
   D. felbamate.

49. Name 2 factors that contribute to childhood seizures.

   ____birth injuries____   ____acute infections____

50. A complex partial seizure is MORE likely than a simple partial seizure to exhibit:
    A. impaired consciousness.
    B. impaired muscle tone.
    C. motor jerking.
    D. short period of staring.

51. One strategy that may provide a clue to the origin of a seizure is to:
    A. attempt to place an airway in the mouth.
    B. gently open the eyes to observe their movement.
    C. provide a clear description of the seizure.
    D. all of the above.

52. Which one of the following types of seizures is MOST common in children between the ages of 4 and 12 years?
    A. Generalized seizures
    B. Absence seizures
    C. Atonic seizures
    D. Jackknife seizures

53. Which one of the following antiepileptic drugs acts only on a developing brain and therefore is used for infantile spasms?
    A. Adrenocorticotropic hormone
    B. Valproic acid
    C. Ethosuximide
    D. Felbamate

54. The drug of choice for the treatment of Lennox-Gastaut syndrome (LGS) is:
    A. nitrazapam.
    B. clonazepam.
    C. felbamate.
    D. valproate.

55. Therapy for epilepsy should begin with:
    A. short-term drug therapy.
    B. combination drug therapy.
    C. only one drug, if possible.
    D. drugs that correct the brain wave pattern.

56. Erythromycin may cause increased side effects and toxicity in children treated for epilepsy with:
    A. carbamazepine (Tegretol).
    B. clonazepam (Klonopin).
    C. valproic acid (Depakote).
    D. felbamate (Felbatol).

57. A new drug used to control seizures that is generally considered safe, well tolerated and does not interfere with other drugs is:
    A. gabapentin (Neurontin).
    B. lamotrigine (Lamictal).
    C. valproate sodium (Depacon).
    D. fosphenytoin (Cerebrex).

58. A poor prognosis for the child with status epilepticus is associated with:
    A. previous developmental delays.
    B. previous neurologic abnormalities.
    C. concurrent serious illness.
    D. all of the above.

59. Nursing intervention for a child during a tonic-clonic seizure should include attempts to:
    A. halt the seizure as soon as it begins.
    B. restrain the child.
    C. remain calm and observe the child.
    D. place an oral airway in the child's mouth.

60. Emergency care of the child during a seizure includes:
    A. giving ice chips slowly.
    B. restraining the child.
    C. putting a tongue blade in the child's mouth.
    D. loosening restrictive clothing.

61. To prevent submersion injuries in children with epilepsy, the child should be instructed to:
    A. never go swimming.
    B. take showers.
    C. wear a bicycle helmet.
    D. all of the above.

62. In most children who have a febrile seizure, the factor that triggers the seizure tends to be the:
    A. rapidity of the temperature elevation.
    B. duration of the temperature elevation.
    C. height of the temperature elevation.
    D. any of the above.

63. When a child has a febrile seizure, it is important for the parents to know that the child will:
    A. probably not develop epilepsy.
    B. most likely develop epilepsy.
    C. most likely develop neurologic damage.
    D. usually need tepid sponge baths to control fever.

64. In most cases chronic recurrent headaches of childhood represent:
    A. tension.
    B. seizures.
    C. intracranial disease.
    D. migraine.

65. Treatment for migraine headaches in children may include:
    A. ergots.
    B. opioids.
    C. acetaminophen.
    D. all of the above.

Critical Thinking • Case Study

Jackson Smith was riding his bike in the street by his house when he was hit by a car. He is 9 years old. He was not wearing a helmet at the time. He has been unconscious since the accident eight hours ago. His mother and father both work full-time and there are 5 other siblings at home ranging in ages from 7 years old to 19 years old.

66. Based on the above information which of the following nursing diagnoses would have the highest priority?
    A. High risk for impaired skin integrity related to immobility
    B. Self care deficit related to inability to feed himself
    C. Altered family process related to a permanent disability
    D. High risk for aspiration related to impaired motor function

67. In order to effectively deal with the altered family process related to the hospitalization the nurse should:
    A. provide information about bicycle safety helmets.
    B. encourage expression of feelings.
    C. encourage the family to provide Jackson's hygiene needs.
    D. provide auditory stimulation for Jackson.

68. In order to help Jackson receive appropriate sensory stimulation the nurse should:
    A. hang a black and white mobile above his bed.
    B. hang a calendar at the foot of his bed.
    C. encourage the family to bring a tape of his favorite music.
    D. administer pain medications as needed.

69. Jackson's parents visit him every day, but never together. The nurse should be concerned about:
    A. marital problems that usually occur during stressful times like this.
    B. whether Jackson's parents are able to receive adequate support for each other with this arrangement.
    C. whether Jackson's siblings are being adequately cared for.
    D. all of the above.

CHAPTER 38
The Child with Endocrine Dysfunction

1. Terms—Hormones

A. cell
B. end organ
C. environment
D. local hormones
E. general hormones

F. target tissues
G. anterior pituitary
H. tropic hormones
I. releasing/inhibitory hormones
J. neuroendocrine system

K. autonomic nervous system
L. parasympathetic system
M. sympathetic system
N. neurotransmitting substances

_____G_____ the master gland

_____E_____ a complex chemical substance produced and secreted into body fluids by a cell or group of cells that exerts a physiologic controlling effect on other cells; produced in one organ or part of the body and are carried through the blood stream to a distant part, or parts, of the body where they initiate or regulate physiologic activity of an organ or group of cells, e.g. thyroid

_____A_____ the component of the endocrine system that sends a chemical message by means of a hormone

_____N_____ acetylcholine and norepinephrine

_____H_____ secreted by the anterior pituitary that regulate the secretion of hormones from various target organs

_____C_____ the component of the endocrine system through which the chemical is transported (blood, lymph, extracellular fluids) from the site of synthesis to the site of cellular action

_____K_____ consists of the sympathetic and parasympathetic systems; control non-voluntary functions specifically smooth muscle myocardium and glands

_____F_____ specific tissues on which hormones produce their effect; e.g. the pituitary hormones stimulate the adrenal glands to secrete adrenocorticotropin

_____I_____ secreted by the hypothalamus and transported by way of the pituitary portal system to the anterior pituitary where they stimulate the secretion of tropic hormones

_____B_____ target cell; the component of the endocrine system that receives the chemical message

_____J_____ the systems that maintain homeostasis; the endocrine and the neuroendocrine system together

_____L_____ primarily involved in regulating digestive processes

_____D_____ a complex chemical substance produced and secreted into body fluids by a cell or group of cells that exerts a physiologic controlling effect on other cells near the point of secretion, e.g. acetylcholine

_____M_____ functions to maintain homeostasis during stress

2. Terms—Pituitary Disorders

A.	idiopathic hypopituitarism	G.	acromegaly	L.	premature thelarche
B.	familial short stature	H.	hypothalamic-pituitary-gonadal axis	M.	premature pubarche
C.	constitutional growth delay	I.	true/complete precocious puberty	N.	premature menarche
D.	Creutzfeldt-Jakob disease (CJD)	J.	functional idiopathic puberty	O.	luteinizing hormone-releasing hormone (LHRH)
E.	biosynthetic growth hormone	K.	precocious pseudopuberty	P.	neurogenic diabetes insipidus
F.	juvenilization			Q.	vasopressin

___J___ constitutional precocious puberty; unusually early activation of the maturation process where no cause can be identified; regarded as a normal course of events at a later age

___Q___ hormone that will alleviate the polyuria and polydipsia in neurogenic diabetes insipidus; other hormones used to treat diabetes insipidus

___C___ refers to individuals (usually boys) with delayed linear growth and skeletal and sexual maturation that is behind that of age-mates

___M___ premature adrenoarch; early development of sexual hair

___E___ prepared by recombinant DNA technology

___O___ regulates pituitary secretions; a synthetic analog is used to manage precocious puberty of central origin

___F___ the frequently occurring phenomenon with growth hormone deficient children where others relate to them in infantile or childish ways

___H___ the sequence of events that stimulate the secretion of gonadotropic hormones from the anterior pituitary at the time of puberty

___A___ growth failure; usually related to growth hormone (GH) deficiency

___I___ results from premature activation of the hypothalamic-pituitary-gonadal axis, which produces early maturation and development of the gonads with secretion of sex hormones, development of secondary sex characteristics, and sometimes production of mature sperm or ova

___D___ a rare and fatal neurodegenerative condition that has been iatrogenically transmitted through human tissue from cadaver-derived growth hormone

___K___ incomplete puberty; pseudosexual precocious puberty; no early secretion of gonadotropin; no maturation of the gonads, but there is appearance of secondary sex characteristics

___G___ the condition that is produced when hypersecretion of growth hormone occurs after epiphyseal closure; growth occurs in a transverse direction

___L___ development of breasts in prepubertal females

___N___ isolated menses without other evidence of sexual development

___P___ hyposecretion of antidiuretic hormone/vasopressin; produces a state of uncontrolled diuresis

___B___ refers to otherwise healthy children who have ancestors with adult height in the lower percentiles and whose height during childhood is appropriate for genetic background

3. Terms—Endocrine Disorders

A. thyroid hormone
B. thyrocalcitonin
C. thyroid stimulating hormone (TSH)
D. Hashimoto disease
E. exopthalmos
F. parathormone (PTH)
G. autoimmune hypoparathyroidism
H. pseudohypopara-thyroidism

I. vitamin D therapy
J. hyperparathyroidism
K. adrenal cortex
L. glucocorticoids
M. mineralocorticoids
N. sex steroids
O. corticotropin-releasing factor (CRF)
P. adrenocorticotropic hormone (ACTH)
Q. aldosterone

R. renin
S. adrenal crisis
T. Waterhous-Friderichsen syndrome
U. congenital adrenogenital hyperplasia (CAH)
V. 21-hydroxylase deficiency
W. 11-hydroxylase deficiency
X. ambiguous genitalia

___X___ most pronounced in the female with masculinization of the external genitalia; the term to use for any infant with hypospadias or micropenis and no palpable gonads

___B___ one of the types of hormones secreted by the thyroid gland

___D___ juvenile autoimmune thyroiditis; lymphocytic thyroiditis; the most common cause of thyroid disease in children and adolescents; accounts for the largest percentage of juvenile hypothyroidism

___C___ produced by the anterior pituitary; controls the secretion of thyroid hormones

___E___ protruding eyeballs; observed in many children with Hashimoto disease; accompanied by a wide-eyed staring expression, increased blinking, lid lag, lack of convergence, and absence of wrinkling of the forehead when looking upward

___I___ treatment used in hypoparathyroidism

___G___ deficient production of PTH; clinical manifestations of decreased serum calcium and increased serum phosphorus are present

___F___ secreted by the parathyroid glands; maintains serum calcium levels

___Q___ the mineralocorticoid that promotes sodium retention and potassium excretion in the renal tubules

___H___ Production of PTH is increased but end-organ responsiveness to PTH is deficient; clinical manifestations of decreased serum calcium and increased serum phosphorus are present.

___O___ androgens, estrogens, and progestins

___N___ causes the pituitary gland to produce adrenocorticotropic hormone (ACTH)

___J___ disorder with clinical manifestations of hypercalcemia, elevated calcium and decreased phosphorus

___L___ cortisol and corticosterone

___S___ the acute form of adrenocortical insufficiency

___K___ secretes the steroid hormones, catecholamines (epinephrine) and norepinephrine

___M___ aldosterone

___U___ excessive secretion of androgens by the adrenal cortex; adrenocortical hyperplasia (ACH), adrenogenital syndrome (AGS) and congenital adrenocortical hyperplasia;

___P___ stimulates the adrenal glands to synthesize glucocorticoids

___R___ converts angiotensinogen to angiotensin I and then to angiotensin II which stimulates the adrenal cortex to secrete aldosterone which preserves sodium, retains water and increases the blood pressure

___T___ the presentation of generalized hemorrhagic manifestations in adrenocortical insufficiency

___V___ the most common biochemical defect associated with congenital adrenogenital hyperplasia (CAH)

___A___ a type of hormone secreted by the thyroid gland that consists of the hormones thyroxine (T4) and triiodothyronine (T3)

___W___ an increase in the mineralocorticoid that leads to hypertension

4. Terms—Diabetes

A. islets of Langerhans
B. alpha cells
C. beta cells
D. delta cells
E. glucagon
F. glycogenolysis
G. somatostatin
H. insulin
I. secondary diabetes mellitus

J. idiopathic diabetes mellitus
K. hyperglycemia
L. glycosuria
M. polyuria
N. polydipsia
O. glucogenisis
P. polyphagia
Q. ketonuria
R. acetone breath

S. ketonemia
T. ketoacidosis
U. ketones
V. Kussmaul respirations
W. nephropathy/retinopathy/ neuropathy
X. glycosylation
Y. hyperglycemic
Z. ketotic
AA. diabetic ketoacidosis (DKA)

___N___ excessive thirst

___H___ the hormone that is characteristically deficient in diabetes mellitus

___C___ produce insulin

___K___ increased concentration of glucose

___B___ produce glucagon

___U___ organic acids that readily produce excessive quantities of free hydrogen ions

___I___ precipitated by exogenous factors including pancreatic trauma hormones and chemicals

___D___ produce somatostatin

___Q___ elimination of b-hydroxybutyric acid, acetoacetic acid and acetone in the urine

___R___ elimination of ketones through the lungs

___F___ the release of stored glucose from the liver and other cells

___M___ osmotic diversion of water, a cardinal sign of diabetes

___E___ causes an increase in the blood glucose by stimulating glycogenolysis

___G___ secreted by the islet cells; believed to regulate the release of insulin and glucagon, but found in greater supply in the hypothalamus where it prevents the release of growth hormone

___O___ protein that is broken down and converted to glucose by the liver

___AA___ dehydration electrolyte imbalance and acidosis from diabetes

___J___ classified into type 1, type 2 and maturity-onset diabetes of youth

___A___ the endocrine portion of the pancreas; contains the alpha cells, the beta cells and the delta cells

___T___ the lowering of the serum pH from ketone bodies in the blood

___L___ glucose in the urine

___X___ proteins from the blood become deposited in the walls of small vessels where they become trapped by glucose compounds; causes narrowing of the microvascular vessels over time

___P___ increased food intake

___Z___ ketones measurable in the blood and urine

___W___ long-term complications of diabetes that involve the microvasculature

___S___ b-hydroxybutyric acid, acetoacetic acid and acetone in the blood

___V___ hyperventilation characteristic of metabolic acidosis

___Y___ elevated blood glucose and glucose in the urine

5. Terms—Diabetes Therapeutic Management

A. regular insulin
B. NPH/Lente insulin
C. multiple daily injection (MDI)
D. insulin pump
E. intranasal insulin administration

F. islet cell/whole pancreas transplant
G. home blood glucose monitoring (HBGM)
H. insulin reaction
I. glucagon

J. Somogyi effect
K. Injectease
L. NovoPen
M. drenergic symptoms
N. neuroglycopenic symptoms

___C___ has been shown to reduce microcvascular complication of diabetes in young, healthy patients who have type 1 diabetes

___B___ intermediate acting

___D___ an electromechanical device designed to deliver fixed amounts of a dilute solution of regular insulin continuously; more closely imitates the release of insulin

___A___ rapid acting

___E___ experimental form of insulin; may be of value for mealtime supplementation

___G___ has improved diabetes management; diabetes management depends on these values

___F___ used in persons who have serious complications, particularly those who require renal transplantation with immunosuppressive therapy

___N___ later signs of hypoglycemia; brain hypoglycemia; difficulty with balance, memory, attention, slurred speech

___I___ releases stored glycogen from the liver; sometimes prescribed for home treatment of hypoglycemia

___K___ a syringe-loaded injector for children to use who do not wish to give themselves injections

___H___ often the most feared aspect of diabetes because severe brain symptoms may develop

___J___ rebound hyperglycemia

___M___ early signs of hypoglycemia; help to raise the blood glucose level; sweating, trembling

___L___ a self contained, compact devise resembling a fountain pen which eliminates conventional vials and syringes

6. Identify the target tissue/gland for each of the following hormones; then match the hormone and gland with its corresponding effect.

Hormone
A. thyroid stimulating hormone
B. luteinizing hormone
C. somatotropic hormone
D. gonadotropin
E. melanocyte-stimulating hormone
F. adrenocorticotropic hormone
G. antidiuretic hormone
H. follicle stimulating hormone
I. oxytocin
J. prolactin

Target Tissue/Gland
A. thyroid gland
B. ovaries, testes
C. _____
D. _____
E. _____
F. _____
G. _____
H. _____
I. _____
J. _____

Hormone's Effect
___G___ increases reabsorption of water
___C___ promotes growth of bone and soft tissue
___F___ stimulates the secretion of glucocorticoids
___H___ initiates spermatogenesis
___A___ regulates metabolic rate
___J___ maintains corpus luteum during pregnancy
___E___ promotes pigmentation of the skin
___I___ causes the let-down reflex
___D___ produces sex hormones
___B___ stimulates the secretion of testosterone in the male

7. A hormone that produces its effect on a specific tissue would be classified as a
_____ hormone.

8. Match the hormone/gland with its corresponding effect.

Hormone

A. parathyroid
B. cortisol
C. aldosterone
D. thyroid
E. androgen
F. glucagon
G. epinephrine
H. progesterone
I. insulin
J. estrogen
K. testosterone

Hormone's Effect

__H__ prepares uterus for fertilized ovum
__E__ influences development of secondary sex characteristics
__J__ promotes breast development during puberty
__F__ inhibits the secretion of insulin
__B__ promotes normal fat protein and carbohydrate metabolism
__G__ produces vasoconstriction and raises blood pressure
__C__ stimulates renal tubules to reabsorb sodium
__K__ stimulates testes to produce spermatozoa
__D__ regulates metabolic rate
__I__ promotes glucose transport into the cells
__A__ promotes reabsorption of calcium and excretion of phosphorous

9. The difference between panhypopituitarism and idiopathic hypopituitarism is that:
   A. panhypopituitarism is often caused by a tumor.
   B. the incidence of idiopathic hypopituitarism is higher in girls.
   C. panhypopituitarism usually has a cause that is unknown.
   D. panhypopituitarism is the cause of short stature in most children whose height is in the lower percentiles.

10. A child with growth hormone deficiency will exhibit the signs of:
    A. retarded height and weight.
    B. abnormal skeletal proportions.
    C. malnutrition.
    D. retarded height, but not necessarily retarded weight.

11. In a child with hypopituitarism, the growth hormone levels would usually be:
    A. elevated after twenty minutes of strenuous exercise.
    B. elevated 45 to 90 minutes after the onset of sleep.
    C. lower in an overnight urine specimen.
    D. rapidly increased in response to insulin.

12. Treatment of choice for the child with idiopathic hypopituitarism may include:
    A. biosynthetic growth hormone.
    B. human growth hormone.
    C. chemotherapy to shrink the tumor.
    D. any of the above.

13. Which one of the following statements about growth hormone replacement therapy in the child with idiopathic hypopituitarism is TRUE?
    A. Therapy will continue for life.
    B. Therapy will not result in achievement of a normal familial height.
    C. Therapy requires subcutaneous injection.
    D. Therapy requires intramuscular injection.

14. Provocative testing for diagnosis of hypopituitarism may require that the nurse monitor the child's:
    A. calcium levels.
    B. phosphorous levels.
    C. glucose levels.
    D. hemoglobin levels.

15. Explain the difference between acromegaly and the pituitary hyperfunction that would not be considered acromegaly.

    _____

    _____

    _____

16. Parents of the child with precocious puberty need to know that:
    A. dress and activities should be aligned with the child sexual development.
    B. heterosexual interest will usually be advanced.
    C. the child's mental age is congruent with the chronological age.
    D. overt manifestations of affection represent sexual advances.

17. Desmopressin acetate may be administered:
    A. by mouth.
    B. intranasally.
    C. topically.
    D. all of the above.

18. The immediate management of syndrome of inappropriate antidiuretic hormone (SIADH) consists of:
    A. increasing fluids.
    B. administering antibiotics.
    C. restricting fluids.
    D. administering vasopressin.

19. The MOST common cause of thyroid disease in children and adolescents is:
    A. Hashimoto disease.
    B. Graves disease.
    C. goiter.
    D. thyrotoxicosis.

20. The initial treatment for the child with hyperthyroidism would MOST likely be:
    A. subtotal thyroidectomy.
    B. total thyroidectomy.
    C. ablation with radioactive iodide.
    D. administration of antithyroid medication.

21. When a thyroidectomy is planned, the nurse should explain to the child that:
    A. iodine preparations will be mixed with flavored foods and then eaten.
    B. he/she will need to hyper extend his/her neck postoperatively.
    C. the skin, not the throat will be cut.
    D. laryngospasm can be a life-threatening complication.

22. The child with hypoparathyroidism will usually exhibit:
    A. short stubby fingers.
    B. dimpling of the skin over the knuckles.
    C. thin, brittle nails.
    D. a short thick neck.

23. A common cause of secondary hyperparathyroidism is:
    A. maternal hyperparathyroidism.
    B. chronic renal disease.
    C. maternal diabetes mellitus.
    D. adenoma of the parathyroid gland.

24. Hypofunction of the adrenal medulla results in:
    A. release of epinephrine and norepinephrine from the sympathetic nervous system.
    B. pheochromocytoma.
    C. adrenal crisis.
    D. myxedema.

25. Diagnosis of acute adrenocortical insufficiency is made based on:
    A. elevated plasma cortisol levels.
    B. the history and physical exam.
    C. depressed plasma cortisol levels.
    D. depressed aldosterone levels.

26. Parent's of a child who has Addison disease should be instructed to:
    A. use extra hydrocortisone only when signs of crisis are present.
    B. discontinue the child's cortisone if side effects develop.
    C. decrease the cortisone dose during times of stress.
    D. report signs of Cushing syndrome to the physician.

27. Which one of the following tests is particularly useful in diagnosing congenital adrenogenital hyperplasia?
    A. Chromosomal typing
    B. Pelvic ultrasound
    C. Pelvic x-ray
    D. Testosterone levels

28. The temporary treatment for hyperaldosteronism prior to surgery would usually involve administration of:
    A. spironolactone.
    B. phentolamine.
    C. furosemide.
    D. phenoxybenzamine.

29. Definitive treatment for pheochromocytoma consists of:
    A. surgical removal of the thyroid.
    B. administration of potassium.
    C. surgical removal of the tumor.
    D. administration of beta blockers.

30. Most children with diabetes mellitus tend to exhibit characteristics of:
    A. maturity-onset diabetes of youth.
    B. gestational diabetes.
    C. type 2 diabetes.
    D. type 1 diabetes.

31. The currently accepted etiology of insulin dependent diabetes takes into account:
    A. genetic factors.
    B. autoimmune mechanisms.
    C. environmental factors.
    D. all of the above.

32. An early sign of insulin dependent diabetes in the adolescent would be:
    A. a vaginal candida infection.
    B. obesity.
    C. Kussmaul respirations.
    D. all of the above.

33. Which one of the following blood glucose levels is most certain to indicate a diagnosis of diabetes?
    A. Fasting blood glucose of 120 mg/dl
    B. Random blood glucose of 140 mg/dl
    C. Fasting blood glucose of 160 mg/dl
    D. Oral glucose tolerance test value of 160 mg/dl

34. State the goal of insulin replacement therapy.

    _____

    _____

35. Glycosolated hemoglobin is an acceptable method to use to:
    A. diagnose diabetes mellitus.
    B. assess the control of diabetes.
    C. assess oxygen saturation of the hemoglobin.
    D. determine blood glucose levels most accurately.

36. The MOST common acute complication of diabetes that a young child encounters is:
    A. retinopathy.
    B. ketoacidosis.
    C. hypoglycemia.
    D. hyperosmolar non-ketotic coma.

37. Describe the treatment for a mild hypoglycemic episode in a young child with diabetes mellitus.

_____

_____

38. Principles of managing diabetes during illness include all of the following EXCEPT:
   A. monitor blood glucose every four hours.
   B. use a sliding scale of regular insulin.
   C. omit insulin when excessive vomiting occurs.
   D. use simple sugars as carbohydrate exchanges.

39. Diabetic ketoacidosis in children with diabetes mellitus is:
   A. the most common chronic complication.
   B. a result of too much insulin.
   C. is a life threatening complication.
   D. rarely requires hospitalization.

40. Which one of the following cardiac wave patterns is indicative of hypokalemia?
   A. Widening of the Q-T interval with a flattened T wave
   B. Shortening of the Q-T interval with an elevated T wave
   C. Shortening of the Q-T interval with a flattened T wave
   D. Widening of the Q-T interval with an elevated T wave

41. The BEST time to effectively teach a child and his/her family the complex concepts of the home management of diabetes mellitus is:
   A. a day or so after diagnosis.
   B. the first 3 or 4 days after diagnosis.
   C. 2 weeks after diagnosis.
   D. a month after diagnosis.

42. The child with diabetes mellitus is taught to weigh and measure food in order to:
   A. receive the nutrients prescribed.
   B. prevent hypoglycemia.
   C. learn to estimate food portions.
   D. prevent hyperglycemia.

43. In regard to meal planning for the child with diabetes mellitus:
   A. fast foods must be eliminated.
   B. foods must be always be weighed and measured.
   C. the exchange list is limited to one type of food.
   D. foods with sorbitol are not recommended.

44. The most efficient rotation pattern for insulin injections involves giving injections in:
   A. one area of the body one inch apart.
   B. different areas of the body each day.

45. In regard to insulin administration:
    A. insulin should never be premixed.
    B. insulin syringes should never be reused.
    C. insulin doses under 2 units should be diluted.
    D. an air bubble in the syringe is insignificant.

46. The child with diabetes mellitus needs to test his/her urine:
    A. for ketones every day.
    B. for ketones at times of illness.
    C. for glucose every day.
    D. for glucose at times of illness.

47. Exercise for the child with diabetes mellitus is:
    A. restricted to non-contact sports.
    B. may require a decreased intake of food.
    C. may necessitate an increased insulin dose.
    D. may require an increased intake of food.

48. Problems with the child adjusting to the self management of diabetes are most likely to occur when diabetes is diagnosed in:
    A. infancy.
    B. adolescence.
    C. the toddler years.
    D. the school age years.

49. Describe the feelings that parents may have when they are raising a child with diabetes mellitus.

_____

_____

_____

Critical Thinking • Case Study

Rebecca Bennett is an 8-year-old who has recently been diagnosed with diabetes mellitus. She is hospitalized with diabetic ketoacidosis and she is beginning to learn about the disease process. Her parents are with her continuously. She has an identical twin sister who is staying with her maternal grandparents.

50. Mrs. Bennett is concerned that Rebecca's sister will also develop diabetes. Based on the above information, an acceptable response for the nurse to make would be to:
    A. reassure the parents that the disease is not contagious.
    B. discuss the hereditary and viral factors of type 1 diabetes.
    C. discuss the hereditary factors of type 1 diabetes.
    D. discuss the viral factors of type 1 diabetes.

51. Which one of the following nursing diagnoses is MOST likely to become a priority after the first few days of Rebecca's hospitalization?
    A. Fluid volume deficit related to uncontrolled diabetes
    B. Fluid volume excess related to hormonal disturbances
    C. Impaired home maintenance management related to lack of knowledge
    D. Impaired respiratory function related to fluid imbalance

52. In preparing the Bennett family for discharge, the nurse should plan to teach:
    A. only Rebecca how to inject insulin.
    B. only Rebecca's parents how to inject insulin.
    C. both Rebecca and her parents how to inject insulin.
    D. the family how to administer oral hypoglycemics.

53. To evaluate Rebecca's progress in relation to her diabetes self management, the BEST measure would be Rebecca's:
    A. parents' verbalizations about the disease process.
    B. blood glucose levels.
    C. glycosolated hemoglobin values.
    D. demonstration of her insulin injection technique.

CHAPTER 39
The Child with Musculoskeletal or Articular Dysfunction

1. What eight topics does the nurse include in the educational plan to promote injury prevention among community children?

   _____   _____

   _____   _____

   _____   _____

   _____   _____

2. The nurse is suspicious for child abuse when:
   1. there is a delay in seeking medical assistance for the injury.
   2. parent's history of the injury is not congruent with the actual injury.
   3. x-rays demonstrate previous fractures in different stages of healing.
   4. child is crying and fearful of separation from parent.

   A. 1, 2, 3, and 4
   B. 1, 2, and 3
   C. 2 and 3
   D. 2, 3, and 4

3. The nurse neighbor of Jimmy, age 5, discovers him lying in the street next to his bicycle. The nurse sends another witness to activate the emergency medical system (EMS) while the nurse begins a primary assessment of Jimmy. Which one of the following BEST describes the primary assessment and its correct sequence?
   A. Body inspection, head-to-toe survey and airway patency
   B. Airway patency, respiratory effectiveness, circulatory status
   C. Open airway, head-to-toe assessment for injuries, and chest compressions
   D. Weight estimation, symptom analysis, blood pressure measurement

4. The nurse suspects Jimmy (question 3 above) has a spinal cord injury. Describe immobilization technique.

   _____

   _____

5. Major consequences of immobilization in the pediatric patient include which one of the following?
   A. Bone demineralization leading to osteoporosis
   B. Orthostatic hypertension
   C. Dependent edema in the lower extremities
   D. Decrease in the metabolic rate

6. What are the three major cardiovascular consequences of immobility?

_____   _____

_____

7. Nursing interventions aimed at preventing problems associated with immobilization include which one of the following?
   A. Encouragement in self-care and allowing patients to do as much for themselves as they are able to perform
   B. Fluid restrictions with strict intake and output
   C. Limitation of active range of motion exercises to once per day
   D. Decreased sensory stimulation to allow adequate rest

8. The fabrication and fitting of braces is termed ___orthotics___.
   The fabrication and fitting of artificial limbs is termed ___prosthetics___.

9. Which one of the following is a complication of immobility that is easily prevented by an appropriate nursing intervention?
   A. Disuse atrophy and loss of muscle mass
   B. Constipation
   C. Hypocalcemia
   D. Pain

10. Which one of the following is NOT included in the teaching plan of a child with a brace or prosthesis?
    A. Frequent assessment of all areas in contact with the brace for signs of skin irritation
    B. Assessment of the stump area before application of the prosthesis
    C. Removal of the prosthesis limited to bedtime unless skin breakage occurs
    D. Protective clothing used under the brace

11. Describe the differences between appropriate patient use for the Stryker frame and the Roto-Rest bed.

_____

_____

_____

12. Bone healing is characteristically more rapid in children because:
    A. children have less constant muscle contraction associated with the fracture.
    B. children's fractures are less severe than adult's.
    C. children have an active growth plate that helps speed repair with less likely occurring deformity.
    D. children have thickened periosteum and more generous blood supply.

13. The method of fracture reduction is NOT determined by which one of the following?
    A. Age of the child
    B. How the fracture occurred
    C. The degree of displacement
    D. The amount of edema

14. Match the following with its description.

A. diaphysis
B. epiphysis
C. epiphyseal plate
D. complete fracture
E. incomplete fracture
F. transverse fracture
G. simple or closed fracture
H. open or compound fracture
I. complicated fracture
J. comminuted fracture
K. greenstick fracture
L. buckle or torus fracture
M. bend fracture
N. osteopenia

__H__ fracture with an open wound from which the bone has protruded

__A__ major portion of the long bone

__D__ fracture fragments are separated

__E__ fracture fragments remain attached

__B__ located at the ends of the long bones

__C__ also called the growth plate because it plays a major role in the longitudinal growth of the developing child

__F__ fracture that is crosswise, at right angles to the long axis of the bone

__J__ small fragments of bone are broken from the fractured shaft and lie in surrounding tissue

__I__ bone fragments cause damage to surrounding organs or tissue

__N__ demineralization of the bone

__L__ appears as a raising or bulging at the site of the fracture

__M__ occurs more commonly in the ulna and fibula and can produce some deformity

__K__ occurs when a bone is angulated beyond the limits of bending

__G__ fracture has not produced a break in the skin

15. What are the five "Ps" of ischemia that are included when assessing fractures to rule out vascular injury?

_____ _____ _____

_____ _____

16. Emergency treatment for the child with a fracture includes:
   A. moving the child to allow removal of clothing from the area of injury.
   B. immobilization of the limb including joints above and below the injury site.
   C. pushing the protruding bone under the skin.
   D. keeping the area of injury in a dependent position.

17. What are the four goals of fracture management?

_____ _____

_____ _____

18. An appropriate nursing intervention for the care of a child with an extremity in a new cast is:
   A. keeping the cast covered with a sheet.
   B. using the fingertips when handling the cast to prevent pressure areas.
   C. using heated fans or dryers to circulate air and speed the cast drying process.
   D. turning the child at least every 2 hours to help dry the cast evenly.

19. To reduce anxiety in the child undergoing cast removal, which one of the following nursing interventions would the nurse expect to be LEAST effective?
    A. Demonstrate how the cast cutter works to the child before beginning the procedure.
    B. Using the analogy of having fingernails or hair cut.
    C. Explain that it will take only a few minutes.
    D. Continual reassurance that all is going well and that their behavior is accepted during the removal process.

20. Julie, age 10, has been placed in a long leg cast for an open fracture. The nurse immediately notifies the physician if assessment findings include which one of the following?
    A. Appearance of blood stained area the size of a quarter on the cast
    B. 2+ pedal pulse
    C. Inability to move the toes
    D. Ability of the nurse to insert one finger under the edge of the cast

21. The three primary purposes of traction for reduction of fractures are:

    _____

    _____

    _____

22. The nurse is caring for 7-year-old Charles after insertion of skeletal traction. Which one of the following is CONTRAINDICATED?
    A. Gently massage over pressure areas to stimulate circulation.
    B. Release the traction when repositioning Charles in bed.
    C. Inspect pin sites for bleeding or infection.
    D. Assess for alterations in neurovascular status.

23. Nursing intervention for the child with an Ilizarov external fixator device includes:
    A. teaching the child to walk with crutches.
    B. observing for the common problem of infection.
    C. allowing full weight bearing once the fixation device has been applied.
    D. allowing full weight bearing following removal of the device.

24. The nurse is assessing Carol, age 8, for complications related to her recent fracture and the application of a flexion cast to her forearm and elbow. Carol is crying with pain, the nurse is unable to locate pulses in the affected extremity, and there is lack of sensitivity to the area as well as some edema. Which one of the following would the nurse suspect as MOST likely to be occurring?
    A. This is a normal occurrence for the first few hours following application of traction.
    B. Volkmann contracture
    C. Nerve compression syndrome
    D. Epiphyseal damage

25. Johnny, a 12-year-old with fracture of the femur, has developed chest pain and shortness of breath. The priority nursing action is:
    A. elevate the affected extremity.
    B. administer oxygen.
    C. administer pain medication.
    D. start an IV infusion of heparin.

26. Match the following types of traction with their best description.

A. Dunlop traction
B. Bryant traction
C. Buck extension
D. Russell traction
E. 90-degree-90-degree traction
F. balance suspension traction
G. Thomas splint
H. Pearson attachment
I. cervical traction
J. manual traction
K. skin traction
L. skeletal traction
M. distraction

_L_ insertion of a wire or pin into the bone

_J_ used to realign bone fragments for cast application

_K_ applied when there is minimum displacement and little muscle spasticity but contraindicated when there is associated skin damage

_A_ treatment of fractures of the humerus when the arm is suspended horizontally

_B_ a type of running traction where the pull is only in one direction

_D_ uses skin traction on the lower leg and a padded sling under the knee

_C_ a type of skin traction with the leg in an extended position; used primarily for short-term immobilization

_E_ skeletal traction where the lower leg is put in a boot cast or supported in a sling and a pin is placed in the distal fragment of the femur

_F_ used with or without skin or skeletal traction; suspends the leg in a flexed position to relax the hip and hamstring muscles

_M_ process of separating opposing bone to regenerate new bone in the created space

_I_ accomplished by insertion of Crutchfield tongs through burr holes

_H_ supports the lower leg

_G_ extends from the groin to midair above the foot

27. Nursing interventions for the child following surgical amputation of a lower extremity include:

A. applying special elastic bandaging to the stump using a circular pattern to decrease stump edema.
B. keeping the stump elevated for at least 72 hours post surgery.
C. encouraging the child to lie prone at least three times a day, increasing the time prone to tolerance of an hour at a time.
D. recognizing that the child is only trying to gain the nurse's attention when the child says there is pain in the missing limb.

28. Match the term with its description.

A. contusion
B. ecchymosis
C. dislocation
D. strain
E. sprain

_____ occurs when the force of stress on the ligament is so great that it displaces the normal position of the opposing bone ends or the bone end to its socket

_____ damage to the soft tissue, subcutaneous structures, and muscle

_____ occurs when trauma to a joint is so severe that a ligament is either stretched or partially or completely torn by the force created as a joint is twisted or wrenched

_____ escape of blood into the tissues

_____ microscopic tear to the musculotendinous unit

29. Immediate treatment of sprains and strains includes:
    A. rest and cold application.
    B. disregarding the pain and "working out" the sprain or strain.
    C. rest, elevation, and pain medication.
    D. compression of the area and heat application.

30. Major sprains or tears to the ligamentous tissue rarely occur in growing children because the
    _____ are stronger than bone. The _____ and the
    _____ _____ are the weakest part of the bone and the usual site of injury.

31. Identify the following as either TRUE or FALSE.
    _____ Athletes who run can experience shin splints, a ligament tear away from the tibial shaft.
    _____ Achilles tendonitis is caused by repeated forcible traction on the short tendon.
    _____ Jumper's knee is caused by epiphysitis of the calcaneus.
    _____ Osgood-Schlatter disease may present with pain and tenderness over the tibial tubercle and an overprominence of involved tubercle.
    _____ Little league elbow presents with pain in the elbow, aggravated by use, and is caused from repetitive strain on lateral epicondylitis.
    _____ Children are less vulnerable to heat injury than adults because of their greater ratio of surface area to body mass and reduced production of metabolic heat for body mass.
    _____ Heat cramps are caused by calcium depletion during vigorous exercise in a hot environment.
    _____ Heat exhaustion occurs from excessive loss of fluids during exercise in a hot environment. Symptoms include thirst, headache, fatigue, dizziness, anxiety or nausea and vomiting.
    _____ The child with heat exhaustion should have external cooling applied with cold towels immediately.
    _____ Heatstroke represents a failure of normal thermoregulatory mechanisms. Onset is rapid and disorientation is present, along with a temperature in excess of 104 degrees F.
    _____ Salt tablets are rarely needed during exercise and may actually do harm by increasing dehydration.
    _____ The optimum diet for an athlete is one that contains the essential food groups and is adjusted to the energy requirements of the sport in which the youngster is engaged.
    _____ It is not necessary to counsel female athletes about pregnancy prevention because they have delayed menarche.
    _____ Drug misuse by athletes most often includes psycho-motor stimulants and anabolic steroids.
    _____ Idiopathic hypertrophic subaortic stenosis as a medical cause of sudden death during a sports activity has a typical triad of severe chest pain with dizziness, prominent pulses and a murmur at the left lower sternal border.

32. Zac, a 16-year-old football star at the local high school, is at the school nurse practitioner's office for acne that is not clearing. During the physical exam it is noted that Zac has achieved a marked increase in muscle and strength in a very short time. Which one of the following would the nurse suspect caused these changes?
    A. Use of ergogenic aid, anabolic steroids
    B. Zac has been working out in the gym more.
    C. Increased protein and vitamins in the diet
    D. Zac is using Ritalin or Preludin.

33. The condition recognized in the infant with limited neck motion, where the neck is flexed and turned to the affected side as a result of shortening of the sterocleidomastodid muscle, is:
   A. torticollis.
   B. paralysis of the brachial nerve.
   C. Legg-Calvé-Perthes disease.
   D. a self-limiting injury.

34. Bob, age 7, is diagnosed with Legg-Calvé-Perthes disease. Which one of the following manifestations is NOT consistent with this diagnosis?
   A. Intermittent appearance of a limp on the affected side
   B. Hip soreness, ache, or stiffness that can be constant or intermittent
   C. Pain and limp are most evident on arising and at the end of a long day of activities
   D. Specific history of injury to the area

35. Slipped femoral capital epiphysis is suspected when:
   A. an adolescent or preadolescent begins to limp and complains of pain in the hip continuously or intermittently.
   B. exam reveals no restriction on internal rotation or adduction but restriction on external rotation.
   C. referred pain goes into the sacral and lumbar areas.
   D. all of the above.

36. An accentuation of the lumbar curvature beyond physiologic limits is termed
   _____. An abnormally increased convex angulation in the curvature of the
   thoracic spine is termed _____. _____ is the forward
   slipping of one vertebral body on another, usually L5 and S1.

37. Diagnostic evaluation is important for early recognition of scoliosis. Which one of the following is the CORRECT procedure for the school nurse conducting this examination?
   A. View the child standing and walking fully clothed to look for uneven hanging of clothing.
   B. View all children from left and right side to look mainly for asymmetry of the hip height.
   C. Completely undress all children before the exam.
   D. View the child who is wearing underpants from behind and when the child bends forward.

38. The surgical technique for the correction of scoliosis consists of:

   _____

   _____

39. Marilyn, age 13, has been diagnosed with scoliosis and placed in a Milwaukee brace. Marilyn asks the nurse about the brace and how long she has to wear it. What is the BEST response?
   A. "The brace will need to be worn only until you have corrective surgery."
   B. "The brace will need to be worn between 16 and 23 hours a day to halt or slow the progression of the curvature."
   C. "The brace will not need to be worn to school, only at home and you will need to sleep in the brace."
   D. "You will need to get specific information about your schedule from your doctor."

40. Nursing implementation directed toward nonsurgical management in a teenager with scoliosis primarily includes:
   A. promoting self-esteem and positive body image.
   B. preventing immobility.
   C. promoting adequate nutrition.
   D. preventing infection.

41. Osteomyelitis acquired from spread of organisms from a pre-existing wound like that of a skin abrasion is termed:
   A. hematogenous.
   B. exogenous.

42. The plan of care for the child during the acute phase of osteomyelitis always includes:
   A. performing wound irrigations.
   B. maintaining IV infusion site.
   C. isolation of the child.
   D. passive range of motion exercises for the affected area.

43. The four goals for therapeutic management of septic arthritis are:

   _____   _____

   _____   _____

44. The most common site for tubercular infection of the bones in older children is:
   A. carpals and phalanges and corresponding bones of the feet.
   B. spine and hip.

45. Nursing considerations for the patient diagnosed with osteogenesis imperfecta include:
   A. preventing fractures by careful handling.
   B. providing non-judgmental support while parents are dealing with accusations of child abuse.
   C. providing guidelines to the parents in planning suitable activities that promote optimum development.
   D. all of the above.

46. Which of the following nursing goals is MOST appropriate for the child with juvenile rheumatoid arthritis?
   A. Child will exhibit signs of reduced joint inflammation and adequate joint function.
   B. Child will exhibit no signs of impaired skin integrity due to rash.
   C. Child will exhibit normal weight and nutritional status.
   D. Child will exhibit no alteration in respiratory patterns or respiratory infection.

47. Clinical manifestations of systemic lupus erythematous among children include:
   A. Raynaud phenomenon, especially of the feet and legs.
   B. development of Herpes Simplex in dry, cracked skin areas.
   C. cutaneous involvement including skin disease as the chief complaint.
   D. patchy areas of alopecia without remission.

48. What are the two objectives of therapeutic management for SLE?

   _____

   _____

49. The principal drugs used in SLE to control inflammation are the _____.

50. The two principal nursing goals for the nurse caring for the child with SLE are:

_____

_____

Critical Thinking • Case Study

Sandy, age 8, has developed joint and leg pain, some joint swelling, fever, malaise and pleuritis. The physician has ordered laboratory testing to include sedimentation rate, rheumatoid factor, and a complete blood count. Tentative diagnosis has been established as juvenile arthritis, systemic onset.

51. If the diagnosis is correct, which of the following would represent the expected laboratory results?
    A. Leukocytosis
    B. Elevated sedimentation rate
    C. Negative rheumatoid factor
    D. All of the above

52. The primary group of drugs prescribed for juvenile arthritis is nonsteroidal anti-inflammatory drugs. Education regarding the use of these drugs should include which of the following?
    A. They produce excellent analgesic and anti-inflammatory effects but little antipyretic effect.
    B. They are administered in the lowest effective dose and given on alternate days rather than daily.
    C. Anti-inflammatory effect occurs 3 to 4 weeks after therapy is begun.
    D. Because there is a narrow margin between effective and toxic dosage, levels need to be monitored regularly until therapeutic dosage is established.

53. Which of the following is the MOST appropriate nursing intervention to promote adequate joint function in the child with juvenile rheumatoid arthritis?
    A. Incorporate therapeutic exercises in play activities.
    B. Provide heat to affected joints by use of tub baths.
    C. Provide written information for all treatments ordered.
    D. Explore and develop activities in which the child can succeed.

54. An expected outcome for the nursing diagnosis of high risk for body image disturbance related to disease process of juvenile arthritis is:
    A. patient/family able to explain disease process.
    B. patient is accepted by peers.
    C. patient will express feelings and concerns.
    D. child will understand and use effective communication techniques.

55. Which of the following are signs of aspirin toxicity?
    A. Tinnitus
    B. Insomnia
    C. Hypoventilation
    D. Vomiting

56. The nutritional goal for Sandy includes:

_____

_____

CHAPTER 40
The Child with Neuromuscular or Muscular Dysfunction

1. Identify the following as TRUE or FALSE.

    __T__ Upper motor neuron lesions produce weakness associated with spasticity, increased deep tendon reflexes, and abnormal superficial reflexes.

    __F__ The primary disorder of lower motor neuron dysfunction is cerebral palsy.

    __T__ Lower motor neuron lesions interrupt the reflex arc, causing weakness and atrophy of the skeletal muscles involved with associated hypotonia or flaccidity with final progression to varying degrees of contracture.

    __F__ Lower motor neuron involvement is most often asymmetric.

    __T__ In most instances the sudden appearance of flaccid paralysis in a previously healthy child can be attributed to an infectious process.

    __T__ Hereditary factors and metabolic disease are more often responsible for muscular weakness and atrophy of gradual onset.

    __T__ The most useful classification of neuromuscular disorders defines the source of the lesion: cerebral cortex, anterior horn cells of the spinal cord, peripheral nerves, myoneural junction, and muscle.

    __T__ Deep tendon reflexes are briskly active in upper neuron disease and diminished or absent in lower motor neuron disease.

2. Match the diagnostic tool with its description.

    A. electromyogram (EMG)   _____ elevated in skeletal muscle disease; most specific test

    B. nerve conduction velocity   _____ present in skeletal and heart muscle

    C. muscle biopsy   _____ Ketamine is used to decrease the pain with this procedure.

    D. CPK   _____ measures electric impulse conduction along motor nerves

    E. aldolase   _____ measures electric potential of individual muscle

3. The nurse knows that the etiology of cerebral palsy is MOST commonly related to which one of the following?
    (A.) Existing prenatal brain abnormalities
    B. Maternal asphyxia
    C. Childhood meningitis
    D. Preeclampsia

4. The nurse is preparing the long-term care plan for a child with cerebral palsy. Which one of the following is included in the plan?
    A. No delay in gross motor development is expected.
    (B.) The illness is not progressively degenerative.
    C. There will be no persistence of primitive infantile reflexes.
    D. All children will need genetic counseling as they get older before planning for a family.

5. Match the term with its description.

A. hemiparesis   _____ pure cerebral paraplegia of lower extremities

B. quadriparesis   _____ involving three extremities

C. diplegia   _____ involves only one extremity

D. monoplegia   _____ similar parts of both sides of the body involved

E. triplegia   _____ most common form of spastic cerebral palsy; motor deficit greater in upper extremity; one side of the body affected

F. paraplegia

G. parietal lobe syndrome   _____ cortical sensory function impairment and therefore impaired two-point discrimination and position sense

H. spastic cerebral palsy

I. dyskinetic cerebral palsy   _____ all four extremities equally affected

J. ataxic cerebral palsy

K. mixed-type cerebral palsy   _____ characterized by abnormal involuntary movement such as athetosis, slow, worm-like, writhing movements that usually involve the extremities, trunk, neck, facial muscles and tongue

    _____ characterized by wide-based gait; rapid repetitive movements performed poorly; disintegration of movements of the upper extremities when the child reaches for objects

    _____ combination of spasticity and athetosis

    _____ may involve one or both sides; hypertonicity with poor control of posture, balance, and coordinated motion; impairment of fine and gross motor skills; abnormal postures and overflow of movement to other parts of the body increased by active attempts at motion

6. Children with cerebral palsy often have manifestations including alterations of muscle tone. Which one of the following is an example of a child with altered muscle tone?
   A. Increased or decreased resistance to passive movements
   B. Development of hand dominance by the age of 5 months
   C. Asymmetric crawl
   D. When placed in a prone position, the child will maintain the hips higher than the trunk with the legs and arms flexed or drawn under the body.

7. Associated disabilities and problems related to the child with cerebral palsy include which one of the following?
   A. All children with cerebral palsy will have intelligence testing in the abnormal range.
   B. There are a large number of eye cataracts associated with cerebral palsy which will need surgical correction.
   C. Seizures are a common occurrence among children with athetosis and diplegia.
   D. Coughing and choking, especially while eating, predispose children with cerebral palsy to aspiration.

8. The nurse is completing a physical exam on 6-month-old Brian. Which one of the following would be an abnormal finding suggestive of cerebral palsy?
   A. Brian is able to hold onto the nurse's hands while being pulled to a sitting position.
   B. Brian has no moro reflex.
   C. Brian has no tonic neck reflex.
   D. Brian has an obligatory tonic neck reflex.

9. The goal of therapeutic management for the child with cerebral palsy is:
    A. assisting with motor control of voluntary muscle.
    B. maximizing the capabilities of the child.
    C. delaying the development of sensory deprivation.
    D. surgical correction of deformities.

10. Which one of the following would be expected in the infant presenting with hypotonia?
    A. When held in horizontal suspension, the infant will respond by slightly raising the head.
    B. When pulled to a sitting position, the infant will demonstrate head lag that is quickly corrected to a normal position.
    C. When placed in horizontal suspension position, the infant's head droops over the examiner's supporting hand and the infant's extremities hang loosely.
    D. The infant presents with a slower weight gain but has a good sucking reflex.

11. The major diagnostic test in diagnosing the infant with hypotonia is _____.

12. The disease inherited only as an autosomal-recessive trait and characterized by progressive weakness and wasting of skeletal muscles caused by degeneration of anterior horn cells is:
    A. Werdnig-Hoffmann disease.
    B. cerebral palsy.
    C. Kugelberg-Welander disease.
    D. Guillain-Barré syndrome.

13. Nursing considerations for the infant with Werdnig-Hoffmann disease should include which one of the following for normal growth and development?
    A. Feeding by nasogastric tube
    B. Use of an infant walker to develop muscle strength
    C. Verbal, tactile, and auditory stimulation
    D. Encouraging the parents to seek genetic counseling

14. A. What are the predominant features associated with juvenile spinal muscular atrophy?

    _____

    B. Describe the management and nursing considerations when treating the child with juvenile spinal muscular atrophy?

    _____

15. Which one of the following is a TRUE statement about Guillain-Barré syndrome?
    A. GBS is a autosomal-recessive inherited disease.
    B. GBS is more likely to affect children than adults with children under the age of 4 years having the higher susceptibility.
    C. GBS is an acute demyelinating polyneuropathy with a progressive, usually ascending, flaccid paralysis.
    D. GBS is an autoimmune disorder associated with the attack of circulating antibodies on the acetylcholine receptors.

16. Diagnostic evaluation for the patient with Guillain-Barré syndrome would include which one of the following results?
    A. Elevated CBC
    B. Cerebrospinal fluid high in protein
    C. Elevated CPK
    D. Sensory nerve conduction time is increased.

17. The priority nursing consideration for the child in the acute phase of Guillain-Barré syndrome is:
    A. careful observation for difficulty in swallowing and respiratory involvement.
    B. prevention of contractures.
    C. prevention of bowel and bladder complications.
    D. prevention of sensory impairment.

18. What are the characteristic symptoms of generalized tetanus?

    _____

    _____

19. Where are the spores of tetanus normally found?

    _____

    _____

20. Terry, age 10 years, received his last tetanus toxoid immunization at the age of 4 years. He now presents to the clinic with a minor laceration sustained while working on his model airplanes. Is a dose of tetanus toxoid booster necessary at this time?
    A. Yes
    B. No

21. Maria, age 5, was born in a South American country and has been in the United States less than one year. While outside playing in the garden, she suffers a minor cut. Since Maria's mother does not think that Maria has ever received immunizations, which one of the following actions would be most appropriate at this time to prevent tetanus?
    A. Have Maria go to the clinic tomorrow for the start of administration of all her needed immunizations.
    B. Administer tetanus immune globulin now.
    C. Administer 1st injection of tetanus toxoid now.
    D. Administer both tetanus immune globulin and tetanus toxoid now.

22. Primary nursing implementations for the child with tetanus include:
    1. control or eliminate stimulation from sound, light, and touch.
    2. maintaining body alignment.
    3. arrange for the child not to be left alone since these children are mentally alert.
    4. knowledge that pancuronium bromide (Pavulon) does not cause total paralysis.
    5. encouraging high intake of fluid.

    A. 1, 2, and 3
    B. 2, 4, and 5
    C. 1 and 2
    D. 1 and 3

23. Risk factors for infant botulism include:
    A. ingestion of honey.
    B. infants with diarrhea before the age of 3 months.
    C. infants living in urban areas.
    D. infants diagnosed with hypertonicity.

24. Infant botulism usually presents with symptoms of:
    A. diarrhea and vomiting.
    B. constipation and generalized weakness.
    C. high fever and decrease in spontaneous movement.
    D. failure to thrive.

25. What is the diagnosis of botulism based on?

    _____

26. Nursing considerations for the pediatric patient with botulism include:
    A. teaching the parents the importance of administering enemas and cathartics for bowel function.
    B. preparing the parents for the fact that the child will have muscular disability after the illness.
    C. using honey as a formula sweetener to increase oral intake.
    D. teaching parents that boiling is not an adequate prevention.

27. Tammy, age 13, is diagnosed with myasthenia gravis. The nurse, in preparing a teaching plan for the family, includes which one of the following as a priority?
    A. Watching for signs of over-medication of anticholinesterase drugs, which include respiratory distress, choking and aspiration
    B. Encouraging strenuous activity
    C. Suggesting to Tammy and her parents to limit Tammy's scholastic accomplishments in school in order to allow for adequate rest
    D. Reducing Tammy's weight to reduce symptom occurrence

28. Spinal cord injury causes three stages of response. The second stage is characterized by which one of the following?
    A. Spinal shock syndrome
    B. Loss of temperature and vasomotor control
    C. Replacement of flaccid paralysis by spinal reflex activity which results in spastic paralysis
    D. Development of scoliosis

29. Diagnostic evaluation of the child who presents with a spinal injury includes a complete neurologic exam. Motor system evaluation is done by:
    A. stimulating peripheral receptors by eliciting the reflexes like the patellar.
    B. observation of gait, noting balance maintenance and noting the ability to lift, flex, and extend extremities.
    C. testing all 12 cranial nerves.
    D. using the blunt end of a safety pin and the sharp point to test each dermatome.

30. What is the general guideline used when determining if the paraplegic has the capacity to be self-helped to walk?

     _____

     _____

31. Management during the first stage of spinal cord injury may include:
    A. steroid administration.
    B. maximizing potential for self-help.
    C. watching for hypotension and hyponatremia.
    D. rehabilitation.

32. Children with neurogenic bladder should be taught:
    A. to keep urine alkaline.
    B. how to perform the Credé maneuver to express urine.
    C. that the bladder that empties periodically by reflex action will not need intermittent catherization.
    D. the necessity of oral antimicrobials administered prophylactically.

33. In discussing sexuality with the teenager that has a spinal injury, the nurse correctly includes which one of the following in the discussion?
    A. Development of secondary sex characteristics will be delayed.
    B. Well-motivated young people can look forward to successful participation in marital and family activities.
    C. If injury occurs before onset of menstruation, ovulation and conception are not possible.
    D. Females can easily experience vaginal or clitoral orgasms.

34. Clinical manifestations of dermatomyositis includes:
    1. proximal limb and trunk muscle weakness.
    2. stiff and sore muscles.
    3. decreased muscle strength and reflex response
    4. red, indurated skin lesions over the malar areas and nose.
    5. skin over extensor muscle surfaces is erythematous, scaly and atopic.

    A. 1, 2, and 3
    B. 1, 2, 4, and 5
    C. 3, 4, and 5
    D. 2, 3, and 4

35. Match the major muscular dystrophy with its characteristics. (Dystrophies may be used more than once.)

    A. pseudohypertrophic (Duchenne)

    B. limb-girdle

    C. facioscapulohumeral (Landouzy-Déjerine)

    _C_ lack of facial mobility; forward shoulder slope

    _B_ weakness of proximal muscles of both pelvic and shoulder girdles

    _A_ lordosis, waddling gait, difficulty in rising from floor and climbing stairs

    _B_ onset in late childhood; autosomal recessive

    _C_ very slow progression and may have periods with no progression

    _A_ onset ages 1-3 years

36. What are the major complications of muscular dystrophy?

Contractures, disuse atrophy, infections, obesity, cardiopulmonary problems

37. Major goals in the nursing care of children with muscular dystrophy include which one of the following?
    A. Promoting strenuous activity and exercise
    B. Promoting large caloric intake
    C. Preventing respiratory tract infection
    D. Preventing mental retardation

38. Diagnostic evaluation of muscular dystrophy includes serum levels of CPK, aldolase, and SGOT. When there is severe muscle wasting and incapacitation related to the disease process, the nurse would expect these serum levels to be:
    A. elevated.
    B. decreased.
    C. normal.
    D. unable to accurately be determined with muscle wasting and incapacitation.

Critical Thinking • Case Study

Kenny, age 4, has a history of premature delivery with cerebral palsy being diagnosed shortly after birth. Assessment findings include quadriplegia, deficient verbal communication skills, but apparently normal levels of intelligence. Kenny has been hospitalized several times in the past because of respiratory infection and gastric reflux. During Kenny's regular follow-up visit, his mother tells the nurse it is becoming harder to care for Kenny because of his needs. Because of Kenny's recent admission to the hospital for pneumonia, she worries that she is not giving Kenny the care he needs.

39. The nurse should explain to Kenny's mother that one of the complications associated with cerebral palsy is respiratory problems. Which one of the following assessment findings could MOST help explain why Kenny is having these problems?
    A. Kenny has constant drooling which contributes to wet clothing and chilling.
    B. Dietary imbalance with poor nutritional intake
    C. The presence of nystagmus and amblyopia
    D. Coughing and choking, especially while eating and history of gastric reflux

40. Kenny's mother asks the nurse how she can improve Kenny's communication skills, and a diagnosis of "impaired verbal communication" is developed. Which one of the following plans would be MOST appropriate for Kenny at this time to improve his communication skills?
    A. Purchase of an electric typewriter or computer to facilitate communication skills.
    B. Enlist the services of a speech therapist.
    C. Teach Kenny the use of nonverbal communications skills like sign language.
    D. Use audio tapes with Kenny to improve his speech abilities.

41. The nurse recognizes that an additional diagnosis is altered family processes related to a child with a lifelong disability. Which of the following implementations should the nurse recognize as being important to include in the plan of care?
    A. Explore potential for additional caregiving support.
    B. Refer the family to a support group of other parents with children with cerebral palsy.
    C. Refer parents to social services for additional suggestions.
    D. All of the above

42. Based on the information given about Kenny, identify the nursing goals that would assist Kenny and his family.

    _____   _____

    _____   _____

    _____   _____

    _____   _____

43. While Kenny is in the hospital, the nurse would plan appropriate play activities that include:
    A. minimized speaking, since Kenny has difficulty with his speech.
    B. solitary play to allow parents to be away from Kenny so that the parents could get rest.
    C. those that help Kenny relax muscles that are tense.
    D. those that require little intellectual functioning.